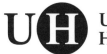
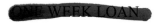

Baillière's
CLINICAL
GASTROENTEROLOGY
INTERNATIONAL PRACTICE AND RESEARCH

Baillière's

CLINICAL

GASTROENTEROLOGY

INTERNATIONAL PRACTICE AND RESEARCH

Volume 2/Number 4
October 1988

Nutritional Support

H. J. G. BURNS FRCS
Guest Editor

Baillière Tindall
London Philadelphia Sydney Tokyo Toronto

− 5 APR 1995

Baillière Tindall   24–28 Oval Road
W.B. Saunders   London NW1 7DX, UK

The Curtis Center, Independence Square West
Philadelphia, PA 19106–3399, USA

1 Goldthorne Avenue
Toronto, Ontario M8Z 5T9, Canada

Harcourt Brace Jovanovich Group (Australia) Pty Ltd
32–52 Smidmore Street, Marrickville, NSW 2204, Australia

Exclusive Agent in Japan:
Maruzen Co. Ltd (Journals Division)
3–10 Nihonbashi 2-chome, Chuo-ku, Tokyo 103, Japan

ISSN 0950–3528

ISBN 0–7020–1296–3 (single copy)

Baillière's Clinical Gastroenterology is published four times each year by Baillière Tindall. Annual subscription prices are:

TERRITORY	ANNUAL SUBSCRIPTION	SINGLE ISSUE
1. UK & Republic of Ireland	£35.00 post free	£15.00 post free
2. USA & Canada	US$68.00 post free	US$25.00 post free
3. All other countries	£45.00 post free	£18.50 post free

The editor of this publication is Seán Duggan, Baillière Tindall, 24–28 Oval Road, London NW1 7DX, UK.

Baillière's Clinical Gastroenterology was published from 1972 to 1986 as *Clinics in Gastroenterology*.

Typeset by Phoenix Photosetting, Chatham.
Printed and bound in Great Britain by Mackays of Chatham PLC, Chatham, Kent.

Contributors to this issue

PHILIP BURGESS MB ChB, BSc, FRCS, FRCS(Ed), First Assistant, Department of Surgery, The Medical School, University of Newcastle upon Tyne, Framlington Place, Newcastle upon Tyne NE2 4HH, UK.

H. J. G. BURNS MB ChB, FRCS, Senior Lecturer, University Department of Surgery, Royal Infirmary, Glasgow G31 2ER, UK.

FORRESTER COCKBURN MD, FRCP(Ed), FRCP(Glasg), DCH, Professor of Child Health and Honorary Consultant Paediatrician, University Department of Child Health, Royal Hospital for Sick Children, Yorkhill, Glasgow G3 8SJ, UK.

T. JOHN EVANS MB BCh, FRCP(Glasg), Consultant Paediatrician, Royal Hospital for Sick Children, Yorkhill, Glasgow G3 8SJ, UK.

KENNETH C. H. FEARON MB ChB, MD, FRCS, Surgical Registrar, Department of Surgery, Royal Infirmary, Glasgow G4 0SF, UK.

LILY FREDRIX DrSc, University Hospital Maastricht, Department of Nutrition, PO Box 1918, 6201 BX Maastricht, The Netherlands.

PETER J. GARLICK MA, PhD, Rowett Research Institute, Bucksburn, Aberdeen AB2 9SB, UK.

WILBERT A. J. J. M. HAAGH BSc, c/o Department of Surgery, University Hospital Maastricht, PO Box 1918, 6201 BX Maastricht, The Netherlands.

MILES IRVING MD, ChM, FRCS(Eng), FRCS(Ed), Professor of Surgery, University of Manchester; Honorary Consultant Surgeon, Hope Hospital, Salford M6 8HD, UK.

MICHAEL JOHN McMAHON MB, ChB, ChM, PhD, FRCS, Senior Lecturer and Honorary Consultant Surgeon, University Department of Surgery, The General Infirmary, Leeds LS1 3EX, UK.

MAARTEN F. VON MEYENFELDT MD, Lecturer in Surgery, University Hospital Maastricht, Department of Surgery, PO Box 1918, 6201 BX Maastricht, The Netherlands.

ROBERT M. PALMER MIBiol, PhD, Rowett Research Institute, Bucksburn, Aberdeen AB2 9SB, UK.

JOHN JASON PAYNE-JAMES MB, BS, FRCS(Eng), FRCS(Ed), Research Fellow in Surgery, Department of Gastroenterology and Nutrition, Central Middlesex Hospital, Acton Lane, London NW10 7NS, UK.

ROSS A. PETTIGREW MB ChB, FRACS, Senior Lecturer in Surgery, University of Otago, Dunedin Hospital, PO Box 913, Dunedin, New Zealand.

JEREMY POWELL-TUCK MD, MRCP, Senior Lecturer, Rank Department of Human Nutrition, London Hospital Medical College, Turner Street, London and The Medical College of St Bartholomew's Hospital, London; Honorary Consultant Physician, The London Hospital and St Mark's Hospital, London, UK.

ALAN SHENKIN MB, ChB, BSc, PhD, MRCPath, MRCP(G), Consultant Clinical Biochemist, Royal Infirmary, Glasgow G4 0SF; Honorary Lecturer, University of Glasgow, Glasgow G12 8QQ, UK.

DAVID B. A. SILK MD, FRCP, Consultant Physician, Co-Director, Department of Gastroenterology and Nutrition, Central Middlesex Hospital, Acton Lane, London NW10 7NS, UK.

A. J. W. SIM MS, FRCS, Professor, University Department of Surgery, Faculty of Medicine and Health Sciences, PO Box 15551, UAE University, Al Ain, United Arab Emirates.

PETER B. SOETERS MD, Professor of Surgery, University Hospital Maastricht, Department of Surgery, PO Box 1918, 6201 BX Maastricht, The Netherlands.

ANGELIE VAN DER AALST BSc, c/o Department of Nutrition, University Hospital Maastricht, PO Box 1918, 6201 BX Maastricht, The Netherlands.

Table of contents

RECENT ISSUE

July 1988
Peptic Ulceration
D. W. PIPER

FORTHCOMING ISSUE

January 1989
Therapy of Liver Disease
M. DAVIS

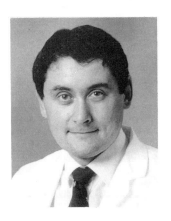

Foreword

The interest of the surgical community in the physiology and technique of nutritional support has waxed and waned over the past 15 years. With increasing experience, it has become obvious that the relationship between illness and malnutrition is not simple and that provision of calories and protein cannot always be relied upon to improve nutritional state or prognosis in stressed patients. With the realization that simple nutritional support will not necessarily provide major clinical gains, many clinicians have lost interest. However, those who have maintained an association with the field have seen a fascinating story develop. Subtle inter-relationships between stress and starvation are now recognized. A new class of mediators of metabolic activity has been discovered and new insights into the control of metabolic processes have been obtained. As a result, research into the nutritional and metabolic problems of clinical medicine is once again at a most exciting stage of development.

It has been a great privilege to be allowed to select topics for this volume, and my intention has been to try to communicate some new concepts to a readership which might not be aware of the changes taking place in the field of clinical nutrition. In addition, I have included chapters on practical aspects of nutritional support. I hope that I have achieved a satisfactory balance between laboratory-based and clinically-based information. I have enjoyed reading the various contributions and have found them stimulating and occasionally provocative. If other readers are stimulated to a greater awareness of nutritional problems in clinical practice and are provoked into action to solve those problems then this volume will have achieved its purpose.

I should like to thank all those authors who provided chapters so promptly. I would also like to thank Margaret Macdonald and the production staff of Ballière Tindall who were extremely patient with the editor when contributions were delayed! The high standard of the finished product is a great testimony to their skill. I would like also to take this opportunity to express my personal gratitude to my teacher, colleague and friend Professor Iain Ledingham. He first stimulated my interest in nutrition and metabolism while I was still a medical student and his enthusiasm and energy continue to be a source of inspiration to many of us working in injury research

H. J. G. BURNS

1

Nutritional consequences of gastrointestinal disease

J. POWELL-TUCK

Gastrointestinal disease affects nutrition through several mechanisms. Nutrient intake is of prime importance. Digestion of food may be impaired; malabsorption may result because of this or because of small bowel disease, resection or bacterial overgrowth. Additionally, diseases or resection of the stomach or the colon may have important nutritional consequences which contribute to the morbidity of the patient. Inflammation, sepsis and nutrient imbalance can affect metabolism. This chapter does not set out to be exhaustive; rather the aim is to illustrate how these various mechanisms can combine in four principal examples. These conditions all have nutritional consequences but have them for different principal reasons. The examples chosen are:

1. Post-gastric surgery.
2. Chronic pancreatic disease.
3. Small bowel resection and intestinal adaptation. (The short bowel syndrome).
4. Inflammatory bowel disease.

GASTRIC SURGERY

Many studies have documented the variable weight loss which occurs after vagotomy, partial gastrectomy and total gastrectomy. Degrees of weight loss seem less with vagotomy with pyloroplasty (where they are minimal) than with gastroenterostomy (Cox, 1969); they are less with Bilroth 1 partial gastrectomy where between 5–42% are below pre-illness weight than with a Polya operation (French and Crane, 1963) where between 50–60% remain below their pre-illness weight. Weight loss is most marked after total gastrectomy where only a third of patients are able to maintain ideal body weight postoperatively (Bradley, 1979). Precise estimates of the amount lost vary so much from study to study as to make them unhelpful. It must be remembered that many of the patients have lost weight *before* the operation or in the immediate postoperative period, so it is important to know with what weight subsequent long-term body weights are being compared.

The weight loss seems, at least in men, to be predominantly from adipose tissue as judged anthropometrically, but a reduction in fat-free mass has been documented in at least one group of women after gastrectomy (Bisballe et al, 1986). The loss of adipose tissue must be due to a change in energy balance, either as a result of decreased intake or because of reduced absorption or theoretically as a result of increased energy consumption. There are no good data on long-term energy consumption in post-gastrectomy patients. Malabsorption of fat (Butler, 1961) occurs and is least marked after Bilroth I, more marked after Bilroth II (Polya) and most marked after total gastrectomy. In total gastrectomy patients faecal fat losses vary typically between 5–30% of intake, an equivalent for a 15% loss on a 100 g intake of between 45–90 kcal per day, but can be as much as 50% (450 kcal). Thus in selected patients at least, malabsorption may be nutritionally important; a loss of 90 kcal per day would account for about 6.5 kg of adipose tissue in a year, allowing 5 kcal per g of adipose tissue.

It has been widely assumed in the literature that diminished intake is responsible for the weight loss. However it has been well known that even patients who have had total gastrectomy are *able* to eat normally. It is interesting to speculate whether the removal of part of the stomach, or the bypassing of the duodenum by ingested food has an effect on the peripheral, peptide-mediated part of appetite/satiety control. Be that as it may, whether or not intake is diminished in these patients is still disputed. A recent study failed to demonstrate a statistically significant difference in energy intake between gastrectomy patients and age-sex matched controls (Bisballe et al, 1986). However the power of the study was such that small, potentially clinically significant differences, could well have been missed – the type 2 error of the study was not considered.

Loss of lean body mass could principally be explained as loss from the body's protein or water compartments. Gastrectomy patients may have considerably raised faecal nitrogen excretion, but bearing in mind the large amount of protein ingested in our diet this alone is unlikely to result in negative nitrogen balance. Fluid losses could result from abnormal sodium handling, and it would be interesting to know more about the compartmental composition of weight loss after gastric surgery. A number of specific nutrient deficiencies arise following such surgery. Of these iron and vitamin B_{12} deficiency are especially important. In addition there is a high incidence of metabolic bone disease.

Iron deficiency

The incidence of iron deficiency anaemia in patients who have undergone vagotomy, partial gastrectomy, and total gastrectomy is similar and thus duodenal bypass does not appear to be an important factor. Any acid-reducing operation is capable of diminishing absorption particularly of non-bound iron salts because at high pH insoluble ferric salts will tend to form. Although absorption of iron from food is impaired, administration of small doses of an iron supplement effectively corrects deficiency. It has been suggested that the predominant cause of iron deficiency in these patients is loss of iron from the remaining stomach or remnant, or the oesophagus (Williams and Hoare, 1979). Gastritis develops very frequently after vagotomy, Bilroth I and Bilroth II (Polya) partial gastrectomies but it is less clear to what extent the degree of gastritis correlates with the iron deficiency.

Vitamin B_{12} deficiency

After total gastrectomy there is no secretion of intrinsic factor so vitamin B_{12} deficiency will ensue after body stores have been exhausted. If there were no depletion of stores before surgery this would take about 3–4 years. After Bilroth II gastrectomy low levels of intrinsic factor are found and these correlate well with the degree of gastritis found on biopsy (Williams and Hoare, 1979).

All acid-reducing operations have the potential for causing reduced B_{12} absorption by virtue of the role of gastric acid in releasing the vitamin from its protein-bound state, the state in which it predominates in the diet. This is thought to be the explanation for the deficiency seen after vagotomy, but its clinical importance is questioned (Lindenbaum, 1980). If bacterial overgrowth occurred in relation to partial or total gastrectomy then this too would be expected to result in vitamin B_{12} malabsorption.

Metabolic bone disease

See review by Jones et al, 1963.

Osteoporosis

Against the background of the rather low calcium intakes of substantial numbers of the general population and its possible relationship with osteoporosis, the appreciable excess of various forms of metabolic bone disease after gastric surgery is interesting. Morgan et al (see Morgan and Pulvertaft, 1969) found cortical thinning in studies of the second right metacarpal bone in about 20% of patients studied more than 10 years after Polya gastrectomy and this figure rose to about 28% in those over 60. The incidence of metabolic bone disease in those who had undergone vagotomy and drainage was similar to that seen in the general population. Among the partial gastrectomy patients there was a higher incidence of cortical thinning in those with a high loss of total body fat relative to body weight. In those whose ratio of total body fat to body weight was diminished by 5% or more dietary calcium was 929 mg compared with 1360 mg in a group of unoperated patients. Achlorhydria (Recker, 1985), but not hypochlorhydria (Bo-Linn et al, 1984) results in impaired absorption of insoluble calcium salts, in particular calcium carbonate, though such salts, when taken with a meal are normally absorbed perhaps because of the low pH of the meal. Correction of impaired calcium absorption in achlorhydria patients is best achieved with a pH adjusted solution of calcium citrate (Recker, 1985).

Osteomalacia

A study estimating dietary vitamin D intake by questionnaire concluded that a higher percentage of patients who had had a previous Polya gastrectomy took less than 50 i.u. daily compared to those who had undergone vagotomy and drainage. This was threefold more likely in females (17%) than in males (5%) (Morgan and Pulvertaft, 1969). The malabsorption of fat which occurs after gastrectomy would make malabsorption of vitamin D a possibility. Among elderly patients diagnosed as having osteomalacia, a high proportion are found to have undergone gastric surgery. A raised alkaline phosphatase is found in patients after gastrectomy. Subclinical osteomalacia has been found in bone biopsies done in a study of 36 patients after gastrectomy. Nevertheless a recent controlled study of asymptomatic patients studied a mean of 8.9 years after gastrectomy did not confirm typical osteomalacia though it showed subclinical vertebral fractures and other bone abnormalities including decreased bone mineral content and hyperosteoidosis. Serum 25-hydroxyvitamin D levels were similar in patients and controls but 1,25-dihydroxyvitamin D levels were significantly higher and 24,25-dihydroxyvitamin D levels were significantly lower in patients. Bone mineral content, as judged by quantitative CT scanning correlated positively ($r=0.73$) with serum 25(OH)-vitamin D levels and negatively ($r=0.63$) with serum 1,25-dihydroxyvitamin D levels (Klein et al, 1987). These results are similar to those of Nilas et al (1985) who compared Bilroth I and Bilroth II operated patients. The 25(OH)-vitamin D concentrations were reduced and 1,25-dihydroxyvitamin D concentrations were increased in both groups but it was only in the Bilroth I patients that bone mineral content was demonstrated to be depleted. Calcium absorption was low–normal in both groups. In practical terms it seems that a clinical trial of calcium with vitamin D is the simplest method for diagnosing and treating patients, who, with a raised alkaline phosphatase, are suspected of having subclinical osteomalacia (Tovey et al, 1985).

Folic acid deficiency

Clark (1973) reviewed the results of five studies and concluded that mild folate deficiency occurs in about 30% of patients after gastrectomy, and severe deficiency occurs in about 5% of such patients. The deficiency is thought to be due principally to deficient dietary intake.

CHRONIC PANCREATIC INSUFFICIENCY

Intake

Nutrient intake has best been documented in children and adolescents with cystic fibrosis. Intake in this condition is influenced not only by the disease (abdominal bloating/cough) but also by the advice given. In some centres a low fat, high calorie diet is advised in order to reduce steatorrhoea and losses of electrolytes, minerals and vitamins while in others it is recognized that it can be very difficult to achieve the high calorie intake needed in the face of severe malabsorption if fat is much reduced in the diet. Dietary studies usually show a substantial subset of patients taking about 80% of Recommended Daily Allowance (RDA) for energy, though with a policy of not limiting fat intake, intakes of 130% are not uncommonly achievable. (Bell et al, 1984; Roy et al, 1984). Reduced energy intake appears to be the principal problem as far as intake is concerned (Parsons et al, 1983).

Most of the studies of nutrient intake in relation to chronic pancreatitis have aimed to characterize risk factors for the disease and therefore concentrate upon the pre-illness diet (Sarles, 1984). The mean daily intake of alcohol is by far the most important dietary risk factor with the logarithm of the risk directly proportional to the intake of alcohol. There is also a relationship, albeit much weaker, between the logarithm of the relative risk and the dietary protein intake. There may also be increased risk of chronic pancreatitis from extremes of fat intake whether high or low. Recurrent abdominal pain reduces nutrient intake and will worsen the undernutrition associated with chronic pancreatitis.

Nutritional status

Although children with cystic fibrosis are born smaller than the general population (Dodge and Yassa, 1980), and the course of their disease is complicated by chronic sepsis, growth of these children can be greatly improved by nutritional treatment. They thus provide us with a remarkable insight into the potential for chronic pancreatic failure to result in undernutrition. In their review Soutter and colleagues (1986) demonstrate in detail the patterns of growth failure which may occur, ranging from chronic stunting with relative preservation of weight for height to more acute loss of weight with wasting but relative preservation of height. In their series 13% of boys and 21% of girls eight or more years old were below the 3rd centile for height with figures of 33% and 42% for weight. Body composition data were also reviewed and demonstrated diminution of both lean body mass and fat stores.

Absorption

Stool nitrogen losses have been assessed in balance studies. Regan et al (1977) showed high mean stool losses of $9 \pm 1\,g$ (SEM) in six patients. Unfortunately nitrogen intake was not given in this paper. Such losses would be nutritionally significant if they occurred on a dietary protein intake of less than 95 g, a level which is unlikely to be achieved in the clinical context of alcoholism or recurrent abdominal pain. Fortunately these high losses appear to be easily corrected by pancreatic enzyme supplementation (Regan et al, 1977).

Steatorrhoea is severe in pancreatic failure and is due not only to failure of pancreatic enzyme secretion but also to reduced secretion of pancreatic bicarbonate and abnormal bile acid physiology (Zentler-Munro and Northfield, 1987). The choice of pancreatic enzyme supplement is beyond the scope of this review but depends upon rates of gastric emptying, duodenal acidity and mixing of the enzyme with the upper intestinal contents. Histamine H_2 antagonists can be synergistic with enzyme supplements. With effective treatment stool fat losses can be reduced from a mean of around 60 g to 10–20 g or so on a constant 100 g fat intake (Regan et al, 1977) thus roughly doubling energy absorption as fat from 360 kcal to 765 kcal. A diet containing a very large amount of fibre (75–80 g), is associated with a 32% higher faecal fat excretion than a diet with a similar content of fat (100 g) but with a fibre content of 12–14 g (Dutta and Hlasko, 1985).

Protein metabolism

A series of undernourished children with cystic fibrosis had elevated urinary excretion of urinary 3–methylhistidine (Miller et al, 1982). Whole body protein turnover studies from the same group of investigators (Holt et al, 1985) showed reduced protein synthesis among patients with acute pulmonary disease and elevated protein breakdown in patients with stable pulmonary involvement. It is not clear from this study (as the authors acknowledged) to what extent nutrient intake varied between the groups and contributed to the results.

Parsons et al (1985) studied the effect of six months protein and energy supplementation on nitrogen balance and protein turnover; during the period of supplementation there was an increased rate of growth. While undergoing nutritional treatment the children were in more positive nitrogen balance and this appeared to be the result of reduced rates of whole body protein breakdown rather than any change in synthesis.

THE SHORT BOWEL SYNDROME AND SMALL INTESTINAL ADAPTATION

For a review on adaptation see Dowling (1982). After resection the remaining small intestine adapts by villous hyperplasia and dilatation. These changes are associated with more rapid cellular turnover in the crypts and an increase in the rates of epithelial cell migration, so that the villus is covered by less mature cells than normal. These cells have diminished individual function but despite this the adaptive hyperplasia which starts within 24 hours or so of resection, but may take many months to be functionally complete, results in an increased segmental absorption of many nutrients including water, electrolytes, mono- and oligosaccharides, and amino acids and oligopeptides. The ileum can adapt to take on jejunal function, but the jejunum cannot adapt to take on the specialist functions of the terminal ileum, namely the absorption of bile acids and vitamin B_{12}.

The mechanisms for such adaptation are complex. They are related to the luminal content of nutrients, especially fat and this trophic effect of food may be mediated through pancreatobiliary secretions or hormones, of which enteroglucagon (Bloom, 1987) remains the prime candidate. The presence of fat in the ileum has a 'braking' effect upon small bowel transit (Spiller et al, 1984), and this may be another adaptive mechanism by increasing the contact time of luminal contents with the absorptive epithelium.

After massive intestinal resection there is very substantial, highly nutritionally relevant, malabsorption even after maximal adaptation. In seven adults with a total small bowel remnant of less than 150 cm jejunum ending in a stoma there was 30–80% malabsorption of energy, with similar results for fat and nitrogen (McIntyre et al, 1986). In 11 children aged 2 months to 9 years with 13 cm (5 in.) to a third of the small intestine remaining, and receiving 55–394 g carbohydrate enterally per day, stool carbohydrate losses ranged between 10.9 and 101 g/day. Carbohydrate loss correlated with stool volume, with an increase of faecal carbohydrate by 1 g associated with an increase in stool weight of about 32 g (Ameen et al, 1987). In addition to calorie and nitrogen malabsorption there is demonstrable malabsorption of other nutrients, for example calcium, magnesium and zinc (Woolf et al, 1987). Losses of water, sodium and other electrolytes are often the earliest determinants of whether nutrition will be able to be maintained by oral or enteral routes or whether parenteral nutrition and fluids will become necessary. Whether or not the colon is still present and in continuity is therefore of importance. Gouttebel et al (1986) found that prolonged parenteral nutrition could be avoided in patients with as little as 50–70 cm of remaining small bowel if the colon was in continuity whereas 110–150 cm was needed if the colon was resected.

Patients with adequate intake and absorption of protein and energy do not need total parenteral nutrition. Their problems may arise from malabsorption of specific nutrients or luminal contents. If 50 cm or more of the terminal ileum has been resected vitamin B_{12} will be poorly absorbed (Lenz, 1975), and there will be malabsorption of bile salts which may have a purgative effect in the colon. Ileal resections of as little as 100 cm can cause steatorrhoea (Hoffmann and Poley, 1972), with resultant potential for loss of fat-soluble vitamins and calcium. Much larger resections of jejunum are tolerated nutritionally, because of the ileum's adaptability, but in the long term malabsorption of iron, calcium and folate are particular problems. B_{12} deficiency may arise if there is bacterial overgrowth. In the presence of high volume diarrhoea, hypomagnesaemia, hypocalcaemia and acid–base disturbances, whether acidosis or alkalosis, may occur. Finally, some other metabolic complications of bowel resection should be mentioned. Gastric hypersecretion occurs in relation to hypergastrinaemia. Gall stones may occur as a result of reduced bile salt absorption. Oxalate renal stones may be related to reduced precipitation of luminal oxalate with calcium in the presence of unabsorbed fat, when the fat binds calcium in competition with the normal calcium–oxalate combination (Chadwick et al, 1972).

INFLAMMATORY BOWEL DISEASE

Patients with inflammatory bowel disease (IBD) may have no or only minor nutritional problems. Those with distal ulcerative colitis, those whose disease is in remission, or in whom the inflammation is effectively suppressed, are unlikely to suffer more than iron or folate deficiency and should pose little problem to the clinician. However there are patients with ulcerative colitis and Crohn's disease who become severely and dangerously undernourished.

The prevalence of undernutrition in IBD is unknown. Hospital-based studies are heavily biased towards the severely ill and take little account of the thousands of patients who seldom if ever need to see a doctor. Such studies depend heavily upon local referral patterns and policies on routine follow up; they can never truly be described as 'unselected'. A study from Leeds (Hill et al, 1977) illustrates the spectrum of nutritional status. Patients with acute colitis or requiring urgent surgery or who were suffering post-operative complications had lost about 10–24% of their body weight, whereas those with disease in remission or attending for routine follow up of an ileostomy or for elective surgery had little or no weight loss.

Energy metabolism

Weight loss may be due to dehydration, loss of adipose tissue or loss of non-water lean body mass. A small study demonstrated anthropometrically a relatively selective depletion of fat stores in a group of 33 patients admitted to hospital for IBD (Powell-Tuck, 1986).

There are no comprehensive estimates of energy expenditure in IBD but intake has been studied. Undernourished out-patients had broadly similar intakes to an unmatched group of normals as judged by a three day semi-weighed dietary assessment, from which it was concluded that reduced food intake is not a common feature in chronically undernourished patients with Crohn's disease (Jones et al, 1984). Giving a nutritionally complete liquid diet to provide a supplement of about 550–750 kcal is, however, effective in causing gains in weight, arm muscle circumference and skin fold thickness (Harries et al, 1983; Lanfranchi et al, 1984). There can be no serious doubt that impaired intake can be a major problem in some patients.

Protein metabolism

This has been more fully reviewed recently (Powell-Tuck, 1986). Protein/ nitrogen losses from the bowel in these conditions (and in the steroid era) seldom exceed 5–7 g N and will usually be adequately provided for by a normal dietary intake of 80 g or so of protein, providing this intake is maintained. The intake of dietary nitrogen is by far the dominant factor in determining the nitrogen balance and the rates of protein synthesis in patients with IBD. Rates of whole body protein turnover are also influenced by sepsis (Long et al, 1977) and disease activity (Powell-Tuck et al, 1984), and there are occasional instances when nitrogen balance remains negative as a result of sepsis despite adequate nutrient intake (Clark and Lauder, 1969).

Growth failure may be associated with IBD in adolescence and several studies have suggested that this can be corrected by increasing nutrient intake (Layden et al, 1976; Kelts et al, 1979). Motil et al (1982) showed that increasing the intake from 2.3 g protein and 67 kcal kg^{-1} per 24h to 3.2 g protein and 96 kcal kg^{-1} per 24h resulted in increased rates of protein turnover and improved nitrogen balance. The relevance of observed diminished growth hormone secretion in IBD remains unclear. Supplementary growth hormone is ineffective in promoting growth in these patients (McCaffery et al, 1974).

There are increased losses of several plasma proteins from the intestine in IBD and the rates of loss correlate with the activity of the disease (Jarnum and Jensen, 1975). That these losses are not the sole cause of the hypo-albuminaemia so commonly associated with moderate to severe IBD is shown by the association of comparable losses of IgG with rises in the plasma concentration of this protein. Other factors which may combine with the intestinal protein losses to result in hypoalbuminaemia are dietary conditions of protein deprivation (which unlike short-term starvation result in reduced albumin synthesis), and abnormal distribution of albumin between intravascular and extravascular spaces, which occurs in response to inflammation, sepsis and trauma (Fleck et al, 1985). Thus hypoalbuminaemia is a poor index of nutritional status in IBD.

Fibre and refined sugar intake

A number of studies have drawn attention to the low intake of fibre and the relatively high intake of refined sugar in IBD (see Table 1). In a prospective trial a high fibre diet low in refined sugar did not favourably influence the course of the illness (Ritchie et al, 1987). On the other hand, elemental diets may have a place in selected patients with Crohn's disease (O'Morain et al, 1984; Sanderson et al, 1987). In controlled trials resting the bowel while providing all nutrients parenterally has been shown to be ineffective in ulcerative colitis (Dickinson et al, 1980; McIntyre et al, 1986).

Nutritional anaemias

Iron deficiency commonly occurs in patients with IBD, presumably as a result of blood loss. Folate deficiency is common also and cannot be attributed to malabsorption alone because it is common in colitis and in distal ileal disease which is unlikely to affect folate absorption. However malabsorption has been documented when the proximal small bowel is involved with Crohn's disease (Hoffbrand et al, 1968). Dietary factors may be important because low fibre diets tend to be depeleted in folic acid, but increased utilization is another likely cause (Dyer et al, 1972). Vitamin B$_{12}$ deficiency is a risk if 50 cm of terminal ileum are resected and will occur if 100 cm are removed. Similarly, disease of the terminal ileum may cause malabsorption of this vitamin. Another cause of B$_{12}$ deficiency in Crohn's disease is bacterial overgrowth complicating a stagnant loop of small intestine in relationship to stricturing, and this may also contribute to hypoalbuminaemia.

Table 1. The diet of patients with Crohn's disease as compared with the general population.

	Controls General population	No. of patients	Pre- illness diet	No. of patients	Diet during illness	No. of patients	Reference
Energy	9.5	*					1
MJ/day	13.4	63	16.4	63	13.4	63	2
	9.6	30	10.4	30			4
	12.3	70	14.4	35			6
Total	273	*					1
carbohydrate	241	30	295	30			4
g/day	261	70	367	70			6
					90	29	5
Total fat	105	*					1
g/day	111	30	112	30			4
	137	70	147	35			6
Total protein	72.3	*					
g/day	74	30	73	30			4
	89	70	96	35			6
Refined sugar	54.5	*					
g/day	65	30	122	30			4
	91	70	156	35			6
	74	63	177	63	116	63	2
	55	34			115	34	3
Total fibre	19.2	30	17.3	30			4
g/day	22.3	70	26.6	35			6

*7696 households.
References: 1 = National Food Survey, 1977; 2 = Martini and Brandes, 1976; 3 = Miller et al, 1976; 4 = Thornton et al, 1979; 5 = Heaton et al, 1979; 6 = Kasper and Sommer, 1979.

Other micronutrient deficiencies

There has been considerable interest in zinc status in IBD. Unfortunately the literature is often difficult to interpret because of the uncertainty as to which methods are best for assessing zinc nutrition. Wolman and his colleagues (1979) demonstrated increased zinc losses from the bowel which correlated with stool volume and could amount to 15 mg or more per day. Zinc deficiency has been documented in Crohn's disease (McClain et al, 1980) and increased zincuria has been shown to occur in active ulcerative colitis (Mills and Fell, 1979). A case of pellagra due to malabsorption of nicotinic acid has been reported in a patient with ileo-colic Crohn's disease. The malabsorption improved with steroid therapy (Pollack et al, 1982). Subclinical vitamin C deficiency is common in Crohn's disease. Deficiency is not related to the activity of the disease but to deficient intake. It may be effectively countered by dietary counselling (Imes et al, 1986). The detection of an abnormal prothrombin in the blood is a sensitive test for vitamin K deficiency; using it Krasinski et al (1985) found deficiency in patients with Crohn's ileo-colitis and ulcerative colitis but not in those with Crohn's colitis alone. Vitamin D deficiency is well documented in Crohn's disease (Driscoll et al, 1982).

REFERENCES

Ameen VZ, Powell GK & Jones LA (1987) Quantification of faecal carbohydrate excretion in patients with short bowel syndrome. *Gastroenterology* **92**: 493–500.

Bell L, Durie P & Forstner (1984) What do children with cystic fibrosis eat? *Journal of Pediatric Gastroenterology and Nutrition* **3 (supplement)**: S137–146.

Bisballe S, Buus S, Lund B & Hessov I (1986) Food intake and nutritional status after gastrectomy. *Human Nutrition: Clinical Nutrition* **40c**: 301–308.

Bloom SR (1987) Gut hormones in adaptation. *Gut* **28 (supplement)**: 31–35.

Bo-Linn GW, Davis GR, Buddrus DJ, Morawski SG, Santa Ana C, Fordtran JS (1984) An evaluation of the importance of gastric acid secretion in the absorption of dietary calcium. *Journal of Clinical Investigation* **73**: 640–647.

Bradley EL (1979) Total gastrectomy. *Clinics in Gastroenterology* **8**: 354–371.

Butler TJ (1961) The effect of gastrectomy on pancreatic secretion in man. *Annals of the Royal College of Surgeons* **29**: 300–327.

Chadwick VS, Modha K & Dowling RH (1972) Mechanism for hyperoxaluria in patients with ileal dysfunction. *New England Journal of Medicine* **289**: 172–176.

Clark CG (1973) Nutritional and metabolic complications of partial gastrectomy. In Cox AG & Williams JA (eds) *Vagotomy on Trial*, pp 53–65, London: Heinemann.

Clark RG & Lauder NM (1969) Undernutrition and surgery in regional illeitis. *British Journal of Surgery* **56**: 736–738.

Cox AG (1969) Effects of vagotomy on nutrition. In Williams JA & Cox AG (eds) *After Vagotomy*, pp 131–136, London: Butterworths.

Dickinson RJ, Ashton MG, Axon ATR, Smith RC, Yeung CK & Hill GL (1980) Controlled trial of intravenous hyperalimentation and total bowel rest as an adjunct to the routine therapy of acute colitis. *Gastroenterology* **79**: 1199–1204.

Dodge JA & Yassa JG (1980) Food intake and supplementary feeding programmes. In Sturgess JM (ed.) *Perspectives in Cystic Fibrosis*, pp 125–135 Toronto Canadian Cystic Fibrosis Foundation. The Imperial Press.

Dowling RH (1982) Intestinal adaptation and its mechanisms. In Jewell DP & Selby WS (eds) *Topics in Gastroenterology 10*, pp 135–156. Oxford: Blackwell.

Driscoll RH, Meridith SC, Sitrin M & Rosenberg IH (1982) Vitamin D deficiency and bone disease in patients with Crohn's disease. *Gastroenterology* **83**: 1252–1258.

Dutta SK & Hlasko J (1985) Dietary fiber in pancreatic disease: effect of high fiber diet on fat malabsorption in pancreatic insufficiency and in vitro study of the interaction of dietary fiber with pancreatic enzymes. *American Journal of Clinical Nutrition* **41**: 517–525.

Dyer NH, Child JA, Mollin DL & Dawson AM (1972) Anaemia in Crohn's disease. *Quarterly Journal of Medicine* **164**: 419–436.

Fleck A, Raines G, Hawker F et al (1985) Increased vascular permeability as a major cause of hypoalbuminaemia in disease and injury. *Lancet* **i**: 781–784.

French JM & Crane CW (1963) Undernutrition, malnutrition and malabsorption after gastrectomy, In Stammers FAR & Williams JA (eds) *Partial Gastrectomy Complications and Metabolic Consequences*, pp 227–262, London: Butterworths.

Gouttebel MC, Saint-Aubert B, Astre C, Joyeux H (1986) Total parenteral nutrition needs in different types of short bowel syndrome. *Digestive Diseases and Sciences* **31**: 718–723.

Harries AD, Jones LA, Danis V et al (1983) Controlled trial of supplemented oral nutrition in Crohn's disease. *Lancet* **i**: 887–890.

Heaton KW, Thornton JW & Emmett PM (1979) Treatment of Crohn's disease with an unrefined carbohydrate rich diet. *British Medical Journal* **2**: 764–766.

Hill GL, Blackett RL, Pickford IR & Bradley JA (1977) A survey of protein nutrition in patients with inflammatory bowel disease – a rational basis for nutritional therapy. *British Journal of Surgery* **64**: 894–896.

Hoffbrand AV, Stewart JS, Booth CC & Mollin DL (1968) Folate deficiency in Crohn's disease: incidence, pathogenesis, and treatment. *British Medical Journal* **1**: 71–75.

Hoffmann AF & Poley JR (1972) Role of bile acid malabsorption in the pathogenesis of diarrhoea and steatorrhoea in patients with ileal resection I Response to cholestyramine or replacement of dietary long chain triglyceride by medium chain triglycerides. *Gastroenterology* **62**: 918–934.

Holt TL, Ward LC, Francis J, Isles A, Cooksley WGE & Shepherd RW (1985) Whole body protein turnover in cystic fibrosis patients and its relationship to pulmonary disease. *American Journal of Clinical Nutrition* **41**: 1061–1066.

Imes S, Dinwoodie A, Walker K, Pinchbeck B & Thomson ABR (1986) Vitamin C status in 137 outpatients with Crohn's disease: Effect of diet counselling. *Journal of Clinical Gastroenterology* **8**: 443–446.

Jarnum S & Jensen KB (1975) Fecal radioiodide excretion following intravenous injection of ^{131}I-albumin and ^{125}I-immunoglobulin G in chronic inflammatory bowel disease. *Gastroenterology* **68**: 1433–1444.

Jones LA, Harries AD, Rhodes J & Heatley RV (1984) Normal energy intake in undernourished patients with Crohn's disease. *British Medical Journal* **288**: 193.

Jones TC, Williams JA & Nicholson G (1963) Disturbances of bone metabolism after partial gastrectomy (post-gastrectomy bone disease), In Stammers FAR & Williams JA (eds) *Patrial Gastrectomy*, pp 190–226, London: Butterworths.

Kasper H & Sommer H (1979) Dietary fiber and nutrient intake in Crohn's disease. *American Journal of Clinical Nutrition* **32**: 1898–1901.

Kelts DG, Grand R, Shen G, Watkins JB, Werlin SL & Boehme C (1979) Nutritional basis of growth failure in children and adolescents with Crohn's disease. *Gastroenterology* **76**: 720–727.

Klein KB, Orwoll ES, Lieberman DA, Meier DE, McClung MR & Parfitt AM (1987) Metabolic bone disease in asymptomatic men after partial gastrectomy with Bilroth II anastomosis. *Gastroenterology* **92**: 608–616.

Krasinski SD, Russell M, Furie BC, Kruger S, Jacques PF & Furie B (1985) The prevalence of vitamin K deficiency in chronic gastrointestinal disorders. *American Journal of Clinical Nutrition* **41**: 639–643.

Lanfranchi GA, Brignola C, Pasquali R et al (1984) Effect of caloric supplementation in malnourished patients with Crohn's disease. *Clinical Nutrition* **3**: 51–53.

Layden T, Rosenberg J, Nemchausky B, Elison C & Rosenberg I (1976) Reversal of growth arrest in adolescents with Crohn's disease after parenteral alimentation. *Gastroenterology* **70**: 1017–1021.

Lenz K (1975) The effect of the site of lesion and extent of resection on duodenal bile acid concentration and vitamin B_{12} absorption in Crohn's disease. *Scandinavian Journal of Gastroenterology* **10**: 241–248.

Lindenbaum J (1980) Malabsorption of vitamin B_{12} and folate. In Winick M (ed.) *Nutrition in Gastroenterology*, pp 105–123, New York: Wiley.

Long CL, Jeevanandam M, Kim BM & Kinney JM (1977) Whole body protein synthesis and catabolism in septic man. *American Journal of Clinical Nutrition* **30**: 1340–1344.

Martini GA & Brandes JW (1976) Increased consumption of refined carbohydrates in patients with Crohn's disease. *Klinische Wochenschrift* **54**: 367–371.

McCaffery TD, Nasr K, Lawrence AM & Kirsner JB (1974) Effect of administered growth hormone on growth retardation in inflammatory bowel disease. *American Journal of Digestive Diseases* **19**: 411–416.

McClain C, Soutor C & Zieve L (1980) Zinc deficiency: a complication of Crohn's disease. *Gastroenterology* **78**: 272–279.

McIntyre PB, Fitchew M & Lennard-Jones JE (1986) Patients with a high jejunostomy do not need a special diet. *Gastroenterology* **91**: 25–33.

McIntyre PB, Lerebours E, Powell-Tuck J et al (1986) A controlled trial of bowel rest in the treatment of severe acute colitis. *Gut* **27**: 481–485.

Miller B, Fervers K, Rohbeck R & Strohmeyer G (1976) Zuckerconsum bei patienten mit morbus Crohn. *Gesellschaft für Innere Medizin* **82**: 922–924.

Miller M, Ward L, Thomas BJ, Cooksley WGE & Shepherd RW (1982) Altered body composition and muscle protein degradation in nutritionally growth-retarded children with cystic fibrosis. *American Journal of Clinical Nutrition* **36**: 492–499.

Mills PR & Fell GS (1979) Zinc and inflammatory bowel disease. *American Journal of Clinical Nutrition* **32**: 2172–2173.

Morgan DB & Pulvertaft CN (1969) Effects of vagotomy on bone metabolism. In Williams JA & Cox AG (eds) *After Vagotomy*, pp 161–171, London: Butterworths.

Motil KJ, Grand RJ, Matthews DE, Bier DM, Maletskos CJ & Young VR (1982) Whole body leucine metabolism in adolescents with Crohn's disease and growth failure during nutritional supplementation. *Gastroenterology* **82:** 1359–1368.

National Food Survey (1977) *Household food consumption and expenditure.* Ministry of Agriculture, Fisheries and Food, London: HMSO.

Nilas L, Christiansen C & Christiansen J (1985) Regulation of Vitamin D and calcium metabolism after gastrectomy. *Gut* **26:** 252–257.

O'Morain C, Segal AW & Levi AJ (1984) Elemental diets in treatment of acute Crohn's disease: a controlled trial. *British Medical Journal* **288:** 1859–1862.

Parsons HG, Beaudry P, Dumas A & Pencharz PB (1983) Energy needs and growth in children with cystic fibrosis. *Journal of Pediatric Gastroenterology and Nutrition* **2:** 44–49.

Parsons HG, Beaudry P & Pencharz PB (1985) The effect of nutritional rehabilitation on whole body protein metabolism of children with cystic fibrosis. *Pediatric Research* **19:** 189–192.

Pollack S, Enat R, Haim S, Zinder O & Barzilai D (1982) Pellagra as the presenting manifestation of Crohn's disease. *Gastroenterology* **82:** 948–952.

Powell-Tuck J (1986) Protein metabolism in inflammatory bowel disease. *Gut* **27 (supplement 1):** 67–71.

Powell-Tuck J, Garlick PJ, Lennard-Jones JE & Waterlow JC (1984) Rates of whole body protein synthesis and breakdown increase with the severity of inflammatory bowel disease. *Gut* **25:** 460–464.

Ritchie JK, Wadsworth J, Lennard-Jones JE & Rogers E (1987) Controlled multicentre trial of an unrefined carbohydrate, fibre rich diet in Crohn's disease. *British Medical Journal* **295:** 517–520.

Recker RR (1985) Calcium absorption and achlorhydria. *New England Journal of Medicine* **313:** 70–73.

Regan PT, Malagelada JR, DiMagno EP, Glanzman SL & Go VLW (1977) Comparative effects of antacids, cimetidine and enteric coating on the therapeutic response to oral enzymes in severe pancreatic insufficiency. *New England Journal of Medicine* **297:** 854–858.

Roy CC, Darling P & Weber AM (1984) A rational approach to meeting macro- and micronutrient needs in cystic fibrosis. *Journal of Pediatric Gastroenterology and Nutrition* **3 (supplement 1):** S154–162.

Sanderson IR, Udeen S, Davies PSW, Savage MO & Walker-Smith JA (1987) Remission induced by an elemental diet in small bowel Crohn's disease. *Archives of Disease in Childhood* **61:** 123–127.

Sarles H (1984) Epidemiology and physiopathology of chronic pancreatitis and the role of the pancreatic stone protein. *Clinics in Gastroenterology* **13:** 895–912.

Soutter VL, Kristidis P, Gruca MA & Gaskin KJ (1986) Chronic undernutrition/growth retardation in cystic fibrosis. *Clinics in Gastroenterology* **15:** 137–155.

Spiller RC, Trotman IF, Higgins BE et al (1984) The ileal brake – inhibition of jejunal motility after ileal fat perfusion in man. *Gut* **25:** 365–374.

Thornton JR, Emmett PM & Heaton KW (1979) Diet and Crohn's disease: characteristics of the pre-illness diet. *British Medical Journal* **2:** 762–764.

Tovey FI, Karamanolis DG, Godfrey J & Clark CG (1985) Post-gastrectomy nutrition: methods of out-patient screening for early osteomalacia. *Human Nutrition; Clinical Nutrition* **39c:** 439–446.

Williams JA & Hoare AM (1979) Partial gastric resection. *Clinics in Gastroenterology* **8:** 321–353.

Wolman SL, Anderson GH, Marliss EB & Jeejeebhoy KN (1979) Zinc in total parenteral nutrition: requirements and metabolic effects. *Gastroenterology* **76:** 458–467.

Woolf GM, Miller C, Kurian R & Jeejeebhoy KN (1987) Nutritional absorption in short bowel syndrome. Evaluation of fluid calorie and divalent cation requirements. *Digestive Diseases and Sciences* **32:** 8–15.

Zentler-Munro PL & Northfield TC (1987) Review: pancreatic enzyme replacement – applied physiology and pharmacology. *Alimentary Pharmacology and Therapeutics* **1:** 575–591.

2

Identification and assessment of the malnourished patient

ROSS A. PETTIGREW

For centuries, it has been recognized that malnutrition has an adverse effect on the well-being and recovery of patients. Hippocrates, in one of his famous aphorisms stated that 'those who are fat about the belly do best; it is bad to be thin and wasted there'. Malnutrition has often been regarded as deficiency of micronutrients such as vitamins or trace elements, but in recent years, deficiencies of the macronutritents (proteins, carbohydrates and fats), commonly called protein-energy malnutrition (PEM), have assumed greater importance and are being recognized more commonly in hospital patients. The importance of PEM in children is undisputed. Retardation of growth and development is evident in children who have had episodes of PEM during early life. The relevance of PEM to hospital patients however is not so clear although it has been assumed that, like children, PEM will have adverse effects on the outcome of illness in adult patients. For this reason, there has been intense interest in identifying patients with PEM by various methods of assessment with a view to demonstrating that they are more likely to have an adverse outcome than normally nourished patients when they undergo 'stress' events such as major surgical procedures.

There is no universally accepted definition by which patients with PEM can be readily identified. Unlike childhood PEM, where the Wellcome classification and definitions, described by Waterlow (1976), based on measurement of weight and clinical features, and related to prognosis and treatment, are generally accepted, there is no consensus on the criteria for defining adult PEM. Definitions based on clinical appearance and supported by measurements of weight, height and weight loss have failed to demonstrate a consistent relationship to outcome after major surgical procedures. Another approach to defining PEM has been based on the assumption that patients with PEM have a greater risk of developing postoperative complications than normally nourished patients. Such high risk or 'malnourished' patients are defined by the 'nutritional' measurements which are associated with outcome variables such as postoperative complications. McLaren and Meguid (1983) have questioned the validity of this approach, as the 'nutritional' measurements used are not solely influenced by the nutritional status of adult hospital patients. Furthermore, it has been shown that less than one half of preoperative patients presenting for major gastrointestinal surgery, defined by high risk 'nutritional' measurement criteria have clear evidence of PEM by the more commonly accepted anthropometric criteria. Many patients who fit the high risk definition appear clinically to be very well nourished, while other very malnourished looking patients are not found to be 'high risk'. The place of nutritional assessment in the clinical management of patients has rightly been said to have reached a crossroads.

ANTHROPOMETRIC ASSESSMENT

Anthropometry is the most commonly used method for the nutritional assessment of animals and children. Recently Jeejeebhoy and Meguid (1986) have pointed out that traditional anthropometric methods of measuring PEM are not appropriate for assessing adult hospital patients because they are not growing. In adults, altered protein and energy intake does not affect anthropometric measurements to the same degree as in growing children. Furthermore, bed rest, protein loss from inflammatory gut disease, fluid changes and other sequelae found in many medical and surgical conditions influence body weight and muscle mass with little alteration in dietary intake. The rate of depletion of nutritional reserves varies throughout an illness. The early adaptive response to decreased intake is for body fat to be used for energy while protein is conserved. Later, as body fat is lost, protein, stored as muscle, is broken down to supply amino acids for vital cellular mechanisms. The addition of 'stress' to this metabolic environment further alters nutritional responses. Finally, studies of pre-operative surgical patients have failed to demonstrate any increased incidence of postoperative complications in anthropometrically depleted patients.

Despite these objections, anthropometric measurements are still used for static (one-off) and dynamic (serial) nutritional assessment of hospital patients. The techniques of anthropometric measurement have been described by Blackburn et al (1977). Gray and Gray (1979) have pointed out that the commonly used World Health Organization standards reported by Jelliffe (1966) are inappropriate because they are based on selected populations of people seeking insurance, military personnel in Italy, Greece and Turkey, and female volunteers. The recent introduction of population-based age, sex and race specific standards for many countries and communities has improved the validity of single assessments, although they still have not been able to be related to postoperative outcome. Weight for height ratios, triceps skinfold thickness and midarm muscle circumference have been the anthropometric measurements most commonly used for static assessment. Although changes detected by serial measurements are limited by the inherent imprecision of the methods, changes in body weight with time are commonly used for dynamic assessment. Forse and Shizgal (1980), using a multiple isotope dilution method to determine body composition in 216 patients, demonstrated significant correlations between body composition and these clinical assessment methods but found wide confidence limits and low sensitivity-specificity which limit the application to individual patients.

Body weight indices

The main components of body weight are water, fat, protein and minerals with smaller contributions from glycogen and other carbohydrates. The relative contribution of each of these components to the development of PEM has been the subject of many studies of body composition as reviewed by Shizgal (1981) using a multiple radioisotope dilution method and by Beddoe and Hill (1985) using in vivo neutron activation analysis (IVNAA). From studies using these methods an understanding of the complex inter-relationships of the nutritional components during illness and the response to various nutritional regimes has been obtained.

At a clinical level, the most important variable influencing body weight is height, with the influence of sex, age and race also being recognized. Goldbourt and Medalie (1974) in a review of weight for height indices concluded that weight divided by height squared (wt/ht^2) was the best index because it showed the least correlation with height. Another reason for using height squared is that it is recognized as an index of lean body mass. The body composition studies of McNeill et al (1979) demonstrated a correlation of total nitrogen content of normal and malnourished patients, determined by IVNAA, with height squared. The ratio wt/ht^2, also called body mass index, quetelets index or relative weight, is now commonly used to compare body weights with modern standards stratified for age, sex and race.

Weight loss, often expressed as a percentage of well weight, is the most commonly used dynamic measurement for the clinical assessment of PEM in hospital patients. If there is no recorded well weight, recalled well weight is preferred to predicted weight for the assessment of weight loss as follows:

$$\% \text{ weight loss} = \frac{\text{recalled weight} - \text{current weight}}{\text{recalled well weight}} \times 100$$

Morgan et al (1980) have shown that errors in determining weight loss from a single measurement of weight are greater if predicted rather than recalled well weights are used. Even so, the weight loss based on recalled weight had a large random error of up to 7.2 kg in their study. There are many other pitfalls in interpreting changes in weight. Acute changes are usually attributable to changes in total body water, although in severe trauma or sepsis losses of wet muscle protein may reach 1 kg/day. Furthermore, patients' recall is not always accurate and some deny ever being weighed. For clinical purposes, patients with a clear recall reporting a weight loss of 5% or greater are probably reliable. Stunkard and Albaum (1981) reported that 70% of their patients could report their weight to within 2 kg or better than 5% of recorded weight. Seltzer et al (1982) have suggested that an absolute weight loss of 10 lb correlates well with mortality of patients in surgical wards, although many of their deaths were from terminal cancer. This approach ignores the fact that a 10 lb weight loss for an obese patient is probably advantageous, but for a malnourished patient the same could be critical.

The combination of a static and dynamic assessment of weight to define nutritionally depleted patients has advantages. A static measurement alone, such as body mass index (wt/ht^2), below a particular percentile of an appropriate population-based standard will include a percentage of patients who normally maintain their weight at a low level. The addition of a dynamic measurement such as weight loss to the assessment will select those who are thin and getting thinner. Furthermore, this combination excludes those patients who are deliberately attempting to lose weight from a higher percentile. Nutritional depletion can be defined as body mass index below the 10th percentile with at least 5% weight loss. We have noted that when this definition is used in surveys of hospital patients, an appropriate proportion of patients below the 10th percentile are excluded by the addition of weight loss criteria. It is important however that any assessment is taken in the clinical context as such a definition may miss identifying the stressed patient whose real weight changes may be masked by water retention as discussed later.

Skinfold thickness

Triceps skinfold (TSF) measurements are made with calipers at the mid-point between the acromion and olecranon processes on the upper arm over the triceps muscle posteriorly. Other skinfold measurements used less commonly include the biceps skinfold, the subscapular skinfold at the lower border of the scapula and the suprailiac skinfold above the iliac crest. Using body density measurements determined by underwater weighing, Durnin and Wormsley (1974) have derived regression equations for the estimation of total body fat from combinations of these skinfold measurements. However, the imprecision of standardizing the site of measurement and the variations between different applications of the calipers and observers has limited the usefulness of skinfold measurements in the clinical assessment of PEM. Hall et al (1980) have reported large coefficients of variation of up to 22.6% for initial measurements of TSF which reduced to 4.9% after many weeks standardizing their techniques. Changes that occur with nutritional repletion are smaller than the errors of measurement and there is no place for skinfolds in the serial assessment of nutritional status. Nevertheless in the clinical setting where population-based standards are available, a one-off measurement, classified by percentile may be helpful in giving a broad idea of body fat stores.

Midarm muscle circumference

The measurement of the circumference of the arm (MAC) at the same point that TSF is measured is used to derive the midarm muscle circumference (MAMC) from the following formula:

$$MAMC = MAC - 2\pi \times TSF$$

Although MAMC is taken as an indirect measurement of the body muscle mass, Collins et al (1979) found that the wide confidence limits made it unsuitable for assessing total protein stores and they were unable to demonstrate a relationship between changes in MAMC and changes in total body nitrogen measured by IVNAA. Klidjian et al (1982) examined both MAMC and a similar measurement made in the forearm and claimed that these measurements were significantly related to postoperative outcome in 120 surgical patients undergoing major abdominal operations. However, similar studies by Mullen et al (1979) and Pettigrew and Hill (1986) have not confirmed this finding. While the coefficient of variation for the measurement of MAMC is less than for TSF, the problems associated with its measurement are similar. Where population-based standards are available, the measurement of MAMC can be useful in classifying patients by percentile but imprecision limits the usefulness of serial measurements for dynamic assessment.

BIOCHEMICAL ASSESSMENT

Serum concentrations of albumin, transferrin, prealbumin and retinol binding protein (RBP) have been the biochemical measurements most commonly used for the assessment of PEM. Because their synthesis is sensitive to altered protein intake, the serum levels of these 'visceral' proteins (as opposed to 'somatic' protein of muscle) are taken as a reflection of total body protein status. Application to the assessment of PEM is related to their half-lives with acute changes being reflected by the proteins with the shorter half-lives (RBP 12 hours, prealbumin 2 days) and more chronic changes reflected by the longer half-life proteins (transferrin 7 days, albumin 21 days). McFarlane et al (1969) found that serum transferrin was particularly accurate at measuring the severity and response to treatment of PEM in Nigerian children. Roza et al (1984) demonstrated a correlation between serum transferrin and total body potassium as an index of body cell mass, but changes in total body potassium with 2 weeks nutritional repletion were not reflected by serum transferrin changes. Shetty et al (1979) reported rapid changes of prealbumin and RBP when changing from high to low energy diets in obese patients, especially if the diet was low in protein. The fact that energy reduction alone also resulted in reduced serum levels of these proteins would argue against their value as markers of protein status, a point made by Golden (1982) in his critical review of transport proteins as indices of protein status. Furthermore, other medical conditions such as chronic liver disease, inflammatory bowel disease and sepsis may also contribute to a low serum albumin concentration.

As pointed out by Fleck et al (1985a), the most important factor altering serum albumin levels in hospital patients is the rate of exchange of albumin between the blood and extravascular space which is, by their calculations, more than 10 times the rates of synthesis and catabolism. This has led them to conclude (Fleck et al, 1985b) that these serum protein changes cannot be accounted for by nutritional and endocrine changes and they should not be assumed to reflect total body protein status. Despite these arguments, many studies have shown that preoperative levels of these serum proteins are most likely to select patients at increased risk of developing postoperative complications. However, the claim that this is related to nutritional status is further refuted by Pettigrew and Hill's study (1986) where more than half the patients identified as high risk by the plasma protein levels were clearly not malnourished. An editorial comment in the Lancet (Editorial, 1986) suggested that the serum proteins were an 'index of severity of illness' rather than nutritional status as a significant proportion of the patients with low plasma protein levels had clinical evidence of sepsis.

IMMUNOLOGICAL ASSESSMENT

Law et al (1974) have shown that both the humoral and cellular immune systems are impaired in patients with PEM and that nutritional repletion will improve immune responses. Tests of the immune status suitable for clinical evaluation of patients have included total lymphocyte count and the delayed hypersensitivity skin test (DHST) with more sophisticated tests reserved for assessment of underlying mechanisms of impaired immunity. Total lymphocyte count is no longer used as a measurement of PEM because it is altered by many non-nutritional factors and correlation with outcome has not been demonstrated. DHST is administered as separate intradermal injections of 4 to 8 recall antigens such as purified protein derivative, mumps, candida and streptokinase-streptodornase. The size of the inflammatory reactions is measured at 24 and 48 hours. The absence of reaction to all the antigens at either reading is classified as 'anergy'. There are variations in the interpretation of intermediate reactions. Pietsch et al (1977) have suggested that because DHST selects patients likely to develop septic complications after surgery, these patients may benefit from a course of nutritional therapy before surgery to reduce the incidence of postoperative complications. However, Brown et al (1982) were not able to demonstrate any relationship of the DHST result to postoperative outcome in their study of 244 patients undergoing major elective surgery and the relationship between nutritional status and the DHST result has been seriously questioned.

In the study by Forse et al (1981) of the relationship between DHST and body composition in 257 patients receiving nutritional support, they showed that, although the majority of anergic patients had a body composition consistent with malnutrition, 21% had normal body composition. Furthermore, only 43% of patients given a two week course of parenteral nutritional repletion improved their DHST result and body composition. They concluded that the DHST response does not accurately reflect nutritional status. Others have shown that infections, uraemia, cirrhosis, trauma, haemorrhage, drugs, anaesthesia and surgery commonly influence the DHST response found in hospital patients. Bates et al (1979) in a review of DHST in general have highlighted the many difficulties in the administration, reading and interpretation of these tests and made recommendations for uniformity. In their critical review, Twomey et al (1982) concluded that the usefulness of DHST for assessing nutritional status remained unproven and reports such as that of Brown et al (1982) have not changed this view.

Combination of assessments

With the unsatisfactory performance of single assessment methods in selecting high risk malnourished patients, attention turned to combinations of these measurements to increase their sensitivity and specificity. In one of the early studies, Mullen et al (1979) using multiple discriminant analysis of the nutritional measurements of patients undergoing major gastrointestinal operations showed that the serum albumin, transferrin and delayed hypersensitivity skin test were the best predictors of postoperative outcome. Later Buzby et al (1980) combined these measurements and TSF into a 'prognostic nutritional index' (PNI) which it was claimed would not only select the high risk patients who might benefit from intensive preoperative nutritional support to reduce their risk but put a figure on that risk. In their prospective study of 100 preoperative patients, they clearly demonstrated a relationship of the PNI to the percentage of patients that developed postoperative complications. Since then, other studies (Table 1) have produced similar prognostic indices for different populations all of which have been shown to select patients who are at increased risk of developing complications after surgery. In the only comparative study of these formulae in 218 patients undergoing major gastrointestinal operations, reported by Pettigrew and Hill (1986), the PNI and two other combinations of assessments correctly selected a high risk patient population. However, it was noted that only a third of these patients selected by the PNI were clearly nutritionally depleted by anthropometric and weight loss criteria. From their data, it was suggested that the PNI was also selecting septic patients and the PNI was not necessarily 'nutritional'. It is noticeable that all the indices rely heavily on plasma protein concentrations and, as Rainey-Macdonald et al (1983) have pointed out, many of the additional variables add little to improving the sensitivity and specificity of the main serum proteins. Therefore, the criticism of the relevance of the plasma proteins in reflecting nutritional status applies to these combined indices as well.

MUSCLE FUNCTION ASSESSMENT

The low sensitivity and specificity of anthropometric, biochemical and immunological measurements of PEM in detecting changes in nutrient intake has led to an exploration of functional changes, particularly in muscle, that occur with PEM. The investigation of grip strength dynamometry in surgical patients preoperatively by Klidjian et al (1982) and the demonstration of a correlation with MAMC, led to the suggestion that it was a form of nutritional assessment. Furthermore, they demonstrated that patients with weak grip strength developed more postoperative complications after surgery. However the correlation of grip strength with MAMC is weak, and non-nutritional factors of age, joint mobility, drug administra-

Table 1. Prognostic indices based on nutritional variables for identifying high risk patients.

Authors	Population	Outcome variable	Index*	High risk	Prospective study‡
Buzby et al (1980) Philadelphia	'Malnourished' major surgery 161 patients	Major postoperative complications	PNI = 158 − 16.8 Alb −0.78 TSF −0.2 Tfn −5.8 DHST	> 50	14 (47%)
Harvey et al (1981) Boston	282 patients referred for TPN†	(a) Deaths	PI = 0.91 Alb − DHST −1.44 Sep +0.98 Dgn −1.09	> 0	—
		(b) Subsequent sepsis	PI = 2.52 −0.99 Dgn −0.01 Tfn	> 0	8 (44%)
Rainey-MacDonald et al (1983) Ontario	55 patients referred for TPN	Major septic complications or death	PI = 1.2 Alb +0.013 Tfn −6.43	< 0	—
Pettigrew and Hill (1986) Leeds	240 gastric colorectal and gallbladder ops	Major postoperative complications or death	PI = 0.099 Alb −0.03 age −2.432	< 0	67 (23%)

* Index variables: Alb = albumin; Tfn = transferrin; TSF = triceps skinfold thickness; DHST = delayed hypersensitivity skin test; Sep = concurrent sepsis (1, no/2, yes); Dgn = diagnosis (1, cancer/2, non cancer).
† TPN = Total parenteral nutrition.
‡ From Pettigrew and Hill (1986). Numbers are the percentage of 218 patients defined as high risk in this study and the complication rate of these high risk patients in brackets.

tion and psychological motivation all influence this test. Another muscle function assessment technique has been the measurement of muscle fatigue in the adductor pollicis muscle. Russell et al (1983) claim that changes in the force frequency curve, obtained by increasing the frequency of stimulation of the ulnar nerve at the wrist and the measurement of the force of contraction of the adductor pollicis muscle, and the maximal relaxation rate are sensitive and specific to alterations in nutritional intake. Church et al (1984) have described histological and biochemical changes occurring in the muscles of malnourished patients which are possibly related to these functional alterations. These changes could explain the decreased respiratory muscle strength in protein-depleted patients observed by Windsor and Hill (1986) and lead to an increased incidence of respiratory complications in malnourished patients. It has yet to be shown that patients with impaired muscle function studies do have an adverse outcome after surgical procedures.

GLOBAL CLINICAL ASSESSMENT

Global clinical assessment is made on the basis of clinical history and examination without anthropometric measurements or the results of laboratory investigations. The fundamentals of a clinical nutritional assessment are a thorough medical history, including a dietary history, the general appearance of the patient and a physical examination directed to particular areas. The clinical history, besides detailing the patient's illness, should include questions on energy, activity, appetite, abnormal losses of fluids such as vomiting, diarrhoea and fistulae, weight changes and the time periods over which symptoms have developed. A dietary history is an important part of the clinical history, with enquiries directed to the pattern of meals, their composition, food fads, the consumption of alcohol and other nutritional supplements and any recent changes. The general appearance of a patient with PEM is illustrated in Figure 1. Physical examination should be directed to assessing the stores of fat in the subcutaneous tissues and protein stores from assessment of muscle bulk.

Muscle wasting is best demonstrated in temporalis muscle, the muscles around the scapulae and in the upper arm, especially if there is overlying wasting of subcutaneous fat. It needs to be remembered that not all patients with reduced fat stores are malnourished, as seen in marathon runners. Conversely, patients with acute weight loss from severe protein catabolism may have fat stores relatively preserved, masking the underlying severe muscle wasting. Furthermore, water retention that often occurs in these patients, further reduces the measured weight loss and obscures the loss of muscle bulk. Other non-specific signs of malnutrition, less frequently observed, include skin rashes, angular conjunctivitis and other eye changes, stomatitis and glossitis, parasthaesiae, peripheral neuropathies and muscular weakness.

In a comparative study of clinical assessment and objective measurements, Baker et al (1982) concluded that a thorough clinical assess-

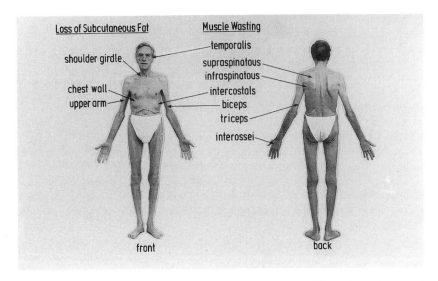

Figure 1. Areas of particular interest in the clinical assessment of fat and muscle stores in patients with protein-energy malnutrition.

ment of patients will identify those patients at greatest risk of developing problems related to their nutritional state better than objective measurements of PEM. They showed that the anthropometric, biochemical and body compositional measurements of 48 surgical patients classified by two clinicians as either normally nourished, mildly malnourished or severely malnourished were significantly different. Comparing the clinical course of these three groups of patients, they reported that the group clinically classified as severely malnourished had significantly increased incidence of hospital infections, more antibiotics prescribed, and a longer hospital stay than the normally nourished. A number of questions raised by Collins (1982) about the background of the observers, the sensitivity of the clinical evaluation, and the endpoints in this study have since been addressed. Pettigrew et al (1984) compared clinical assessment with anthropometric and immunological assessment of 198 surgical patients and noted that the clinician trained in nutritional assessment was more sensitive and specific in identifying nutritionally depleted and anergic patients than an untrained clinician. However, less than two thirds of patients in this study were correctly classified as anthropometrically depleted by either clinician. In another study, Pettigrew and Hill (1986) compared the ability of the operating surgeon to select preoperatively those patients at high risk of developing postoperative complications with the predictive ability of objective measurements. In a population of 218 patients about to undergo major gastrointestinal operations, they demonstrated that measurements of plasma proteins were better at predicting outcome than the surgeons, few of whom had any training in nutritional assessment. However, a clinical assessment, which noted medical as well as nutritional risk factors, made by one surgeon trained in nutritional assessment did predict patients developing complications as well as did the use of plasma protein levels. Comparisons of the sensitivity and specificity of these assessments, reported by Detsky et al (1984) and Pettigrew and Hill (1986), also demonstrate the relevance of training, endpoints and the population under study. Detsky's report found that global clinical assessment was the most sensitive and specific for predicting in-hospital infections in 48 surgical patients, although 25% of their patients did not have a surgical procedure. In contrast, Pettigrew and Hill's study of 218 patients, all of whom had a major abdominal operation, found that plasma proteins, especially prealbumin, were more sensitive and specific in predicting the more important postoperative complications than the surgeon's assessment. Depending on the endpoints chosen and the training of the physician, global clinical assessment can identify patients who have an increased risk of an adverse outcome, many of whom have other features of PEM. However, in clinical practice, nutritional assessment is not given high priority and objective measurements are needed to raise the clinician's awareness to the potential for nutritional problems.

STRESS AND MALNUTRITION

The adaptive response to reduced dietary intake is to use body energy stores (i.e. fat) and preserve protein stores (i.e. muscle). If carbohydrate intake is insufficient to meet the necessary requirement of certain tissues for glucose, the conversion of protein to glucose in the liver is initiated. The consequent attrition of protein is limited in starving patients by the adaptation of some glucose-obligated tissues to ketones as a substrate, slowing but never halting the loss of protein conversion to glucose. This adaptive response results in the wasting of fat and muscle in a controlled fashion while preserving the important functions of proteins in plasma transport and immuno-competence.

The classical studies of injury by Cuthbertson (1936) demonstrated the metabolic sequelae of stress in normally nourished patients. The loss of nitrogen along with other products of protein catabolism reaches a peak at 5–10 days after injury and is followed by a longer anabolic phase. The source of the nitrogen loss is mainly muscle protein and is dependent on the severity and duration of the stress. The increased nitrogen loss and rise in energy expenditure is limited after the stress of major operative procedures but is dramatically increased by more major stresses of severe sepsis and trauma such as burns. Increased levels of catecholamines, cortisol, and glucagon induce hyperglycaemia, without suppressing fatty acid oxidation while insulin levels remain relatively low. Protein breakdown serves not only to supply amino acids for acute phase proteins but also to supplement the hyperglycaemia through their conversion to glucose by gluconeogenesis in the liver. The overall effect is to increase the availability of energy substrates, especially glucose, to the injured tissues many of which are glucose obligated.

The addition of this stress response to the metabolic environment of a malnourished patient can seriously compromise their ability to survive the dual insults. The acceleration of protein breakdown from an already diminished store and the poor handling of energy substrates results in rapid clinical deterioration. In contrast to the slow nutritional depletion of the starving patient, the depleted, stressed patient shows more rapid weight loss, greater nitrogen losses and increased fluid retention which may mask many of the areas where fat and muscle wasting would be found clinically. The difference between depletion alone and stressed depletion have been likened to the differences seen in marasmus and kwashiorkor of childhood PEM. Coward and Lunn (1981) have described the pathophysiological changes of childhood marasmus as an adaptive response to energy deficit which is similar to the response of the starving adult patient. On the other hand, kwashiorkor children have severe muscle wasting, oedema and low plasma proteins that is thought to be related to a relative deficiency of protein in the diet. The contribution of infection, that often accompanies this form of malnutrition, to the pathogenesis of kwashiorkor is debated. The overall picture is similar to the stressed depleted adult patient.

McLaren and Meguid (1983) have suggested that a classification of adult PEM, based on the childhood PEM concepts may be useful in assessing type and severity of PEM. The nutritional profiles of adult 'marasmic' and 'kwashiorkor' patients described by Blackburn et al (1977) have proved too complex for wide acceptance in clinical practice. A simpler classification of PEM suitable for hospital patients and based on the concepts of depletion and stress is illustrated in Figure 2. The X axis represents protein stores and the Y axis, metabolic expenditure. Normally nourished patients, who are

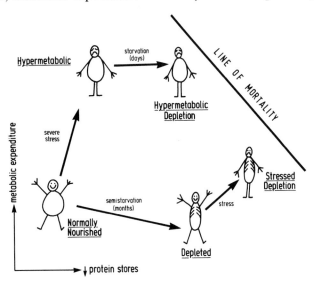

Figure 2. Schematic representation of the nutritional and stress events that affect hospital patients, their influence on protein status and metabolic expenditure, and their relationship to mortality.

starved over a period of time (usually months) gradually lose protein stores with a reduction in resting metabolic expenditure as their body cell mass shrinks. This state is labelled 'depleted'. If there is an added stress, metabolic expenditure and protein loss is increased, the kwashiorkor-like state of 'stressed depletion' is observed and the mortality line approached more quickly. The other pathway from normally nourished to the line of mortality occurs in the severely stressed patient, who becomes 'hypermetabolic' and, over a period of days, loses protein stores to reach 'hypermetabolic depletion'. Clearly, there are many scenarios between these pathways but the implications for outcome are illustrated. Small degrees of stress at the nutritionally depleted end of the spectrum are more devastating than similar degrees of stress at the normally nourished end. From clinical experience, the majority of malnourished patients do well after uncomplicated surgery, but where the stress is severe or a continuing metabolic response to trauma exists, the outcome in malnourished patients is compromised.

Hill and Church (1984) have used a similar classification for determining the energy and protein requirements of surgical patients. The relationship of this classification to outcome is given in Table 2 using data from 218 patients in Pettigrew and Hill's study (1986). Nutritional depletion was defined by body mass index below the 10th percentile of New Zealand standards specific for age, sex and race and weight loss greater than 5% of well weight. Plasma albumin of 32 g/l or less was used to indicate stress. The complication rate for depleted non-stressed patients was slightly, but not significantly, lower than for normally nourished patients. However, the complication rate of 54% for non-depleted stressed patients is significantly higher than for their non-stressed colleagues. It is these anthropometrically 'well nourished' patients with hypoalbuminaemia who contribute significantly to the high risk population of surgical patients. Examining the preoperative factors contributing to the stress of this group revealed that six patients had clinical evidence of sepsis. The implications for management are clear in that such patients need adequate treatment of their sepsis, such as drainage of abscesses, to improve the metabolic environment before the nutritional problems can be successfully treated. However, patients who are depleted with serum protein levels above 32 g/l have a low complication rate and delaying surgery for nutritional repletion is not indicated.

Table 2. Preoperative classification of 218 patients undergoing major gastrointestinal operations into stressed and depleted categories and their major postoperative complication rates.

| | Depletion category | | | |
| | Not depleted | | Depleted* | |
Stress category	n	Complications	n	Complications
Not stressed	Normal		Depleted	
(Albumin > 32 g/l)	129	20 (16%)	64	8 (13%)
Stressed	Stressed		Stressed depleted	
(Albumin ≤ 32 g/l)	13	7 (54%)	12	4 (33%)

* Weight/height^2 below 10th percentile and weight loss.
n, Number of patients.

THE PREVALENCE OF PEM IN WESTERN HOSPITAL PATIENTS

The reported prevalence of PEM in western hospitals, summarized in Table 3, varies according to the population under study and the criteria chosen to define PEM. Bollet and Owens (1973) reported low extractable protein levels in the hair roots of 23% of their minor medical and surgical patients

Table 3. Prevalence of protein-energy malnutrition in hospital patients using various nutritional measurements.

Authors (year)	Population studied	n	Nutritional measurement	Abnormal and standard*	Percentage abnormal
Bollet and Owens (1973)	Medical & surgical (minor)	144	wt/ht albumin	< 90% ML < 35 g/l	12 24
	Medical (major)	351	wt/ht albumin	< 90% ML < 35 g/l	24 35
Bistrian et al (1974)	Surgical patients	131	wt/ht TSF MAMC albumin	<90% J < 90% J < 90% J < 35 g/l	22 56 49 54
Bistrian et al (1976)	Medical patients	204	wt/ht TSF MAMC albumin	< 90% J < 90% J < 90% J < 35 g/l	39 74 50 45
Hill et al (1977)	Minor surgery	40	MAMC albumin transferrin	> 2 sd PC < 36.9 g/l < 231 mg%	19 13 26
	Preop. major surgery	21	MAMC albumin transferrin	> 2 sd PC < 36.9 g/l < 231 mg%	35 20 36
Weinsier et al (1979)	Medical patients	134	wt/ht TSF MAMC albumin	< 90% ML < 90% J < 90% J < 35 g/l	16 28 13 46
Mullen et al (1979)	Elective preop. major surgery patients	64	TSF MAMC albumin transferrin	< 90% J < 90% J < 30 g/l < 220 mg%	33 36 16 50
Klidjian et al (1982)	Elective preop. major surgery patients	120	wt/ht MAMC Grip Str albumin	< 85% ML < 85% J < 85% PC < 35 g/l	21 25 60 10
Pettigrew and Hill (1986)	Elective preop. major surgery patients	218	wt/ht² TSF MAMC albumin transferrin prealbumin	< 3rd %tile PC < 3rd %tile PC < 3rd %tile PC < 32 g/l < 200 mg% < 14 mg%	24 20 18 11 27 25

* Standards: J = Jelliffe (1966); ML = metropolitan life tables; PC = population-based controls; sd = standard deviation; %tile = percentile.
n, Number of patients.

which they suggested was indicative of PEM. In their more seriously ill medical patients, 32% had low hair root protein levels. Overestimates of the prevalence of PEM have been reported when anthropometric measurements are used with inappropriate population-based standards. A survey of 131 patients in surgical wards at Boston City Hospital by Bistrian et al (1974) classified patients as severely malnourished if measurements were less than 60% below their standard, and moderately malnourished if between 60 and 90% of the standard. By their criteria, up to two thirds of their patients were moderately or severely malnourished on measurements of TSF, MAMC and albumin. They claimed that the significant correlation demonstrated between MAMC and serum albumin indicated that over half the surgical population in their hospital had evidence of protein depletion. A similar survey of 251 patients in the medical wards of the same hospital by Bistrian et al (1976) found that almost three quarters of their patients surveyed were moderately or severely malnourished by TSF measurements and they concluded that medical patients had an energy depletion in contrast to surgical patients' protein depletion.

In a more carefully controlled study, Hill et al (1977) surveyed 105 general surgical patients at Leeds General Infirmary using staff and patients undergoing daycase procedures as controls. Patients were placed in four categories: minor operations (40), preoperative major operations (21), less than 1 week postoperative (17) and 1 week or more postoperative (27). Using the 95% confidence limits of the control population, they reported that the percentage of patients outside these limits were 33% for weight loss, 30% for MAMC, 26% for plasma albumin, 20% for haemoglobin, and 41% for plasma transferrin. For all but weight loss, the differences between controls and patients 1 week or more postoperatively were significant and differences between controls and patients less than 1 week postoperatively for haemoglobin and transferrin were also significant. They also noted that in only a few cases was there reference to the patient's nutritional status in the hospital notes and they concluded that PEM was a significant but largely unrecognized problem in their hospital. The prospective study of Weinsier et al (1979) of patients in medical wards also reported a significant deterioration in the nutritional status in over 50% of their patients during a 2 week hospital stay.

The prevalence of patients with poor prognostic indices varies with the population studied. In their prospective study of the PNI, Buzby et al (1980) found that 39% of their patients had a PNI greater than 50 but they acknowledge that their patients were preselected by their clinicians as being malnourished by referral for nutritional assessment. Other studies of preoperative patients have indicated a lesser prevalence of a high PNI. Only 14% of the 218 patients undergoing major gastrointestinal operations in Pettigrew and Hill's study (1986) had a modified PNI greater than 50. The prevalence of patients with other high risk indices in their study are shown in Table 1.

There have been no published studies of the prevalence of malnutrition as defined by the depleted/stress classification. In the single day survey of 198 hospital surgical patients reported by Pettigrew et al (1984) 15% of their hospital population were depleted only, 13% were classified as stressed depletion, and 23% were not depleted and stressed. Many of the patients in the last two groups were septic or had recently undergone an operation. In their later study of 218 preoperative patients undergoing major abdominal surgery (Table 2) depletion was found in 35% of patients. In 12% of patients, plasma albumin concentrations were below 32g/l but only half of these were also depleted.

It would appear, therefore, that between 20 and 30% of hospital patients have some evidence of PEM which is likely to become more apparent during hospitalization. This is not necessarily indicative of the quality of dietary services because it often is a reflection of ongoing disease processes or postoperative complications for which oral nutritional support alone is unable to compensate adequately. Whether other forms of nutritional support can alter this progression of PEM is debatable.

TECHNICAL OR NUTRITIONAL COMPLICATIONS?

The conclusion that the serum proteins were 'nutritional' indicators of postoperative complications in early studies of surgical patients was based on the false assumption that these proteins reflected total body protein status. It is now recognized that many other conditions, such as sepsis, also lower these serum protein concentrations and predispose patients to an increased complication rate. Nevertheless, the demonstration that these so called 'nutritional' measurements select patients who develop postoperative complications after surgery has resulted in a tendency to classify certain complications as 'nutritional'. Support for this approach has come from studies of the biological effects of PEM in animals and patients. Thus sepsis is considered a 'nutritional' complication because there is clear evidence of impaired immune responses in PEM as reviewed by Law et al (1974). Wound dehiscence is also labelled 'nutritional' as studies such as that of Irvin and Hunt (1974) have demonstrated a significant delay in restoration of wound strength in protein-depleted rats compared with well fed controls. Likewise respiratory complications, venous thrombosis and cardiac problems are 'nutritional' on the basis of studies showing impaired muscle performance in malnourished patients. However, direct evidence for the association of nutritional status with these complications in clinical studies is lacking and surgeons have remained sceptical, especially as the reduction of many of these complications in recent years has occurred without preoperative nutritional support. For example, the reduction in the rate of wound dehiscence after laparotomy is attributable to a better understanding of the mechanical factors in suturing technique as highlighted by Jenkins (1976) and to better suture materials. Furthermore, it is naive to suggest that among the factors of preoperative bowel preparation, use of drains, faecal loading and contamination, blood loss, local ischaemia, local sepsis and anastomotic tension that are known to contribute to the development of anastomotic leaks, correction of malnutrition will override all. In fact, the converse is more likely. The delay in wound healing of patients with PEM will not become clinically apparent when wounds have been correctly closed with strong non-absorbable sutures. Much of the morbidity associated with impaired respiratory muscle function in patients with PEM can be reduced by attention to pre and postoperative chest physiotherapy. The clinical impression of many surgeons that even severely depleted patients often do very well after major surgical procedures cannot be ignored. The biological effects of PEM must be weighed against the technical ease of operating on malnourished patients where fat does not obscure vital structures. For these reasons, many practising surgeons consider that the clinical importance of nutritional status to the development of postoperative complications has been overestimated.

The view that it is technical events that occur during operation that contribute to postoperative outcome more than nutritional status is supported by the study of Pettigrew et al (1987). Their operating surgeon's preoperative assessment of 103 patients undergoing major gastrointestinal resections did not identify patients at significantly increased risk of developing postoperative complications whereas a medical risk assessment and assessment by plasma albumin concentration did. However, immediately after the operation, the surgeon's prediction of those patients likely to develop complications improved dramatically, especially if compared with his preoperative assessment. Of 27 patients selected as high risk preoperatively, 10 developed major complications. Postoperatively, the surgeon assessed the risk as less in 11 of these patients and only one developed a complication. Similarly, in the 76 patients assessed as low risk preoperatively, 16 developed complications but, postoperatively, the surgeon increased the assessment of risk in 22 of these patients of which 11 developed complications. Of 38 patients who remained high risk or who increased their risk assessment postoperatively, 53% developed major postoperative complications compared with 9% of 65 patients who remained low risk or decreased their postoperative risk assessment. When the reasons why the surgeon had changed his assessment of risk were evaluated, it was found that in 82% technical factors occurring at operation were identified. In the remaining 18%, findings of advanced malignancy or abscess altered the postoperative assessment. A comparison of assessments is demonstrated in Figure 3 using receiver operating characteristic (ROC) curves as described by Detsky et al (1984). For preoperative serum albumin and medical assessment, the selection of high risk patients is only significant at the very left of the curve. In contrast to the surgeon's preoperative assessment which at no point is significant, the surgeon's postoperative assessment is significant for almost all points on the curve. The combination of the pre and postoperative surgeon's assessments as described above (53% versus 9% complication rate) gave the highest sensitivity/specificity, represented as a single point on the ROC graph rather than a curve because it is a logical expression rather than variable quantity.

It has become clear that preoperative nutritional support cannot compensate for poor technical performance and the nutritional assessment of patients is unlikely to predict accurately postoperative complications where good operative technique is evident. It may yet be shown that where preoperative nutritional assessment indicates depletion, and technical prob-

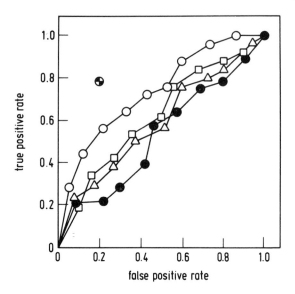

Figure 3. Receiver operating characteristic curves for comparing pre and postoperative assessment of 103 patients undergoing elective major gastrointestinal resections. (See text for details.) △, serum albumin level; ●, medical assessment; □, preoperative assessment; ○ postoperative assessment; ◐, combination of pre- and post-operative assessment.

lems are encountered at operation that early postoperative nutritional therapy may expedite patient recovery from anticipated postoperative complications.

SUMMARY

The assessment of protein-energy malnutrition has become important for identifying patients whose nutritional status increases their risk of an adverse outcome during hospitalization. Anthropometric, biochemical and immunological measurements, used either alone or in combination are not sensitive or specific enough for monitoring short-term nutritional changes, although some of these variables are associated with an increased incidence of postoperative complications after surgical procedures. The sensitivity of clinical assessment is dependent on the training of the clinician and the outcome variable being sought. For most clinicians, objective measurements are needed to raise their awareness to potential nutritional problems. The relationship of nutritional status to clinical events, particularly stress events during hospitalization, is critical to the interpretation of nutritional measurements and relating them to outcome variables. A classification based on the concepts of nutritional depletion and stress is presented. The prevalence of PEM has been shown to be between 20 and 30% in western hospitals, depending on the population studied and the criteria used to define PEM. In studies which have claimed an association between nutritional status and outcome, the contribution of nutritional variables to the development of postoperative complications has been overestimated and the relevance of technical factors underestimated.

REFERENCES

Baker JP, Detsky AS, Wesson DE et al (1982) Nutritional assessment: a comparison of clinical judgement and objective measurements. *New England Journal of Medicine* **306:** 969–972.

Bates SE, Suen JY & Tranum BL (1979) Immunological skin testing and interpretation. A plea for uniformity. *Cancer* **43:** 2306–2314.

Beddoe AH & Hill GL (1985) Clinical measurement of body composition using in vivo neutron activation analysis. *Journal of Parenteral and Enteral Nutrition* **9:** 504–520.

Bistrian BR, Blackburn GL, Hallowell E & Heddle R (1974) Protein status of general surgical patients. *Journal of American Medical Association* **230:** 858–860.

Bistrian BR, Blackburn GL, Vitale J, Cochran D & Naylor J (1976) Prevalence of malnutrition in general medical patients. *Journal of American Medical Association* **235:** 1567–1570.

Blackburn GL, Bistrian BR, Maini BS, Schlamm HT & Smith MF (1977) Nutritional and metabolic assessment of the hospitalized patient. *Journal of Parenteral and Enteral Nutrition* **1:** 11–22.

Bollet AJ & Owens S (1973) Evaluation of nutritional status of selected hospital patients. *American Journal of Clinical Nutrition* **26:** 931–938.

Brown R, Bancewicz J, Hamid J et al (1982) Failure of delayed hypersensitivity skin testing to predict postoperative sepsis and mortality. *British Medical Journal* **284:** 851–853.

Buzby GP, Mullen JL, Matthews DC, Hobbs CL & Rosato EF (1980) Prognostic nutritional index in gastrointestinal surgery. *American Journal of Surgery* **139:** 159–167.

Church JM, Choong SY & Hill GL (1984) Abnormalities of muscle metabolism and histology in malnourished patients awaiting surgery: effects of a course of intravenous nutrition. *British Journal of Surgery* **71:** 563–569.

Collins JA (1982) Clinical judgement versus the laboratory. *New England Journal of Medicine* **306:** 987–988.

Collins JP, McCarthy ID & Hill GL (1979) Assessment of protein nutrition in surgical patients – the value of anthropometrics. *American Journal of Clinical Nutrition* **32:** 1527–1530.

Coward WA & Lunn PG (1981) The biochemistry and physiology of kwashiorkor and marasmus. *British Medical Bulletin* **37:** 19–24.

Cuthbertson DP (1936) Further observations on the disturbance of metabolism caused by injury, with particular reference to the dietary requirements of fracture cases. *British Journal of Surgery* **23:** 505–520.

Detsky AS, Baker JP, Mendelson RA et al (1984) Evaluating the accuracy of nutritional assessment techniques applied to hospitalized patients: Methodology and comparisons. *Journal of Parenteral and Enteral Nutrition* **8:** 153–159.

Durnin JVGA & Womersley J (1974) Body fat assessed from total body density and its estimation from skinfold thickness: measurements on 481 men and women aged from 16 to 72 years. *British Journal of Nutrition* **32:** 77–97.

Editorial (1986) Indicators of surgical risk. *Lancet* **i:** 1422–1423.

Fleck A, Raines G, Hawker F et al (1985a) Increased vascular permeability: a major cause of hypoalbuminaemia in disease and injury. *Lancet* **i:** 781–784.

Fleck A, Colley CM & Myers MA (1985b) Liver export proteins and trauma. *British Medical Bulletin* **41:** 265–273.

Forse RA & Shizgal HM (1980) The assessment of malnutrition. *Surgery* **88:** 17–24.

Forse RA, Christou N, Meakins JL, MacLean LD & Shizgal HM (1981) Reliability of skin testing as a measure of nutritional state. *Archives of Surgery* **116:** 1284–1288.

Goldbourt U & Medalie JH (1974) Weight-height indices. *British Journal of Preventative and Social Medicine* **28:** 116–126.

Golden MHN (1982) Transport proteins as indices of protein status. *American Journal of Clinical Nutrition* **35:** 1159–1165.

Gray GE & Gray LK (1979) Validity of anthropometric norms used in the assessment of hospitalized patients. *Journal of Parenteral and Enteral Nutrition* **3:** 366–368.

Hall JC, O'Quigley J, Giles GR, Appleton N & Stocks H (1980) Upper limb anthropometry: the value of variance studies. *American Journal of Clinical Nutrition* **33:** 1846–1851.

Harvey, KB, Moldawer LL, Bistrian BS & Blackburn GL (1981) Biological measures for the formulation of a hospital prognostic index. *American Journal of Clinical Nutrition* **34:** 2013–2022.

Hill GL & Church JM (1984) Energy and protein requirements of general surgical patients requiring intravenous nutrition. *British Journal of Surgery* **71:** 1–9.

Hill GL, Blackett RL, Pickford I et al (1977) Malnutrition in surgical patients- an unrecognised problem. *Lancet* **i:** 689–692.

Irvin TT & Hunt TK (1974) Effect of malnutrition on colonic healing. *Annals of Surgery* **180:** 765–772.

Jeejeebhoy KN & Meguid MM (1986) Assessment of nutritional status in the oncologic patient. *Surgical Clinics of North America* **66:** 1077–1090.

Jelliffe DB (1966) *The assessment of the nutritional status of the community.* Geneva: World Health Organization.

Jenkins TPN (1976) The burst abdominal wound: a mechanical approach. *British Journal of Surgery* **63:** 873–876.

Klidjian AM, Archer TJ, Foster DM & Karran SJ (1982) Detection of dangerous malnutrition. *Journal of Parenteral and Enteral Nutrition* **6:** 119–121.

Law DK, Dudrick SJ & Abdou NI (1974) The effects of protein calorie malnutrition on immune competence of the surgical patient. *Surgery Gynecology and Obstetrics* **139:** 257–266.

McFarlane H, Ogbeide MI, Reddy S et al (1969) Biochemical assessment of protein-calorie malnutrition. *Lancet* **i:** 392–395.

McLaren DS & Meguid MM (1983) Nutritional assessment at the crossroads. *Journal of Parenteral and Enteral Nutrition* **7:** 575–579.

McNeill KG, Mernagh JR, Jeejeebhoy KN, Wolman SL & Harrison JE (1979) In vivo measurements of body protein based on the determination of nitrogen by prompt gamma analysis. *American Journal of Clinical Nutrition* **32:** 1955–1961.

Morgan DB, Hill GL & Burkinshaw L (1980) The assessment of weight loss from a single measurement of body weight: the problems and limitations. *American Journal of Clinical Nutrition* **33:** 2101–2105.

Mullen JL, Gertner MH, Buzby GP, Goodhart GL & Rosato EF (1979) Implications of malnutrition in the surgical patient. *Archives of Surgery* **114:** 121–125.

Pettigrew RA & Hill GL (1986) Indicators of surgical risk and clinical judgement. *British Journal of Surgery* **73:** 47–51.

Pettigrew RA, Charlesworth PM, Farmillo RW & Hill GL (1984) Assessment of nutritional depletion and immune competence: a comparison of clinical examination and objective measurements. *Journal of Parenteral and Enteral Nutrition* **8:** 21–25.

Pettigrew RA, Burns HJG & Carter DC (1987) Evaluating surgical risk: the importance of technical factors in determining outcome. *British Journal of Surgery* **74:** 791–794.

Pietsch JB, Meakins JL & MacLean LD (1977) The delayed hypersensitivity response: application in clinical surgery. *Surgery* **82:** 349–355.

Rainey-Macdonald CG, Holliday RL, Wells GA & Donner AP (1983) Validity of a two-variable nutritional index for use in selecting candidates for nutritional support. *Journal of Parenteral and Enteral Nutrition* **7:** 15–20.

Roza AM, Tuitt D & Shizgal HM (1984) Transferrin – a poor measure of nutritional status. *Journal of Parenteral and Enteral Nutrition* **8:** 523–528.

Russell DMcR, Leiter LA, Whitwell J, Marliss EB & Jeejeebhoy KN (1983) Skeletal muscle function during hypocaloric diets and fasting: a comparison with standard nutritional assessment parameters. *American Journal of Clinical Nutrition* **37:** 133–138.

Seltzer MH, Slocum BA, Cataldi-Betcher EL et al (1982) Instant nutritional assessment: absolute weight loss and surgical mortality. *Journal of Parenteral and Enteral Nutrition* **6:** 218.

Shetty PS, Watrasiewicz KE, Jung RT & James WPT (1979) Rapid-turnover transport proteins: an index of subclinical protein-energy malnutrition. *Lancet* **ii:** 230–232.

Shizgal HM (1981) The effect of malnutrition on body composition. *Surgery Gynecology and Obstetrics* **152:** 22–26.

Stunkard AJ & Albaum JM (1981) The accuracy of self-reported weights. *American Journal of Clinical Nutrition* **34:** 1593–1599.

Twomey P, Ziegler D & Rombeau J (1982) Utility of skin testing in nutritional assessment: a critical review. *Journal of Parenteral and Enteral Nutrition* **6:** 50–58.

Waterlow JC (1976) Classification and definition of protein-energy malnutrition. In *Nutrition in Preventative Medicine* pp 530–555 Geneva: World Health Organization monograph series No. 62.

Weinsier RL, Hunker EM, Krumdieck CL & Butterworth CE (1979) Hospital malnutrition. A prospective evaluation of general medical patients during the course of hospitalization. *American Journal of Clinical Nutrition* **32:** 418–426.

Windsor JA & Hill GL (1986) Does organ disfunction occur in protein depleted preoperative patients? *Australian and New Zealand Journal of Surgery* **56:** 257.

3

Perioperative nutritional support

MICHAEL J. McMAHON

A proportion of patients who undergo surgical operations display the clinical and metabolic characteristics of malnutrition, and these patients appear to be more likely to develop postoperative complications related to infection or poor healing than those who are normally nourished. Since the evolution of techniques which enable effective nutrition to be delivered during the perioperative period, even when the gastrointestinal tract is unavailable, many attempts have been made to test the hypothesis that perioperative nutritional support can reduce postoperative complications in the 'malnourished' patient. There is ample attestation to the beneficial influence of nutritional support upon postoperative complications based upon uncontrolled clinical experience, but verisimilitude is not proof. It appears possible to test the hypothesis relatively simply using the well established technique of the randomized clinical trial, but clear-cut answers have not emerged, probably because nutrition is often a minor component of the many determinants of operative outcome, and because precise and specific end-points by which to judge the efficacy of nutritional support are not available. Nevertheless, for both humanitarian and economic reasons, it is important to establish the role of perioperative nutritional support.

THE CASE FOR PERIOPERATIVE NUTRITIONAL SUPPORT

Malnutrition and the risk of postoperative complications

In 1936, Studley described a consecutive series of patients who underwent surgical treatment for peptic ulceration. There was a 33% mortality in patients who had lost more than 20% of body weight compared to a mortality rate of 4% in patients without such extensive weight loss. Since Studley's report, increased risk of postoperative complications has been associated with other manifestations of malnutrition, such as low plasma albumin levels (Bistrian et al, 1974), low levels of short-half-life proteins such as transferrin (Mullen et al, 1979a), anergy to skin test antigens (Meakins et al, 1977), and impaired grip strength (Klidjian et al, 1982). Malnutrition is not a precisely defined condition, and a working definition, such as that provided by Dempsey et al (1988), 'A state of *relative* nutrient deprivation and/or metabolic perturbation which compromises host defences and increases the risk of complications and death', whilst encompassing most circumstances and embracing the spirit of common usage, provides no assistance to those who wish to measure it. There is no consensus about which of the individual variables associated with malnutrition is most appropriate to allow identification of the malnourished patient undergoing an operation, to what extent the variables are disease-specific, and what threshold levels are appropriate to the definition of malnutrion. Even if the influence of disease can be disregarded, difficulties of definition still exist because there is probably a continuum of anthropometric and functional change between the extremes of obesity and inanition, and no particular 'cut-off' point which identifies malnutrition. Thus the definition of malnutrition is to a large extent arbitrary and relates to the purpose for which the term is being used. In order to attempt to increase the precision of nutritional assessment, multiple variables have been considered. Probably the best known are those first reported by Mullen et al (1979b). One hundred and sixty-one patients who underwent major surgery were extensively studied preoperatively by measurement of anthropometric variables, plasma proteins and aspects of white cell function and immunity. Postoperative complications were recorded and a linear predictive equation known as the Prognostic Nutritional Index (PNI) was developed.

PNI (percentage risk) = 158−16.6 (ALB) −0.78 (TSF) −0.2 (TFN) −5.8 (DH)

Where: ALB = albumin (g/dl)
        TSF = Triceps skinfold (mm)
        TFN = Serum transferrin (mg/dl)
        DH   = Maximum cutaneous delayed hypersensitivity reactivity to any of three recall antigens.

The PNI was applied prospectively to 100 consecutive patients undergoing operations for gastrointestinal disease. There was a highly significant correlation between PNI and postoperative complications or death. If the PNI was greater than 40% then postoperative sepsis was predicted with a sensitivity of 89% and death with a sensitivity of 93% (Buzby et al, 1980). Baker et al (1982) showed that when an experienced clinician classified patients as well nourished, mildly malnourished or severely malnourished on the basis of a careful history and physical examination, it was possible to predict postoperative complications related to infection with a similar degree of precision to that obtained by the measurement of nutritional variables such as anthropometrics, plasma proteins or delayed cutaneous hypersensitivity. Thus, it is possible to select measurable variables which will give an approximate estimate of the risk of postoperative complications. What remains unclear is the relationship of the variables to nutrition.

Interrelationships of disease and nutrition

Sepsis and malignant disease can induce similar changes in body composition, plasma protein status and immune function to those attributed to malnutrition, an effect which is probably mediated by cytokines and related substances. In the majority of surgical patients, observed abnormalities of 'nutrition-related' variables are usually the result of the influence of both disease and undernutrition, and the magnitude of the contribution of each is difficult to assess, even if a careful history of food intake is recorded, markers of sepsis measured, and the stage of disease carefully estimated. The inclusion of factors related to disease, e.g. the presence or absence of cancer, can help to improve the accuracy of predictive equations to assess the magnitude of the risk of postoperative complications (Harvey et al, 1981). The relative contribution of disease and nutrition to the genesis of postoperative complications is important and fundamental to the concept of preoperative nutritional support. If complications are due, partly or wholly, to a relative deficiency of nutrient intake, then it is reasonable to expect that nutritional support will influence their frequency. If the disease process itself, independent of influences upon appetite or the ability to ingest, digest or absorb food, is the major determinant of changes in 'nutrition-related' variables and of postoperative complications, then nutritional support is less likely to help.

The response to perioperative nutritional support

Are abnormalities of 'nutrition-related' variables reversible by preoperative nutrition, and is the risk of postoperative complications thereby diminished?

Ching et al (1980) studied a total of 34 patients who were given nutritional support using intravenous nutrition or an elemental diet. Plasma albumin was less than 35 g/litre in 26 patients, 18 of whom (69%) exhibited a rise in serum albumin and were thus considered to have responded to therapy. There was a highly significant correlation between rise in albumin and survival ($P < 0.001$). Starker et al (1986) studied 43 patients who had lost 10% or more of body weight, who had a plasma albumin of < 35 g/litre and who were scheduled for a major abdominal procedure. Preoperative intravenous nutrition was supplied for approximately one week, and in 23 patients (53%) there was a response to nutritional therapy characterized by a rise in plasma albumin and a loss in body weight due to diuresis. In this study, and in that of Ching et al (1980), postoperative complications appeared to be more common in patients who did not show a response to nutritional support. In Starker's study, an additional 16 patients who failed to show a response to intravenous nutrition after 1 week were fed for a total of 4–6 weeks preoperatively. The postoperative complication rate in the 16 patients was similar to that of those who had responded to intravenous nutrition after 7 days of feeding. It is probable that the additional patients were a highly selected group and it is uncertain that the apparently reduced complication rate was due solely to the influence of a longer period of intravenous nutrition. Nevertheless, these studies, and others, do suggest that only a proportion of patients fed preoperatively will show a response to nutritional support.

In animal models, protein depletion caused by dietary restriction, even of relatively short duration, leads to a diminished bursting strength of colonic anastomoses (Daly et al, 1972). The effect of malnutrition can be reversed by refeeding preoperatively, and diminished by postoperative nutritional supplementation (Ward et al, 1982). Studies by Haydock and Hill (1987) suggest that an analogous situation exists in man. They assessed wound healing by measuring the accumulation of hydroxyprolene during a 7-day period in fine tubes of thin-walled gortex which were implanted in the subcutaneous tissue of the arm. Wound healing was found to be significantly poorer in patients with various degrees of malnutrition than in normally nourished individuals. Preoperative intravenous feeding improved hydroxyprolene accumulation.

The relationship between abnormalities of 'nutrition-related' variables and postoperative complications, the influence of nutritional support upon the variables, at least in a proportion of patients, and experimental evidence concerning the influence of nutritional deprivation and refeeding upon wound healing, build a *prima facie* case to support the beneficial effect of perioperative nutrition upon postoperative complications.

PRACTICAL APPLICATION OF NUTRITIONAL SUPPORT IN THE PERIOPERATIVE PERIOD

Which route to select?

The availability of the alimentary tract for nutritional support is the principal determinant of the most appropriate technique to use. In general terms, the gastrointestinal tract is available for the nutritional support of patients pre- and postoperatively, except when the primary disease causes obstruction to, or inflammation of, part of the gastrointestinal tract, or when there is gastrointestinal dysfunction such as postoperative paralytic ileus. Encouragement to eat might be successful for patients who have been unable to eat as a result of environmental or economic circumstances, but in my experience it does not constitute effective preoperative nutritional support in patients who have lost weight. Meguid and Meguid (1985) showed that even if there was no complication after an intra-abdominal procedure, it was more than a week before oral intake provided 60% of predicted energy needs in most patients. If a complication developed, or if the patient was malnourished prior to operation, the period of inadequate food intake was considerably lengthened. Bastow et al (1983) demonstrated a similar pattern in elderly women who had sustained a fracture of the femoral neck. Food intake was significantly less in the patients who were thin and undernourished. The conclusion to be drawn from these studies is that when nutritional support is needed in the perioperative period, it must be delivered by the enteral or parenteral routes, although some recent, as yet unpublished, work from Aarhus in Denmark suggests that the careful use of liquid food supplements can be effective postoperatively. It is a general principle that intravenous nutrition is appropriate to patients for whom enteral nutrition would be unavailable or ineffective. Preoperatively, intravenous nutrition has been used extensively in patients with gastrointestinal disease, particularly carcinoma of the gastrointestinal tract, and postoperatively in patients who develop complications such as obstruction, ileus or fistula. It is usually possible to pass a fine bore nasoenteric feeding tube beyond an obstructing carcinoma of the oesophagus, and to place a fine bore jejunostomy catheter at the time of laparotomy in order to deliver enteral feed into the small bowel during the recovery stage even though the patient has had an operation which involves the oesophagus, stomach or pancreas. The modern concept of the feeding jejunostomy was developed by Delaney and Garvey (1973) and has since been embraced enthusiastically, with advocacy of immediate postoperative nutritional support (Hoover et al, 1980). Recently the feeding jejunostomy has received something of a bad press, but with careful selection of patients, meticulous attention to the technique of placement of the jejunostomy catheter, and a few days' delay before feeding is commenced, complications such as peritonitis and aspiration pneumonia appear to be preventable (Heberer and Harder, 1986). The use of a polymeric diet as opposed to an elemental diet appears to reduce the troublesome complication of diarrhoea which has frequently been recorded (Hinsdale et al, 1985).

Comparative efficacy of enteral and intravenous nutrition

Starving patients undergo villous atrophy of the small bowel and a reduction in size and secretory output from the pancreas. These changes might reduce the efficacy of nutritional support delivered by the enteral route. Lim et al (1981) compared parenteral nutrition with feeding via a Witzel type of gastrostomy (which needed a small laparotomy) preoperatively in patients with carcinoma of the oesophagus. The patients who were fed intravenously gained more weight and achieved earlier positive nitrogen balance. Nevertheless, the gastrostomy patients were usually in positive nitrogen balance after 5 days of feeding. McArdle et al (1981) compared enteral and parenteral feeding in a variety of malnourished patients. They also reported more positive nitrogen balance in the parenterally fed patients but the differences were not significant, and in contrast to the study of Lim et al (1981) there was no apparent delay in the achievement of nitrogen balance in the enteral group. Yeung et al (1979) compared the body composition of surgical patients fed for 2 weeks parenterally or enterally. They also noted a greater weight gain in the parenterally fed patients, but by studying body composition using in vivo neutron activation analysis, they were able to demonstrate that the major component of the weight gain was water. When used postoperatively, enteral feeding achieves significantly better nitrogen balance than conventional management (Sagar et al, 1979). Randomized studies which have compared enteral and parenteral nutrition after operation or trauma have failed to show any significant difference between the two methods with respect to nitrogen balance or changes in the concentrations of plasma proteins (Adams et al, 1986; Bower et al, 1986; Fletcher and Little, 1986).

CLINICAL EFFECTS OF PERIOPERATIVE NUTRITIONAL SUPPORT

Anecdotes, wider experience and initial randomized trials

Studies by Hadfield (1965) and Mogissi et al (1977) suggested that intravenous nutrition provided before and after operation led to a smoother and less complicated postoperative course in patients who had undergone oesophagectomy, oesophagogastrectomy or pancreaticoduodenectomy. Holter and Fischer (1977) reported the first randomized study of pre- and postoperative intravenous nutrition. Patients with carcinoma of the gastrointestinal tract and weight loss of more than 10 lbs were randomized to receive intravenous nutrition (8.4 MJ/day; 13 gN/day) for 3 days preoperatively and for up to 10 days postoperatively, or to receive routine hospital food preoperatively, and routine fluid management and hospital food postoperatively. Thirty patients were randomized to receive intravenous nutrition and 26 conventional management; two patients died in each group. The incidence of major complications such as ileus, gastrointestinal obstruction or fistula or wound dehiscence, and of minor complications such as respiratory and urinary infections, was similar in both groups. Mullen et al (1980) reported an extensive but unrandomized experience. They applied the PNI to 144 patients who were due to undergo major intra-abdominal or intrathoracic procedures. The decision whether or not to feed intravenously was made by a clinician who was unaware of the PNI score. Fifty patients were given intravenous nutrition $(147 \text{ kJ kg}^{-1} \text{ day}^{-1}; 0.24 \text{ gN kg}^{-1} \text{ day}^{-1})$ for 7 days preoperatively and during the postoperative period, and 95 patients were managed routinely without nutritional support. There were quite marked differences between the two groups with respect to postoperative complications. There were ten complications and two deaths in 50 patients who received perioperative intravenous nutrition compared to 31 complications and 27 deaths in 95 patients who did not. In fact, 89% of the routinely managed patients were given intravenous nutrition postoperatively for clinical reasons. The authors compared the results with the complication rate they would expect for a given PNI score. Patients who had not received preoperative nutritional support suffered the expected rate of complications, but those who received preoperative intravenous nutrition had significantly fewer postoperative complications than predicted. Criticisms of this study concern the comparability of the patients and the lack of precise details about the manner in which the decision to feed was made, and by whom.

Heatley et al (1979) reported a further randomized study of preoperative intravenous nutrition in 74 patients who were admitted for operation upon an oesophageal or gastric carcinoma. There were significantly fewer infected wounds amongst the 38 patients who were fed preoperatively compared to 36 controls ($P < 0.05$). There were no differences in the rates of anastomotic leakage or death. Nutritional criteria were not used to select patients for randomization and only 36 patients received a resection. Fourteen of the patients were found to have a benign lesion or no abnormality at all at the time of laparotomy. Thompson et al (1981) randomized 21 patients with gastrointestinal cancer and weight loss which exceeded 10 lbs, to 5 more days of preoperative intravenous nutrition ($168–210\,kJ\,kg^{-1}\,day^{-1}$) or to hospital food only. Intravenous nutrition was continued postoperatively until the patients were able to take a normal diet. There were no deaths in either group and only one major complication in the nine patients randomized to diet compared to two complications in the patients who received intravenous nutrition. The authors' conclusion that preoperative intravenous nutrition did not alter the rate of postoperative complications was not justified from such a small study. Sako et al (1981) randomized 69 patients with head and neck cancer to receive postoperative intravenous nutrition ($147\,kJ\,kg^{-1}\,day^{-1}$) or to receive a diet of food or enteral nutrition delivered by nasogastric tube. Nitrogen balance was significantly greater in patients who received intravenous nutrition but there were no differences in the incidence of postoperative complications and no evidence that intravenous nutrition prolonged survival. In fact, survival was poorer in the patients who received intravenous nutrition but the differences were not significant when postoperative deaths were excluded.

Does enteral feeding have a beneficial influence upon the outcome from operations? In a randomized study of 30 patients who underwent major gastrointestinal operations, Sagar et al (1979) concluded that enteral feed delivered via a double lumen tube could improve recovery compared to conventional management. This conclusion was based upon a difference in hospital stay but there was no significant difference in the incidence of complications. A randomized trial of fine-bore jejunostomy feeding versus conventional management carried out in patients who underwent laparotomy and resection or anastomosis for gastrointestinal cancer was reported by Smith et al (1985). Patients were well matched and the incidence of postoperative complications was similar in both groups, but 20 complications and one death were attributed to the jejunostomy, and the fed patients were in hospital longer. A randomized study of postoperative jejunostomy feed versus routine intravenous fluid management in patients who underwent extensive oesophageal, gastroduodenal, biliary or pancreatic procedures was reported by Hoover et al (1980). Jejunostomy feeding resulted in more rapid weight gain and more positive nitrogen balance but no clinical benefits were evident. Thirty-four per cent of the patients fed via jejunostomy suffered diarrhoea, but an enteral diet was used (Vivonex). In a randomized study of patients undergoing total cystectomy, feeding via a jejunostomy appeared to be without obvious clinical advantages (Daly et al, 1987). Other recent papers have pointed out the limited efficacy and considerable dangers of early routine postoperative jejunostomy feeding (Hayashi et al, 1985; Bruining et al, 1983; Adams et al, 1986a).

Requirements for trials of perioperative nutritional support

A clear and unequivocal advantage of perioperative nutritional support, whether delivered by the enteral or parenteral routes, has not emerged from the foregoing studies. This may be because nutritional support has little if any beneficial influence, but it is also possible that the studies have failed to demonstrate the true value of nutritional support because of small numbers of patients, heterogeneous and perhaps inappropriate clinical groups, and variable, if any, criteria of undernutrition. The importance of nutrition as a determinant of outcome from surgical operations is unknown but it may be secondary to factors such as type and extent of disease, age of the patient, presence or absence of concurrent disease, type and magnitude of the operation, skill of the surgeon and the use of prophylactic antibiotics. In order to investigate the value of nutritional support it is necessary to design a randomized trial with minimization of variables by careful selection of patients on the basis of disease, intended treatment, nutritional depletion, standardization of treatment and classification of complications according to carefully defined criteria. It is important that patients are chosen in whom there is a high probability that nutrition will influence outcome. It would be inappropriate to include patients undergoing repair of a simple groin hernia because even severe malnutrition might have little impact upon outcome, but apposite to include patients scheduled to undergo gastric resection for carcinoma, for whom impaired healing can have disastrous consequences. It is obviously important to know the expected complication rate, and to assume the influence of nutrition in order that the number of patients needed to achieve a reasonable probability that the real effect of the treatment will be demonstrated, can be calculated. This may pose a problem, because the tighter the protocol the more difficult it is to recruit sufficient patients. The nutritional regimen which is chosen must be of sufficient duration and intensity to influence some of the markers of nutritional depletion, but not of such prolonged duration that it causes unreasonable delay. It should be possible to quantify the degree of response to the nutritional regimen preoperatively. This topic is extensively discussed by Buzby et al (1988).

Extensive randomized studies

Two studies have been reported which appeared to have sufficient power to address the topic. Muller et al (1982) reported the results of a randomized study of 10 days of preoperative intravenous nutrition ($185 \, kJ \, kg^{-1} \, day^{-1}$; $0.24 \, gN \, kg^{-1} \, day^{-1}$) versus routine management in 125 patients who underwent operation for gastrointestinal cancer. Intravenous nutrition was discontinued at the time of operation and instituted thereafter in either group only if it was needed to treat a postoperative complication. Nutritional status was not included in the entry criteria and 63% of the patients in the control group and 67% of those in the intravenous nutrition group respectively had a carcinoma of the upper gastrointestinal tract. Approximately three-quarters of the patients in each group underwent potentially curative resections. Several 'nutrition-related' variables were measured at the commencement of treatment and at the time of operation; the mean levels of some plasma proteins were lower in the control group. There was little difference between the groups with respect to the incidence of wound infections or respiratory complications but there were 19 major complications (intra-abdominal abscess, peritonitis, anastomotic leakage or ileus) in the routinely managed patients compared to 11 in those given preoperative intravenous nutrition. This difference, 32% versus 17%, was significant at the 5% level. Mortality was 19% in the control group compared to 5% in the intravenously fed patients. This was also significant at the 5% level. Widespread acceptance of the general application of the results of this study is limited by the level of significance of the differences (which might be expected by chance once in every 20 studies), by the fact that a second treatment group was dropped from the study before its completion but not mentioned in the paper, and by the fact that anastomotic leakage, a major cause of mortality and morbidity in the study, disappeared from both groups when an anastomotic stapler was used (Koretz, 1986).

Bastow et al (1983) studied a total of 744 elderly women with a fracture of the neck of the femur. Patients were divided into three groups according to arm circumference and triceps skinfold thickness: well nourished, thin, and very thin. Patients who fell into the thin and very thin groups (with the exception of those who were severely demented or who had severe concomitant physical disorders) were randomized to receive the hospital ward diet or the ward diet plus supplementary feeding by a nasoenteric tube at night. Feeding was started within 5 days of the operation and was continued for approximately one month. Nine of the 58 control patients (16%) died compared to seven of the 64 tube-fed patients (11%). Tube feeding reduced the time to reach specified goals and was associated with a shorter hospital stay ($P = 4\%$). When the very thin patients alone were considered, there was no significant effect of tube feeding upon the return of plasma albumin concentrations to normal, but thyroid-binding prealbumin levels were significantly higher in the patients who received tube feeding than in controls.

These two studies lend cautious support to the concept that nutritional support influences the outcome from surgical operations. They also demonstrate the difficulty involved in attempts to demonstrate nutritional efficacy in such a multivariate situation. The importance of a homogeneous diagnostic group was illustrated in the study by Muller et al (1982). When the patients were stratified according to tumour site, differences between the fed and control groups were only present in patients with gastric and oesophageal malignancies (Koretz, 1986). The study of Bastow et al (1983) indicated very clearly the need for strict criteria of nutritional depletion.

CURRENT STATUS OF PERIOPERATIVE NUTRITIONAL SUPPORT

Nutritional regimens for the patient undergoing operation

At the present time it is difficult to argue convincingly for the routine use of perioperative nutritional support for any specific disease or operation. However, in my view there is sufficient evidence to suggest that in patients who are grossly malnourished, and anergic to skin test antigens, nutritional support is appropriate and potentially beneficial. The type of operation and the estimate of the duration of postoperative starvation are clearly important factors to include in the equation. It is not possible to make recommendations about specific nutritional criteria which need to be met before feeding is introduced. It is probably most appropriate that the skilled clinician takes into account 'nutritional' evidence such as weight loss, plasma protein concentrations and perhaps hand grip strength, together with the magnitude of the operation and his prediction of the future course of the patient, in order to reach a judgement.

Where possible, enteral nutrition should be the preferred choice. Preoperatively, this will normally need to be delivered via a nasoenteral feeding tube, although techniques such as endoscopic percutaneous gastrostomy may be of value (Ponsky et al, 1985; Wu et al, 1987). There is no evidence that elemental diets or specialized diets such as those enriched by high concentrations of branched-chain amino acids offer advantages over a standard polymeric diet for tube feeding (Hinsdale et al, 1985; Fick et al, 1986; Daly et al, 1987). Intravenously, it seems usual to employ a feed containing about $147 \text{ kJ kg}^{-1} \text{ day}^{-1}$ and about $0.23 \text{ gN kg}^{-1} \text{ day}^{-1}$ as synthetic amino acid. There is little evidence to support the use of specialized amino acid solutions such as those containing a high proportion of branched-chain amino acids and no evidence to suggest that the so-called peripheral protein sparing amino acid therapy is effective nutrition in the perioperative patient (Hensle, 1978; Garden et al, 1983; Hogbin et al, 1984). Similarly, there is little evidence to suggest that the use of nutritional regimens providing large amounts of energy or nitrogen (hyperalimentation) is either beneficial or safe for use in the perioperative period. Controversy continues regarding the relative values of glucose and lipid emulsion as fuel sources. As long as a small amount of lipid is provided in order to prevent essential fatty acid deficiency, glucose is probably a satisfactory fuel source for use preoperatively, and in the postoperative patient who is without sepsis. Fat emulsion is more readily utilized as a fuel source after trauma or in patients with sepsis, but I prefer to limit the infusion of lipid emulsion to 50% of the total infused energy. At the present time, I prefer to provide perioperative nutrition through a tunnelled central venous catheter, but in some patients, who have good peripheral veins and in whom the need for nutritional support is not critical, peripheral venous feeding probably has a role. Its disadvantage is a limitation upon the infusion of hypertonic glucose solutions, but it is probable that even if only 2000–3000 kJ are provided as glucose, nitrogen sparing can be considerable.

Time and duration of perioperative nutritional support

When and how long to feed are further points of uncertainty. In severely malnourished patients it seems logical to attempt to achieve an element of nutritional restitution prior to operation and to continue nutritional support postoperatively. I do not think it is important to be obsessional about the provision of energy immediately after the operation, and if preoperative nutrition has been provided, management may be simplified if nutritional considerations can be ignored for the initial day or two following operation.

If preoperative nutrition brings benefit to the patient the mechanisms by which it does so are unclear. The duration of feeding that is usually employed is certainly insufficient to make substantial differences to body composition, and changes in the concentrations of plasma proteins are relatively small. Other factors, such as the induction of enzyme systems, the accumulation of glycogen stores and normalization of membrane function, might be more important. Ignorance of the mechanisms makes it difficult for measurements to be made that will predict the response to feeding, and thus it is difficult to determine the optimum duration of nutritional support. It has been suggested that the response is variable from one patient to another, and that a positive response, indicated by a rise in albumin and a fall in weight, could predict patients who would derive clinical benefit from intravenous nutrition (Starker et al, 1983). In non-responders, extension of the period of preoperative intravenous nutrition to 4–6 weeks resulted in similar reduction in postoperative complications (Starker et al, 1986). These studies are important, because they suggest that the optimum period of preoperative nutrition may be very variable. They were not randomized studies and will probably require independent validation before the concept of the variable response receives widespread practical support. Preoperative nutrition is unavailable for some patients, particularly those who have an emergency operation. A fixed duration of postoperative nutrition is probably inappropriate; the usual guideline is to continue nutritional support until the patient is able to take an adequate oral intake. I frequently switch the patient to night-time only feeds before stopping nutritional support altogether. Both enteral and parenteral nutrition can be provided at home, but the former is much simpler to arrange.

With modern technology, nutritional support can be provided to all patients. In view of the evidence linking malnutrition to an increased risk of postoperative complications, it is folly to deny the severely malnourished patient undergoing a major procedure the potential benefits of perioperative nutritional support, even though its role has not been convincingly demonstrated in the setting of a randomized clinical trial. It is difficult to justify specialized nutritional support for patients who are mildly malnourished and scheduled for a relatively minor procedure. Between these two extremes there lies a wide variety of opinion. Ultimately, it is for the clinician to consider the merits of each individual case and decide accordingly.

REFERENCES

Adams MB, Seabrook GR, Quebbeman EA & Condon RE (1986a) Jejunostomy. A rarely indicated procedure. *Archives of Surgery* **121:** 236–238.

Adams S, Dellinger EP, Wertz MJ et al (1986b) Enteral versus parenteral nutritional support following laparotomy for trauma: a randomised prospective trial. *Journal of Trauma* **26:** 882–891.

Baker JP, Detsky AS, Wesson DE et al (1982) Nutritional assessment. A comparison of clinical judgement and objective measurements. *New England Journal of Medicine* **306:** 969–972.

Bastow MD, Rawlings J & Allison SP (1983) Benefits of supplementary tube feeding after fractured neck of femur: a randomised controlled trial. *British Medical Journal* **287:** 1589–1592.

Bistrian BR, Blackburn GL, Hallowell E & Heddle R (1974) Protein status of general surgical patients. *Journal of the American Medical Association* **230:** 858–860.

Bower RH, Talamini MA, Sax HC, Hamilton F & Fischer JE (1986) Postoperative enteral vs parenteral nutrition. *Archives of Surgery* **121:** 1040–1945.

Bruining HA, Schattenkerk ME, Obertop H & Ong GL (1983) Acute abdominal pains due to early postoperative elemental feeding by needle jejunostomy. *Surgery, Gynecology and Obstetrics* **157:** 40–42.

Buzby GP, Mullen JL, Mathews DC, Hobbs CL & Rosato EF (1980) Prognostic nutritional index in gastrointestinal surgery. *American Journal of Surgery* **139:** 160–167.

Buzby GP, Williford WO, Peterson OL et al (1988) A randomised clinical trial of total parenteral nutrition in malnourished surgical patients: the rationale and impact of previous clinical trials and pilot study on protocol design. *American Journal of Clinical Nutrition* **47:** 357–365.

Ching M, Grossi CE, Angers J et al (1980) The outcome of surgical treatment as related to the response of the serum albumin level to nutritional support. *Surgery, Gynecology and Obstetrics* **151:** 199–202.

Daly JM, Vars HM & Dudrick SJ (1972) Effects of protein depletion on strength of colonic anastomoses. *Surgery, Gynecology and Obstetrics* **134:** 15–21.

Daly JM, Bonau R, Stofberg P et al (1987) Immediate postoperative jejunostomy feeding. Clinical and metabolic results in a prospective trial. *American Journal of Surgery* **153:** 198–206.

Delany HM & Garvey JW (1973) Jejunostomy by a needle catheter technique. *Surgery* **73:** 786–790.

Dempsey DT, Mullen JL & Buzby GP (1988) The link between nutritional status and clinical outcome: can nutritional intervention modify it? *American Journal of Clinical Nutrition* **47:** 352–356.

Fick TE, van Rooyen W, Schattenkerk ME et al (1986) A nonelemental versus an elemental diet for early postoperative enteral feeding by needle catheter jejunostomy. *Clinical Nutrition* **5:** 105–107.

Fletcher JP & Little JM (1986) A comparison of parenteral nutrition and early postoperative enteral feeding on the nitrogen balance after major surgery. *Surgery* **100:** 21–24.

Garden OJ, Smith A, Harris NWS et al (1983) The effect of isotonic amino acid infusions on serum proteins and muscle breakdown following surgery. *British Journal of Surgery* **70:** 79–82.

Hadfield JIH (1965) Preoperative and postoperative intravenous fat therapy. *British Journal of Surgery* **52:** 291–298.

Harvey KB, Moldawer BS, Bistrian BR et al (1981) Biologic measures for the formulation of a hospital prognostic index. *American Journal of Clinical Nutrition* **34:** 2013–2022.

Hayashi JT, Wolfe BM & Calvert CC (1985) Limited efficacy of early postoperative jejunal feeding. *American Journal of Surgery* **150:** 52–56.

Haydock DA & Hill GL (1987) Improved wound healing response in surgical patients receiving intravenous nutrition. *British Journal of Surgery* **74:** 320–323.

Heatley RV, Williams RHP & Lewis MH (1979) Preoperative intravenous feeding—a controlled trial. *Postgraduate Medical Journal* **55:** 541–545.

Heberer M & Harder F (1986) Alternative methods of nutrition in the postoperative phase. *World Journal of Surgery* **10:** 95–101.

Hensle TW (1978) Protein-sparing in cystectomy patients. *Journal of Urology* **119:** 355–358.

Hinsdale JG, Lipkowitz GS, Pollock TW, Hoover EL & Jaffe BM (1985) Prolonged enteral nutrition in malnourished patients with nonelemental feeding. *American Journal of Surgery* **149:** 334–338.

Hogbin BM, Smith AM & Craven AH (1984) Evaluation of peripheral essential aminoacid infusion following major surgery. *Journal of Parenteral and Enteral Nutrition* **8:** 511–514.

Holter AR & Fischer JE (1977) Effects of peri-operative hyperalimentation on complications in patients with carcinoma and weight loss. *Journal of Surgical Research* **23:** 31–34.

Hoover HC, Ryan JA, Anderson EJ & Fischer JE (1980) Nutritional benefits of immediate postoperative jejunal feeding. *American Journal of Surgery* **139:** 153–159.

Klidjian AM, Archer TJ, Foster KJ & Karren SJ (1982) Detection of dangerous malnutrition. *Journal of Parenteral and Enteral Nutrition* **6:** 119–121.

Koretz RL (1986) Nutritional support: how much for how much? *Gut* **27:** 85–95.

Lim STK, Choa RG, Lam KH, Wong J & Ong GB (1981) Total parenteral nutrition versus gastrostomy in the preoperative preparation of patients with carcinoma of the oesophagus. *British Journal of Surgery* **68:** 69–72.

McArdle AH, Palmason C, Morency I & Brown RA (1981) A rationale for enteral feeding as the preferable route for hyperalimentation. *Surgery* **90:** 616–623.

Meakins JL, Pietsch JB, Rubenick O et al (1977) Delayed hypersensitivity: indicator of acquired failure of host defences in sepsis and trauma. *Annals of Surgery* **186:** 241–250.

Meguid MM & Meguid V (1985) Preoperative identification of the surgical cancer patient in need of postoperative supportive total parenteral nutrition. *Cancer* **55:** 258–262.

Moghissi K, Hornshaw J, Teasdale PR & Dawes EA (1977) Parenteral nutrition in carcinoma of the oesophagus treated by surgery: nitrogen balance and clinical studies. *British Journal of Surgery* **64:** 125–128.

Mullen JL, Gertner MH, Busby GL, Goodhart GL & Rosato EF (1979a) Implications of malnutrition in the surgical patient. *Archives of Surgery* **114:** 121–125.

Mullen JL, Buzby GP, Waldman TF et al (1979b) Prediction of operative morbidity and mortality by preoperative nutritional assessment. *Surgical Forum* **30:** 80–82.

Mullen JL, Buzby GP, Mathews DC, Smale BF & Rosato EF (1980) Reduction of operative morbidity and mortality by combined preoperative and postoperative nutritional support. *Annals of Surgery* **192:** 604–613.

Muller JM, Brenner U, Dienst C & Pichlmaier H (1982) Preoperative parenteral feeding in patients with gastrointestinal carcinoma. *Lancet* **1:** 68–71.

Ponsky JL, Gauderer MWL, Stellato TA & Aszodi A (1985) Percutaneous approaches to enteral alimentation. *American Journal of Surgery* **149:** 102–105.

Sagar S, Harland P & Shields R (1979) Early postoperative feeding with elemental diet. *British Medical Journal* **1:** 293–295.

Sako K, Lore JM, Kaufman S et al (1981) Parenteral hyperalimentation in surgical patients with head and neck cancer: a randomised study. *Journal of Surgical Oncology* **16:** 391–402.

Smith RC, Hartemink RJ, Hollinshead JW & Gillett DJ (1985) Fine bore jejunostomy feeding following major abdominal surgery: a controlled randomised clinical trial. *British Journal of Surgery* **72:** 458–461.

Starker PM, Lasala PA, Askanazi J et al (1983) The response to TPN. A form of nutritional assessment. *Annals of Surgery* **198:** 720–724.

Starker PM, Lasala PA, Askanazi J et al (1986) The influence of preoperative total parenteral nutrition upon morbidity and mortality. *Surgery, Gynecology and Obstetrics* **162:** 569–574.

Studley HO (1936) Percentage of weight loss: a basic indicator of surgical risk in patients with chronic peptic ulcer. *Journal of the American Medical Association* **106:** 458–460.

Thompson BR, Julian TB & Stremple JF (1981) Peri-operative total parenteral nutrition in patients with gastrointestinal cancer. *Journal of Surgical Research* **30:** 497–500.

Ward MWN, Danzi M, Lewin MR, Rennie MJ & Clark CG (1982) The effect of subclinical malnutrition and refeeding on the healing of experimental colonic anastomoses. *British Journal of Surgery* **69:** 308–310.

Wu TK, Pietrocola D & Welch HF (1987) A new method of percutaneous gastrostomy using anchoring devices. *American Journal of Surgery* **153:** 230–252.

Yeung CJ, Smith RC & Hill GL (1979) Effect of an elemental diet on body composition. Comparision with intravenous nutrition. *Gastroenterlogy* **77:** 652–657.

4

Clinical aspects of vitamin and trace element metabolism

ALAN SHENKIN

It is customary in reviews of this type to group all the micronutrients together, whether organic (vitamins) or inorganic (essential trace elements), and to keep them quite separate from discussions of the major nutrients of amino acids, fats and carbohydrates. Although this brings benefits of simplicity of presentation, in that many micronutrients can be covered relatively briefly, the classification is arbitrary and potentially misleading. Individual micronutrients have more relevance when considered together with the effects which they have on the metabolism of the major nutrients, such as the role of thiamine in carbohydrate metabolism, or of zinc in protein metabolism. Moreover, in the context of clinical nutrition of hospital patients, deficiencies of individual micronutrients are unlikely to occur in isolation, being more commonly found in association with deficiency of many components of the diet, including protein energy malnutrition as well as other vitamins or trace elements.

Interactions between the micronutrients themselves may be especially important, and a wide range are now recognized, such as zinc and vitamin A, selenium and vitamin E, and iron and vitamin C (Levander and Cheng, 1980). However, for clarity, the metabolism of each element and the effects of deficiency are usually described as though they exist independently.

GENERAL CONCEPTS

The usual definition of an essential trace element is that if it is removed from the diet, it will cause reproducible pathological changes (either structural or biochemical) which can be uniquely reversed by addition of the element to the otherwise complete diet. A similar definition holds for the vitamins, although with some slight variations to account for those vitamins which can be produced in the body under certain conditions, such as vitamin D or vitamin K.

An important feature of micronutrient metabolism is the progressive nature of the abnormalities. Thus, although they are characterized by the end result of the 'full blown' deficiency picture, this usually represents the end result of prolonged depletion of the nutrient. As Brubacher (1982) pointed out, stages of deficiency progress from an early depletion of the body pool, to reduced synthesis of metabolites and vitamins, to lowering of the activity of vitamin (or trace element) dependent enzymes and hormones, to biochemical and functional disturbances and finally to the morphological changes. Only at these later stages do clinical signs of deficiency become evident, passing from relatively non-specific to relatively characteristic and ultimately irreversible changes. It is therefore important to detect vitamin or trace element depletions early, so that intermediary metabolism can be maintained and the progression of the deficiency state prevented. For many of the micronutrients, the clinical penalty of the early biochemical abnormality may not be apparent, but it is logical to assume that it would be beneficial to the patient to maintain a normal tissue pool of the micronutrient together with normal coenzyme activity.

NUTRITIONAL REQUIREMENTS

As a general rule, the requirements of the micronutrients are linked to the amount of the major nutrients provided. This is particularly the case for the water-soluble vitamins when the recommended dietary allowances (RDA) in health specifically relate vitamin B_1 and vitamin B_2 intake to energy requirement and the vitamin B_6 requirement to the amino acid content of the diet (Food and Nutrition Board, 1980). There is a less close association of certain other vitamins and trace elements with the major nutrients, because of the wider range of functions of these micronutrients in areas not directly related to intermediary metabolism. However, the extent of net anabolism is very important, deficiency status often being precipitated by a period of rapid tissue regeneration but without adequate micronutrient provision. Other sources of loss of micronutrients from the body should also be borne in mind, especially malabsorption states, loss of gut contents due to diarrhoea or fistula, or losses of trace elements or vitamins during dialysis. Any of these may lead to depletion of one or more of the micronutrients.

SCOPE OF THIS CHAPTER

In this chapter, the various micronutrients are briefly summarized in terms of their normal metabolism and the effects of acute illness or chronic deficiency. The provision of micronutrients to adult patients is discussed, but special aspects of requirements in premature infants and neonates are described elsewhere.

FAT-SOLUBLE VITAMINS

Vitamin A (retinol)

Normal metabolism

Vitamin A has two main roles, firstly to stimulate rod vision (dark adaptation), and secondly to maintain membrane stability in epithelial cells. This latter function may be achieved by enhancing glycosylation in mucopolysaccharide synthesis or by direct action on cellular DNA to increase protein synthesis.

Vitamin A is usually obtained in the diet from carotene in plants or retinol esters in fish or dairy products. After absorption in lymph from the gut (which requires bile and lipase), retinol esters are transported to the tissues, where they are stored primarily in the liver, with small amounts in other tissues. In the well nourished individual, there is 6–12 months of retinol requirements stored (about 150–300 mg/g liver). Vitamin A is mobilized from liver stores as retinol, and is solubilized by binding to retinol-binding protein (RBP). The retinol–RBP complex is normally bound to prealbumin. Both RBP and prealbumin have short half-lives (about 11 hours and 48 hours respectively), and the amount of circulating retinol is very dependent on the synthetic rates of these proteins. This, in turn, depends partly on protein nutritional status. Plasma retinol in health is maintained within fairly narrow limits over a range of liver vitamin A concentrations, and hence the plasma concentration of retinol is not a good index of vitamin A status.

Effects of acute illness

Since RBP and prealbumin are both 'negative acute-phase proteins', their concentrations fall rapidly in acutely ill patients, often to about 50% of normal values (Shenkin et al, 1980). Plasma retinol is therefore low in such situations and increased vitamin A supplements are not indicated. On the other hand, patients in renal failure, especially if chronic, tend to have high plasma retinol concentrations, possibly as a result of reduced catabolism of RBP by renal tubular cells. Although vitamin A toxicity can occur with typical gastrointestinal and skin changes, this is unlikely in such patients unless vitamin A supplements are also taken.

Long-term deficiency syndromes

Chronic vitamin A deficiency is well characterized. The clinical symptoms include night blindness (slow dark adaptation), corneal conjunctival changes (xerophthalmia), and smell, taste and hearing changes. In Western countries, it is most likely to occur in patients with chronic fat malabsorption syndromes, e.g. coeliac disease, Crohn's disease, or short bowel syndrome (Main et al, 1983). Alternatively, patients receiving long-term intravenous nutrition have been reported to develop vitamin A deficiency with symptoms of impaired dark adaptation (Howard et al, 1980). There have also been many reports of low plasma vitamin A during intravenous nutrition, but these have rarely been associated with clinical symptoms and were probably due to reduced RBP concentration.

Provision of vitamin A

Vitamin A intake for healthy individuals eating an oral diet ranges from

Table 1. Vitamin requirements and supply in selected enteral nutrition products.

	Units	RDA[a] (UK 1979)	RDA[a] (USA 1980)	Ensure[d]	Enrich[d]	Clinifeed[e] Iso	Fortison[f]	Wyeth[g] Standard	Liquisorbon[h] MCT	Reabilan[e]	Vivonex[i]
Vitamin A	µg	750	800–1000	1500	1730	900	1400	728	1150	1600	1680
Vitamin D	µg	b	b	10.0	13.0	8.5	10.0	10.0	10.5	10.0	11.5
Vitamin E	mg	—	7–10	46	73	20	63	35	12	30	34
Vitamin K	µg	—	70–140[c]	72	92	—	—	437	150	100	75
Vitamin C	mg	30	60	300	230	80	100	73	90	200	67
Vitamin B_1	mg	0.9–1.3	1.0–1.5	3.0	3.0	2.0	1.4	1.7	1.5	3.0	1.7
Vitamin B_2	mg	1.3–1.6	1.2–1.7	3.4	3.3	2.4	2.0	1.9	1.7	3.0	1.9
Vitamin B_6	mg	—	1.9–2.2	4.0	4.0	3.0	2.0	2.9	2.0	4.0	2.2
Vitamin B_{12}	µg	—	3.0	12.0	11.5	5.0	4.0	2.9	6.0	4.0	6.7
Folic acid	µg	300	400	400	770	277	500	388	400	500	467
Niacin	mg	15–18	13–19	40	38	24	20	20	20	40	22
Biotin	mg	—	0.1–0.2[c]	0.3	0.6	0.1	0.3	0.1	0.3	0.2	0.3
pantothenate	mg	—	4–7[c]	10	19	18	10	5	11	10	11

[a]RDA is age-dependent—values are shown for adults.
[b]RDA dependent upon exposure to sunlight.
[c]Estimated safe and adequate daily intake.
[d]Abbott Laboratories (Berkshire).
[e]Roussel (Middlesex).
[f]Cow and Gate (Wiltshire).
[g]Wyeth Nutrition (Berkshire).
[h]E. Merck (Hampshire).
[i]Eaton Laboratories (London).

750 μg retinol equivalents (2475 IU vitamin A) (DHSS, 1979) to 800 μg retinol equivalents (2640 IU vitamin A) for females and 1000 μg retinol equivalents (3300 IU vitamin A) for males (Food and Nutrition Board, 1980). This amount is amply provided by 2 litres of most commonly used tube feeds (Table 1). The Expert Committee of the AMA (American Medical Association, 1975) recommended 1000 μg (3300 IU) as the intake for patients requiring intravenous nutrition. A number of studies have now indicated that this amount is probably adequate for patients requiring either short-term nutrition in hospitals or longer-term nutrition at home. Vitamin A is usually provided in intravenous nutrition as retinol or as retinol palmitate.

When vitamin A is provided together with water-soluble nutrients, it is susceptible to absorption onto the plastic tubes of the administration set (Gillis et al, 1983). This absorption is variable, and may lead to substantial loss of vitamin (about 50–60% of retinol, or about 10–15% of retinol palmitate) from the infusion. Infusion of the vitamin within a fat emulsion may reduce the amount of absorption in this way (Greene et al, 1987). Moreover, the opacity of fat emulsion reduces the photodegradation of vitamin A by UV light.

Monitoring adequacy of supply

There are no satisfactory simple tests for assessment of adequacy of vitamin A provision. Measurement of plasma vitamin A is of limited value, although if taken in conjunction with the plasma RBP concentration and C-reactive protein (to obtain an estimate of the acute-phase response), and other estimates of visceral protein nutritional status (serum transferrin and albumin), it is possible to exclude chronic under- or overprovision of vitamin A.

Vitamin D

Normal metabolism

Vitamin D is required for the normal metabolism of the major minerals calcium, phosphorus and magnesium. It also appears to have an important role in differentiation and control of growth of red and white blood cells (Editorial, 1984; Manolagas et al, 1986). Cholecalciferol (vitamin D_3) is synthesized in man under the action of UV light on 7-dehydrocholecalciferol in skin. The main dietary source is ergocalciferol (vitamin D_2) from vegetables. Both forms of vitamin D are converted to the active form of 1,25-dihydroxy vitamin D, first by 25-hydroxylation in the liver, and subsequently by 1-hydroxylation in the kidney, under the control of parathyroid hormone.

Vitamin D circulates bound to a specific α-globulin and is stored in its unaltered form in adipose tissue, from which it is released as required for hydroxylation. Stores of vitamin D in health are sufficient to last several months.

Effects of acute illness

There are no clear effects of acute illness on vitamin D metabolism, although in acute renal failure serum 25-hydroxy vitamin D concentration falls after 1–2 weeks. As a result of the impaired 1-hydroxylation, patients in chronic renal failure may require vitamin D supplements (1-α-hydroxy vitamin D or 1,25-dihydroxy vitamin D) but these should be used with caution because of concern that they may contribute to the progression of the disease.

Long-term deficiency syndromes

The effects of vitamin D deficiency are well characterized and include rickets in children and osteomalacia in adults. Deficiency states most commonly occur either as a result of decreased dietary intake or where there is fat malabsorption.

Osteomalacia due to vitamin D deficiency has not been observed in adults receiving intravenous nutrition, although aluminium-induced bone disease has occurred in patients receiving solutions heavily contaminated with aluminium (Koo et al, 1986). Rickets, however, has occurred in some premature infants receiving intravenous nutrition (Leape and Valae, 1976). A more common problem in adults receiving long-term intravenous nutrition has been a form of metabolic bone disease characterized by hypercalciuria, intermittent hypercalcaemia and severe bone pain. These findings improved within 1–2 months after stopping the vitamin D supplementation of the intravenous regimen in some patients (Shike et al, 1980). On the other hand, Klein et al (1982) found no relationship between vitamin D and metabolic bone disease of intravenous nutrition. This controversy remains unresolved, but it would seem prudent not to provide excess vitamin D.

Provision of vitamin D

The recommended dietary allowance for vitamin D for healthy individuals is 10 μg (400 IU vitamin D) orally per day. This amount is present in 2 litres of most tube feeds. Because of the reduced requirement for gastrointestinal absorption of calcium and phosphorus during intravenous nutrition, the Nutritional Advisory Group of the AMA recommended 5 μg (200 IU) intravenously per day for patients receiving intravenous nutrition. Vitamin D_2 (ergocalciferol) is usually provided intravenously. Various studies have indicated that vitamin D_2 5 μg/day is adequate to correct 25-hydroxy vitamin D_2 and 1,25-dihydroxy vitamin D_2 concentrations (Shils et al, 1985). As with the other fat-soluble vitamins, vitamin D may be absorbed from the infusate onto the administration set and tubing (Gillis et al, 1983).

Monitoring adequacy of supply

The main way to assess vitamin D status is by measuring serum calcium, phosphorus and alkaline phosphatase, together with urinary excretion of calcium and phosphorus. When abnormalities of mineral metabolism are detected, a more precise estimate of vitamin D status can be obtained by measuring serum 25-hydroxy vitamin D concentration (reference range 10–50 μg/litre), although measurement of 1,25-hydroxy vitamin D, if technically feasible, is a more accurate measurement of functional activity.

Vitamin E

Metabolism

Vitamin E is a group of seven related biological substances, tocopherols, which have powerful antioxidant properties. Vitamin E is therefore closely associated with selenium in removing free radicals and superoxides, and thus preventing peroxidation of fatty acids within cell membranes. In this way, it promotes membrane integrity, and is especially important in erythrocyte membranes in the newborn.

Vitamin E is derived largely from plants and vegetable oils. It is absorbed with the other fat-soluble vitamins, and is found in blood associated with low-density lipoprotein. Adipose tissue is the main site of storage.

Effects of acute illness

There are no specific effects associated with acute illness, although it is probable that any patient with severe hypercatabolism and increased neutrophil activity will have an increased rate of production of free radicals.

Long-term deficiency syndromes

Deficiency of vitamin E in man is less common than in animals but a number of syndromes are recognized. In premature infants, vitamin E deficiency is related to retrolental fibroplasia (Johnson et al, 1974) and to haemolytic anaemia (Ritchie et al, 1968). In adults and children with severe malabsorption, neuromuscular syndromes with elevated creatine kinase and creatinuria occur, probably due to skeletal muscle damage (Bieri and Farrell, 1976). Vitamin E deficiency has been observed in a patient during intravenous nutrition, the main clinical features being ataxia and visual disturbance (Howard et al, 1982).

Provision of vitamin E

Vitamin E activity is measured in terms of milligram α-tocopherol equivalents, which makes allowance for the different activities of the various forms of tocopherol in the diet. There is a close relationship between the requirement for vitamin E and that for polyunsaturated fatty acids (PUFAs). It is estimated that approximately 7–13 mg D-α-tocopherol per 24 hours is usually adequate, but 17 mg/24 h or more may be necessary if there is a high PUFA intake (Horwitt, 1974).

The AMA recommendation for intravenous nutrition is 10 mg α-tocopherol per 24 hours. Patients receiving intravenous fat emulsions will receive an intake of vitamin E which is present as a component of the intravenous triglyceride extract. However, emulsions based on soya bean oil (e.g. Intralipid®) contain only about 8% of the vitamin E as α-tocopherol, the remainder being less potent β- and γ-tocopherols, whereas emulsions based on sunflower oil (e.g. Liposyn®) contain a very much higher proportion of α-tocopherol. To allow for this variability in supply and also for the fact that patients do not always receive fat emulsion daily, the AMA recommended an additional provision of 10 mg D-α-tocopherol per day. About 35% of the vitamin E infused can be lost in the intravenous tubing (Gillis et al, 1983).

Monitoring adequacy of supply

Assessment of vitamin E status is complicated by its binding to circulating lipoproteins. It has therefore been suggested that plasma α-tocopherol levels should be expressed as a ratio to β-lipoprotein, cholesterol or total lipid (Sokol et al, 1984). Moreover, measurement of total vitamin E may be misleading if there are large amounts of relatively inactive β- and γ-tocopherol isomers present. If assessment is required, HPLC separation of isomers is necessary together with measurement of plasma lipids.

Vitamin K

Metabolism

Vitamin K occurs naturally as vitamin K_1 (phylloquinone) in green plants and as vitamin K_2 (menaquinones) in bacteria and animals. It is required for the hepatic synthesis of the blood-clotting factors prothrombin and factors VII, IX and X.

In man, the half-life of intravenously injected vitamin K is relatively short, with about 40–50% excretion in bile and 20% excretion in urine within 3 days (Shearer et al, 1972). There is little storage of vitamin K, and hence a regular source of supply is necessary. Absorption of dietary vitamin K is dependent on bile salts and occurs with other fat-soluble vitamins in the small bowel. Of the vitamin K synthesized in the colon, the proportion absorbed is not known (Shearer et al, 1974).

Deficiency syndromes

Vitamin K deficiency may be induced by antibiotic therapy which alters the intestinal flora. Deficiency is also likely in any condition leading to decreased intake or fat malabsorption, or when hepatocellular damage may prevent the normal utilization of vitamin K (Ansell et al, 1977).

Provision of vitamin K

The minimum daily adult requirements for vitamin K range from 0.03 to 1.5 µg/kg body weight (Frick et al, 1967), corresponding to about 2–100 µg/

day. Because of the contribution of intestinal bacteria, no specific recommended dietary allowance is made, although the suggested safe and adequate level of intake is 70–140 µg/24 h. The Expert Panel of the AMA do not recommend routine provision of vitamin K intravenously as part of the vitamin supplements for patients receiving intravenous nutrition, because of difficulties if they are simultaneously receiving anticoagulants. However, relatively few patients fall into this category, and it would seem reasonable to provide a regular intake of vitamin K, especially since many patients receiving intravenous nutrition have abnormalities of intestinal function which may affect the intestinal flora. A recent study has indicated that daily provision of 1 mg vitamin K intravenously is as effective as a once-weekly 10 mg intramuscular injection (Schepers et al, 1988). This is, however, quite a large dose, and we have found that provision of 150 µg/day intravenously is adequate to maintain normal blood coagulation (Shenkin et al, 1987).

Monitoring adequacy of supply

The main method of assessing vitamin K status is the one stage prothrombin time, although this is an assessment of the effectiveness of vitamin K status rather than the status itself. Specific methods for vitamin K measurement in blood are now available by HPLC, although these are not yet in widespread use (Shearer, 1983).

WATER-SOLUBLE VITAMINS

Thiamine (vitamin B₁)

Metabolism

Thiamine is required in the diet as a precursor of thiamine pyrophosphate, a coenzyme with a key role in oxidative decarboxylation of pyruvic acid, and also for transketolation reactions in the pentose phosphate pathway. Thiamine is therefore of special importance in carbohydrate metabolism. It is absorbed efficiently in the upper small intestine and is transferred to the tissues, where little is stored, there being only about 30 mg thiamine in the whole body compared with the daily requirement of 1–2 mg.

Effects of acute illness

Since thiamine is closely linked with carbohydrate metabolism, any acute illness which increases resting energy expenditure also increases the requirement for thiamine, e.g. any severe infection, fever, trauma or hyperthyroidism.

Deficiency syndromes

Signs of thiamine deficiency may develop early in patients receiving an inadequate intake. The clinical picture appears to depend upon the severity of the illness, together with the duration and magnitude of the inadequacy of supply. In relatively mild but chronic deficiency, symptoms are primarily neurological, with paraesthesia and peripheral neuropathy. In more severe cases, which usually include deficiencies arising in patients requiring intravenous nutrition, cardiovascular features develop, including high-output cardiac failure and oedema. Cardiac beriberi may also present as a low-output failure (Shoshin beriberi) and this has also been observed during intravenous nutrition (La Selve et al, 1986). We have found a high incidence of biochemical thiamine depletion in patients in intensive care units (about 20%) and this is associated with a higher mortality (Cruickshank et al, 1988).

The most acute form of deficiency is Wernicke's encephalopathy, in which symptoms may extend from confusion to coma and death. Although this is usually found in alcoholics with severe deficiency, it has also been frequently observed during intravenous nutrition (Nadel and Burger, 1976). Thiamine deficiency in such patients may only be diagnosed at post mortem, but this is a potentially preventable complication and hence adequate thiamine provision is essential.

Provision of thiamine

The requirement for thiamine has usually been related to energy intake, and in the oral diet the RDA is for a minimum intake of 1 mg/day or 0.5 mg/ 4.2 MJ (1000 kcal), whichever is the greater. However, it is recognized that severe illness causes additional requirements for thiamine, and the recommendation of the AMA for patients receiving intravenous nutrition is for 3.0 mg/24 h. Although this level of provision is probably adequate for most patients requiring intravenous nutrition, in the severely stressed patient in intensive care we recommend that patients receive an additional 50–250 mg once-weekly in addition to the above standard dosage.

Monitoring adequacy of supply

The most widely used test in clinical practice is probably the measurement of erythrocyte transketolase before and after in vitro addition of exogenous thiamine pyrophosphate (Bayoumi and Rosalki, 1976). Normal values are less than 25% activation. Although it is a useful screening method, quantitation is difficult, and measurement of serum thiamine may also be helpful in determining thiamine status (reference range 25–70 µg/litre). In the less acute situation, measurement of blood pyruvate and lactate after a loading dose of glucose is a sensitive test of thiamine status.

Riboflavin

Metabolism

Riboflavin is phosphorylated in the intestinal mucosa during absorption and is transferred to the tissues where it combines to form the coenzymes flavin mononucleotide (FMN) and flavin adenine dinucleotide (FAD). These form the prosthetic groups of enzyme systems involved in hydrogen transport and which are vital to normal oxidative metabolism.

After absorption in the upper gastrointestinal tract, riboflavin is distributed to all tissues with little capacity for storage. Riboflavin is excreted mainly in the urine, which is a good guide to the amount of intake.

Effect of acute illness

As with thiamine, any serious illness causing an increase in resting energy expenditure is likely to promote riboflavin deficiency. Acute deficiency is therefore more likely following severe accidental trauma and surgery. We have recently observed a poorer riboflavin status in patients admitted to our Intensive Care Unit who subsequently died than in those who recovered. Less than 10% of the patients had biochemical evidence of deficiency and none had clinical signs. This observation suggests that a deterioration of riboflavin status even within normal limits may have a detrimental effect on clinical outcome.

Long-term deficiency syndromes

Clinical signs of riboflavin deficiency are difficult to recognize, since such a deficiency rarely occurs in isolation. Cheilosis and angular stomatitis are prominent features, together with glossitis and a seborrhoeic dermatitis which particularly affects the nose and face. Normochromic, normocytic anaemia may also occur. Such deficiency has been observed in patients during intravenous nutrition (Duhamel et al, 1979), but is more common in patients with chronic debilitating diseases or during periods of increased demand due to rapid anabolism, such as childhood and pregnancy (Jeppsson and Gimmon, 1985).

Provision of riboflavin

The RDA for riboflavin in the oral diet has been estimated as 0.6 mg/4.2 MJ (1000 kcal) for persons of all ages, with a minimum intake of 1.2 mg/day. This amount is present in 2 litres of commercial tube feeds (Table 1).

The Nutritional Advisory Group of the AMA recommended an intake of 3.6 mg/24 h during intravenous nutrition, to allow for the increased requirements due to disease, together with the anticipated increased urinary loss (American Medical Association, 1975). Riboflavin is very sensitive to photodegradation by UV light, and hence the amount actually provided to the patient may differ from the amount initially added to the regimen. Care must be taken to try to protect the added vitamin prior to its infusion (Allwood, 1984a). This can be achieved by either covering the infusion bag or adding the water-soluble vitamins into the fat emulsion, where the opacity of the solution offers protection.

Monitoring adequacy of supply

The most commonly used test to assess riboflavin status clinically is measurement of erythrocyte glutathione reductase activity before and after the addition of FAD in vitro (Bayoumi and Rosalki, 1976). Normal values are less than 60% activation. Methods for measurement of riboflavin both in blood and in urine have also been reported, although these are of less value in assessing the intracellular content of the vitamin in the individual patient.

Pyridoxine (vitamin B_6)

Metabolism

Vitamin B_6 is a group of three related substances, pyridoxine, pyridoxal and pyridoxamine, which after absorption are converted in the liver to the metabolically active form, pyridoxal phosphate. This is distributed throughout body tissues, where it plays a key role in amino acid metabolism as coenzyme for deamination and transamination reactions. Requirements for vitamin B_6 are therefore related to protein and amino acid intake. About 70% of the vitamin is excreted in urine as the inactive metabolite 4-pyridoxic acid.

Long-term deficiency syndromes

Deficiency of vitamin B_6 is rare and has been seen most commonly in infants who develop a hypochromic microcytic anaemia, gastrointestinal disturbances and progressive nervous system involvement leading ultimately to seizures. In adults and children, a non-specific dermatitis, cheilosis and angular stomatitis may also occur. Deficiency has been associated with severe malabsorption, chronic liver disease or alcoholism, and also with drugs which affect the metabolism of vitamin B_6 (e.g. isoniazid or hydralazine). There have been no reports of vitamin B_6 deficiency during intravenous nutrition.

Provision of vitamin B_6

The average adult requirement for pyridoxine is at least 1.25 mg/day with an intake of 100 g protein. To allow sufficient margin for variation in diet, the RDA has been suggested at 2.2 mg/day for males and 2.0 mg/day for females. There is considerable variation in the amount of vitamin B_6 present in synthetic tube feeds (Table 1), some feeds barely providing this recommended intake.

The AMA recommendation for intravenous nutrition was 4.0 mg/24 h, this amount taking account of the requirement for increased amino acid metabolism during intravenous nutrition.

Monitoring adequacy of supply

For routine clinical use, the best functional assay is measurement of the activity of erythrocyte glutamic–oxaloacetic transaminase before and after addition of pyridoxal phosphate. The lower the activation of enzyme activity, the better the vitamin B_6 status (normal values less than 150% activation). Specific assays of blood levels of pyridoxine, pyridoxal and pyridoxal phosphate are now available, and together with urinary losses these may be useful on a research basis to quantify more accurately the requirements during intravenous nutrition.

Niacin

Metabolism

Niacin is present in small amounts in most plant and animal food products and is absorbed throughout the small intestine. It is converted in the tissues to the coenzymes NAD and NADP, which are of fundamental importance in dehydrogenase reactions involving glycolysis, citric acid cycle and fatty acid oxidation. Niacin is excreted in the urine in the form of the hepatic metabolites N-methyl niacinamide and N-methyl-3-pyridone-5-carboxylamide, which can be used as indices of niacin intake. Dietary tryptophan can be converted to some extent to niacin, about 60 mg tryptophan being equivalent to 1 mg niacin.

Deficiency syndromes

Niacin deficiency results in pellagra, a complex clinical syndrome characterized by weakness, a painful erythematous rash, especially on the face and back of the hands, stomatitis, glossitis and gastrointestinal symptoms. In severe cases, delirium, dementia and coma may ensue.

Clinical deficiency in hospitals is most commonly due to inadequate intake in chronic alcoholism, but also occurs in patients with severe malabsorption or chronic debilitating disease (Moran and Greene, 1979). Pellagra may also occur in patients receiving isoniazid due to reduced conversion of tryptophan to niacin. Although deficiency has not been observed during intravenous nutrition, a syndrome of acute encephalopathy probably due to niacin deficiency has been observed in malnourished subjects receiving intravenous glucose infusions (Goldsmith, 1977).

Provision of niacin

The recommended allowances for niacin are commonly related to energy expenditure because of the close relationship of the coenzymes with enzymes of oxidative metabolism. The RDA for adults is 6.6 mg/4.2 MJ (1000 kcal) (or 6.6 niacin equivalents, allowing for the contribution from tryptophan) and not less than 13 mg/day. This amount is present in all proprietary tube feeds (Table 1).

To allow for the increased requirements in disease, the AMA recommendation is for 40 mg/24 h during intravenous nutrition.

Monitoring adequacy of supply

Monitoring niacin status is rarely necessary in the clinical context. However, for assessment of individuals or in research studies, whole-blood niacin measurements (Shils et al, 1985) or excretion of urinary metabolites (Dempsey et al, 1987) have been found to be useful.

' Folate

Metabolism

Folic acid (pteroyl glutamic acid) is present in a wide variety of vegetable and animal foods, usually as the polyglutamate form. Free folic acid is formed by hydrolysis in the small intestine and is readily absorbed. During absorption, the folic acid is reduced and methylated to form the main active form, methyl tetrahydrofolic acid. Folate is active throughout tissues of the body in transferring one-carbon units (methyl groups) from amino acids to purine and pyrimidine precursors. Megaloblastic changes in folate and vitamin B_{12} deficiency result from the consequently impaired DNA synthesis.

Total body folate stores amount to about 50 mg, of which 1% turns over each day (Brody et al, 1984). Folate is excreted primarily in urine but also in bile, there being an enterohepatic circulation of about 100 µg/day.

Effects of acute illness

There have been a number of reports of critically ill patients developing severe folic acid deficiency shortly after commencing intravenous nutrition. Thus Wardrop et al (1977) observed a marked fall in serum folate within 48 hours of commencing amino acid/sorbitol/ethanol infusion and although the ethanol may have been particularly involved in this, Tennant et al (1981) had a similar result with amino acid infusions. Pancytopenia developed in some patients within one week. The mechanism of these rapid changes is not clear but probably relates to increased folate metabolism. Acute deficiency is most likely in patients with severe infections plus renal failure (Beard et al, 1980) or hepatic failure (Steinberg, 1972). Apart from the pancytopenia, jaundice may be a notable feature which resolves rapidly on folate therapy.

Long-term deficiency syndromes

Because of the relatively slow turnover of folate, signs of folic acid deficiency may take several months to develop if intake is inadequate. The sequence of events is a reduction in serum folate concentration by 3 weeks, hypersegmentation of polymorphonuclear leukocytes at about 7 weeks, increased urinary formiminoglutamic acid at 14 weeks, reduced red cell folate by 17 weeks, and bone marrow megaloblastosis and anaemia at 19 weeks (Goldsmith, 1975). Patients may also develop glossitis, listlessness, irritability and weight loss.

Patients more likely to develop folate deficiency include those with severe folate malabsorption due to inflammatory bowel disease, increased folate requirements due to serious illness, and decreased hepatic stores due to inadequate intake or hepatic disease, and those on haemodialysis who have increased loss of the vitamin.

Provision of folate

Usually about 25–50% of dietary folic acid is nutritionally available, and 400 µg/day are normally recommended in the oral diet. Not all tube feeds achieve this level of supply, although absorption from such artificial feeds may be more efficient. During intravenous nutrition, as little as 200 µg/24 h may be enough for maintenance (Stromberg et al, 1981) but the recommendation of the AMA was for a daily supply of 400 µg/day to allow for increased requirements and repletion of folate stores.

Monitoring adequacy of supply

Folate is one of the easier vitamins to assess nutritionally, since relatively simple competitive protein-binding assays are now available to measure serum folate and therefore obtain an estimate of recent intake, and also red cell folate to provide an index of total body status.

Vitamin B_{12}

Metabolism

Vitamin B_{12} is a group of cobalt-containing substances known as cobalamins. It is present in food of animal origin only, particularly liver. The glycoprotein intrinsic factor, secreted in the gastric juice, is necessary for absorption in the terminal ileum. Vitamin B_{12} in the blood is bound to transport proteins, transcobalamins I, II and III. The total body content of vitamin B_{12} is about 1–10 mg, up to 90% of which is present in the liver. There is also an enterohepatic circulation of vitamin B_{12} which minimizes losses from the body.

Vitamin B_{12} has widespread actions on cells. These include the regeneration of folic acid from the 5-methyl tetrahydrofolate pool, and this explains the interrelationship of signs and symptoms of folate and vitamin B_{12} deficiencies. Moreover, coenzymes which require cobalamin play an important role in methylation of homocystine to methionine (and therefore choline and betaine synthesis) in the pathway for metabolism of odd chain length fatty acids. Vitamin B_{12} therefore has a role in fat, protein and nucleic acid metabolism.

Long-term deficiency syndromes

Because of the extensive stores and minimal excretion, vitamin B_{12} deficiency is very rare and may take several years to develop even on a minimal vitamin B_{12} intake. Pernicious anaemia is, of course, the most common deficiency disease, resulting from lack of secretion of intrinsic factor in the stomach and intestinal failure in absorption of dietary B_{12}. Deficiency may also result from chronic alcoholism or from folate deficiency, since folate is required for vitamin B_{12} absorption (Jeppsson and Gimmon, 1983).

Vitamin B_{12} deficiency is characterized by macrocytic anaemia with megaloblastosis and glossitis. In severe cases, neurological complications develop, including paraesthesia of hands and feet, muscle weakness and personality changes. No deficiency states have been described in patients receiving intravenous nutrition.

Provision of vitamin B_{12}

The RDA for vitamin B_{12} is 3 µg/day for adults, assuming at least 50% absorption of dietary vitamin B_{12}. The AMA advised 5 µg/day for adults receiving intravenous nutrition, again making an allowance for the increased requirement anticipated if energy expenditure is increased (Anderson, 1977). Various authors have provided from 2 µg/day to 1000 µg/week, testifying to the safety of parenteral vitamin B_{12} (Jeppsson and Gimmon, 1983).

Monitoring adequacy of supply

Vitamin B_{12} status can be readily checked by measurement of the serum concentration, using competitive protein binding or microbiological assays.

Biotin

Metabolism

Biotin is a water-soluble sulphur-containing vitamin which is a coenzyme for many carboxylase reactions. It plays an important role in linking the metabolism of carbohydrate and fat through the reactions of pyruvate carboxylase and acetyl coenzyme A carboxylase enzymes.

It is present in most foods, especially those of animal origin. Biotin is also synthesized by the intestinal flora, but the proportion absorbed is not known. Biotin is water-soluble and is excreted as free biotin in the urine.

Long-term deficiency syndromes

Deficiencies in man have most often been associated with excessive ingestion of avidin from raw egg whites, which bind to the vitamin and make it unavailable for absorption. Deficiency symptoms have included a dry scaly dermatitis, anorexia, nausea and vomiting, and mental depression (Moran and Greene, 1979). Cases of biotin deficiency have been reported during long-term total parenteral nutrition in adults (Innis and Allardyce, 1983) as well as in children (Mock et al, 1981). Although an unusual complication, since biotin is not always provided to patients receiving intravenous nutrition, the combination of scaly dermatitis and alopecia together with depression and other neurological signs should raise the possibility of biotin deficiency.

Provision of biotin

The human requirement is not known, but the Food and Nutrition Board have suggested an intake of 100–200 µg/day in the oral diet. The Nutrition Advisory Group of the AMA recommended 60 µg/day for adults receiving intravenous nutrition, and this level of intake has been found adequate to maintain whole-blood biotin concentration in patients receiving home parenteral nutrition (Shils et al, 1985) and also urinary biotin excretion in short-term intravenous nutrition post-surgery (Dempsey et al, 1987).

Monitoring adequacy of supply

Assays for biotin are rarely available, although microbiological assays for urinary or plasma biotin have been developed and are useful on a research basis (Bonjour, 1977).

Vitamin C (ascorbic acid)

Metabolism

Vitamin C exists as both ascorbic acid and dehydroascorbic acid, both of which are effective in man. The main source of vitamin C in the diet is fruit and vegetables, vitamin C being readily absorbed from the upper small bowel. It is distributed throughout the tissues of the body where it is effective in a range of hydroxylation reactions. In collagen synthesis it plays a key role in hydroxylation of proline and lysine. It is also involved in the metabolism of tyrosine and other amino acids, and in microsomal drug metabolism. Ascorbic acid may also have a role as a biological antioxidant (Levine, 1986).

The body pool of vitamin C in healthy adults is about 1500 mg, with a turnover rate of about 3%/day. Thus deficiency might be expected after about 30–40 days on an inadequate intake. The renal threshold for vitamin C is about 1.4 mg/100 ml, above which vitamin C appears in the urine (Burns, 1974).

Effects of acute illness

In patients with acute infectious disease or following severe trauma, plasma ascorbic acid falls rapidly. This is thought to be due to a shift of ascorbic acid from serum to the wound (Goldsmith, 1977). It has been suggested that vitamin C requirements are markedly increased (by as much as 100-fold in major trauma) and that normal body stores can be exhausted as early as 48 hours after injury (Burns, 1974).

Long-term deficiency syndromes

Classically, vitamin C deficiency results in scurvy, which is characterized at first by non-specific symptoms of weakness, lassitude and muscle pains, which progress to weight loss and eventually to bleeding into the skin and gums. The signs in children may be more apparent.

There is a long list of conditions said to be associated with an increased requirement for vitamin C, including infectious diseases, thyrotoxicosis, neoplastic disease, surgical stress, trauma, pressure sores and renal failure. However, apart from the biochemical evidence of depletion, clear-cut evidence of a clinical deficiency state with signs and symptoms have rarely been described. Nonetheless, subclincial effects of vitamin C deficiency may be important before such signs develop. One patient has been described with a coagulation defect associated with vitamin C deficiency during intravenous nutrition (Robson et al, 1980).

Provision of vitamin C

A daily intake of 10 mg ascorbic acid can prevent scurvy, although this does not provide for adequate reserves. Additional vitamin C is also required to sustain other tissue functions. The RDA for the oral diet is 30 mg/day in the UK (DHSS, 1979) and 60 mg/day in the USA (Food and Nutrition Board, 1980). Commercially available tube feeds provide a wide range of vitamin C intakes, although all exceed 60 mg in 2 litres (Table 1).

The Nutrition Advisory Group of the AMA suggested 100 mg as the intake during intravenous nutrition, to allow for the anticipated increased requirements during stress. One potential problem during intravenous nutrition is the rapid oxidation of vitamin C in the presence of copper when all nutrients are mixed together in a 3-litre bag (Allwood, 1984b). We have found that vitamin C status is maintained during short-term intravenous nutrition when such a complete nutritive mixture is used (Shenkin et al, 1987), but losses of vitamin C may occur and if necessary during long-term feeding further steps should be taken to infuse vitamins and trace elements separately. This problem requires further evaluation.

Monitoring adequacy of supply

There are a number of methods available for measuring ascorbic acid. Plasma ascorbic acid gives a reasonable index of the adequacy of recent intake (reference range $>10\,\mu$mol/litre; >0.2 mg/100 ml), whereas measurement of leukocyte or platelet ascorbic acid is a better index of tissue stores.

VITAMIN PROVISION DURING ENTERAL AND PARENTERAL NUTRITION

Proprietary feeds for use in enteral nutrition contain widely differing amounts of the various vitamins, although in a volume of 2 litres or in 8.4 MJ (2000 kcal) virtually all of the feeds provide an excess of each vitamin (Table 1). Moreover, vitamin supplements in both tablet or liquid form are available, and can be used to supplement intake if required. Similarly, a number

Table 2. Vitamin requirements and supply in total parenteral nutrition.

	Units	RDA[a]	AMA[b]	Multibionta[c]	Solivito[d] + Vitlipid Adult	Solivito N[d] + Vitlipid N Adult	MVI-12[e] (2 amps)
Thiamine	mg	1.5	3.0	50	1.2	3.0	3.0
Riboflavine	mg	1.7	3.6	10	1.8	3.6	3.6
Nicotinamide	mg	19	40	100	10	40	40
Pyridoxine	mg	2.2	4.0	15	2	4.0	4.0
Folic acid	μg	400	400		200	400	400
Cyanocobalamin	μg	3.0	5.0		2	5.0	5.0
Pantothenic acid	mg	7	15	25	10	15	15
Biotin	μg	300	60		300	60	60
Ascorbic acid	mg	60	100	500	300	100	100
Retinol	mg	1.0	1.0	3	0.75	1.0	1.0
Cholecalciferol	μg	10	5		3	5	5
Phytylmenaquinone	mg	0.14			0.15	0.15	
Tocopherol	IU	15	10	5		10	10

[a]USA recommended dietary allowance (Food and Nutrition Board, 1980)—upper limit.
[b]Expert Panel of AMA Recommendations (American Medical Association, 1975).
[c]E. Merck (Hampshire).
[d]Kabi Vitrum (Middlesex).
[e]USV Laboratories (New York).

of multivitamin preparations for intravenous use are available, and some of those widely used in the UK are summarized in Table 2. A large number of intravenous preparations are available in the USA, and these have been tabulated and compared (Jeppsson and Gimmon, 1983). It is essential that an adequate intake of all vitamins should be provided to patients requiring nutritional support. One major problem continues to be loss of vitamins from the nutritional preparations, whether due to degradation by UV light, interaction of vitamins with essential trace elements, or loss of vitamins onto the infusion bag or giving set. The fact that patients have theoretically received an adequate vitamin intake does not therefore ensure maintenance of vitamin status. If a suspicion of vitamin deficiency arises, appropriate tests should be carried out to confirm the adequacy of vitamin status.

ESSENTIAL INORGANIC MICRONUTRIENTS—TRACE ELEMENTS

Zinc

Metabolism

Zinc is one of the most diverse of the essential elements, since it is a component of more than 100 metalloenzymes. These play a part in virtually all aspects of metabolism, including acid–base balance (carbonic anhydrase), bone and liver metabolism (alkaline phosphatase) and several steps of protein and nucleic acid biosynthesis. Adequate zinc nutrition is therefore essential for normal tissue function, growth and repair.

Zinc is ingested in the diet in most foodstuffs, the best sources being good-quality animal or plant protein. Zinc is absorbed throughout the small intestine to a total extent of 20–40% of the intake. This proportion is markedly affected by other dietary components, phytate (from flour), fibre and phosphate all reducing absorption (Shenkin et al, 1987). Moreover, zinc absorption may be reduced by iron intake since both compete for the same absorption mechanism in the upper small intestine (Solomons, 1986).

Absorbed zinc is bound to plasma albumin in the portal blood and is initially concentrated in the liver in the form of metallothionein, before being released to the tissues. Most zinc is excreted in the faeces via the bile, urinary output normally consisting of less than $10\,\mu mol/24\,h$ ($650\,\mu g/24\,h$) and being independent of dietary intake.

Effects of acute illness

Total plasma zinc concentration is lowered by stressful stimuli such as injury, organic disease, inflammatory disease, infection and corticosteroid pharmaceuticals. This fall is mediated primarily by the cytokines such as interleukin 1, which stimulate metallothionein synthesis in the liver (Kampshmidt, 1980).

Urine zinc also increases after injury, the duration and extent being related to the magnitude of trauma (Davies and Fell, 1974). The extra zinc originates from catabolism of skeletal muscle protein and is paralleled by increases in urinary nitrogen and potassium.

Long-term deficiency syndromes

The extent of symptoms of zinc deficiency depend upon the severity and duration of the deficiency state. Relatively mild forms occur in patients with chronic malabsorption due to dietary factors, alcoholic liver disease, or other chronic debilitating illness. They are characterized by anorexia, lethargy, rough skin, delayed wound healing, and growth retardation in adolescents (Prasad, 1988).

More severe forms of deficiency occur in the zinc deficiency of intravenous nutrition, in severe alcoholism which promotes zinc loss in the urine, following penicillamine therapy, and in the inborn error of zinc absorption acrodermatitis enteropathica. Such patients develop a bullous pustular dermatitis, alopecia, diarrhoea and impaired healing. Zinc also has an important role in T lymphocyte function, and zinc-deficient patients are susceptible to severe bacterial or fungal infections. This reduced immunocompetence may in part be due to the role of zinc in stimulating the biological activity of the thymic hormone, thymulin (Bach et al, 1988).

Zinc deficiency during intravenous nutrition has been widely reported when zinc supplementation is inadequate. This is particularly likely during the recovery period of anabolism which may follow an episode of severe catabolism with loss of body protein and zinc (Kay et al, 1976). Wolman et al (1978) demonstrated that adequate zinc during intravenous nutrition is necessary for insulin activity and to achieve a positive nitrogen balance.

Table 3. Essential element requirements and supply in selected enteral nutrition products.

	Units	RDA[a]	Ensure[c]	Enrich[c]	Clinifeed[d] Iso	Fortison[e]	Wyeth[f] Standard	Liquisorbon[g] MCT	Reabilan[d]	Vivonex[h]
							Approximate composition per 8.4 MJ (2000 kcal)			
Iron	mg	10–18	18	24	13	20	13	15	20	20
	(µmol)	(180–320)	(320)	(430)	(240)	(360)	(240)	(270)	(360)	(360)
Iodine	µg	150	150	190	NS	120	150	120	150	165
	(µmol)	(1.2)	(1.2)	(1.5)	NS	(0.9)	(1.2)	(0.9)	(1.2)	(1.3)
Zinc	mg[b]	15	23	30	18	14	19	12	20	16.5
	(µmol)	(229)	(353)	(459)	(277)	(214)	(290)	(185)	(306)	(252)
Copper	mg[b]	2–3	2.0	2.5	2.0	2.0	2.0	2.5	2.0	2.2
	(µmol)	(31–47)	(31)	(40)	(31)	(31)	(31)	(40)	(31)	(35)
Manganese	mg[b]	2.5–5	5.0	6.4	4.2	8.0	0.4	2.5	4.0	3.1
	(µmol)	(46–91)	(91)	(115)	(77)	(146)	(8)	(46)	(73)	(56)
Selenium	µg[b]	50–200	NS	NS	NS	NS	76	50	100	NS
	(µmol)	(0.6–2.5)	NS	NS	NS	NS	(1.0)	(0.6)	(1.3)	NS

[a] Taken from the USA Recommended Dietary Allowances (Food and Nutrition Board, 1980). RDA is age-dependent—values shown are for adults.
[b] Safe and adequate dietary supply (Food and Nutrition Board, 1980).
[c] Abbott Laboratories (Berkshire).
[d] Roussel (Middlesex).
[e] Cow and Gate (Wiltshire).
[f] Wyeth Nutrition (Berkshire).
[g] E. Merck (Hampshire).
[h] Eaton Laboratories (London).
NS: Not stated by manufacturer—no information available as to Cr, Mo and F content.

Provision of zinc

The recommended 'safe and adequate dietary supply' of the Food and Nutrition Board (1980) is for 15–25 mg (250–400 µmol) zinc per day. There is considerable variation between different commercial tube feeds with respect to zinc provision, some being barely adequate (Table 3). The fibre containing feed (Enrich®) contains additional zinc to compensate for the anticipated reduction in zinc absorption.

Patients receiving intravenous nutrition usually have increased urinary losses as a result of increased protein catabolism and also due to the formation of zinc–amino acid complexes (Berthon et al, 1980). In addition, there may be increased losses due to fistula or other gastrointestinal fluids. Most patients therefore require 50–100 µmol/day intravenously, although some may have an even greater requirement.

Monitoring adequacy of supply

Since about 90% of zinc is bound to albumin, plasma zinc is particularly affected by changes in plasma albumin concentration. Moreover, plasma zinc is affected by the acute-phase response, and hence interpretation of serum changes is difficult in stressed patients. Nonetheless, a persistently low serum concentration of less than 8 µmol/litre (50 µg/100 ml) may indicate inadequate provision. Measurement of leukocyte zinc may be a more sensitive and specific test of zinc status (Prasad, 1988) but this is technically difficult.

Copper

Metabolism

Cuproenzymes also have a wide range of activities. Cytochrome c oxidase is critical for electron transfer, and superoxide dismutase is involved in free radical scavenging, tyrosinase in melanin synthesis, ferroxidase in iron metabolism, and lysyl oxidase in elastin and collagen synthesis.

About 30% of copper is absorbed from the average diet but this is strongly influenced by other dietary constituents, especially zinc, iron and phytate, all of which reduce absorption. Synthesis of caeruloplasmin occurs in the liver, and more than 90% of plasma copper is bound to caeruloplasmin. Copper homeostasis is maintained by the liver, excess being excreted in the bile.

Effects of acute illness

Caeruloplasmin is an acute-phase protein whose concentration increases in plasma after the stress of infection or injury. This rise occurs later than the depression of iron, zinc and amino acid concentrations in serum. Failure to show such an increase in serum copper after severe stress may indicate inadequate copper stores in the liver.

Urinary copper excretion is increased during catabolic illness although to a lesser extent than urine zinc. Carr and Wilkinson (1975) demonstrated increased urine copper in children for up to two months following burn injury.

Long-term deficiency syndromes

Apart from Menkes syndrome, which is an inborn error of copper absorption, the best documented evidence of human deficiency is in malnourished infants receiving exclusively a cows' milk diet. They develop hypochromic anaemia, which is resistant to iron therapy, and neutropenia. Children fed intravenously with copper-deficient regimens have developed similar signs and symptoms, but in addition there are bone abnormalities related to defects of collagen synthesis and abnormalities of smell and taste (Karpel and Peden, 1972). In adults the bone changes are not observed (Dunlap et al, 1974). Clinically apparent copper deficiency is a late complication of prolonged depletion and is preceded by many weeks of low serum copper and caeruloplasmin.

Provision of copper

The recommended 'safe and adequate dietary supply' of copper is 2–3 mg (31–47 μmol) per day. This amount is contained in 2 litres of most proprietary tube feeds. For patients receiving intravenous nutrition, the AMA recommendation is 8–24 μmol (500–1500 μg) per day. Shike et al (1981) found that 5–10 μmol/day was adequate to maintain balance in relatively stable patients. However, since patients requiring intravenous nutrition may already have developed a negative copper balance, and also since there may be increased copper losses in biliary or intestinal fluid, an intake of 20 μmol/day is reasonable for most patients. We have used this routinely in medical and surgical patients with no evidence of overprovision. Since copper is excreted largely by the liver, patients with impaired liver function may be less able to cope with a copper load, and supplements should be used with caution.

Monitoring adequacy of supply

Although serum copper and caeruloplasmin are affected by the acute-phase reaction, measurement of serum copper (reference range 15–25 μmol/litre) can nonetheless give a guide to gross under- or overprovision of copper, especially if interpreted in the light of other acute-phase proteins, such as C-reactive protein.

Iron

Metabolism

Of the 3–5 g (60–100 mmol) of iron present in the adult human, 65% is in the circulating blood as the haem prosthetic group, 30% is stored in the reticulo-endothelial sytem (RES) and bone marrow as ferritin and haemosiderin, and about 5% is present in other ferroproteins, such as myoglobin and the cytochrome system. Although 30 mg (600 µmol) of iron is released each day from the destruction of ageing red cells, most of this is reutilized and only 1 mg (20 µmol) is excreted, mainly in the bile. This is balanced by the usual oral intake of 10–20 mg (200–400 µmol), of which a variable amount is absorbed. More than 20% of haem iron is absorbed, whereas non-haem iron absorption ranges from 3% to 8%, depending upon the dietary ascorbic acid content. Iron absorption occurs in the upper small intestine, is particularly affected by fibre content and may be reduced by zinc supplements (Solomons, 1986). Since absorption of iron into mucosal apoferritin is associated with oxidation from ferrous to ferric iron, a reaction at least partly controlled by caeruloplasmin, the copper stores of an individual may also affect iron status. Transport of iron from the intestine to iron stores and thence to bone marrow is brought about by the globulin, transferrin.

Effect of acute illness

Acute infection, surgical trauma, or accidental injury all cause a fall in serum iron, due to a redistribution of iron into cells of the RES and the reaction of interleukin 1 and other cytokines (Kampschmidt, 1980). There is also a fall in serum transferrin due to reduced synthesis of this short-half-life protein (about 8 days), and its increased transcapillary escape (Fleck, 1988), but the fall in serum iron is greater and hence transferrin saturation is reduced. This appears to be due largely to an increase in RES ferritin, and therefore an increase in storage iron (Konijn et al, 1981). These factors all lead to a reduced delivery of iron to the bone marrow and reduced utilization of iron, leading to anaemia.

In the acutely ill individual, these changes are, on balance, believed to be beneficial by reducing the amount of iron which might otherwise be available in the circulation for bacterial growth (Weinberg, 1978). On the other hand, iron is needed by neutrophils and lymphocytes for optimal function (Chandra and Dayton, 1982) and hence reduction in total body iron should be prevented.

Long-term deficiency syndromes

Iron provision during nutritional support is often neglected, due to uncertainty about optimal requirements and technical difficulties in provision. Norton et al (1983) indicated that as much as 200 µmol (10 mg) per day may be necessary to maintain iron balance is some patients receiving intravenous nutrition. On the other hand, Cook (1984) has suggested that regular iron need not be provided, since blood can be transfused when required. Most patients receiving long-term nutritional support are probably iron-deficient, due to inadequate intake, malabsorption and repeated venepuncture.

Provision of iron

The RDA for iron is 10–18 mg (180–320 μmol) in the average oral diet, and this is variably met by commercial tube feeds (Table 1). One fibre-containing feed (Enrich®) contains additional iron to compensate for the expected reduction in iron absorption.

In patients receiving intravenous nutrition, the trace element supplement Additrace® provides a maintenance level of iron, but this may need to be supplemented by total dose iron infusion (although this may have side-effects) or by blood transfusion.

Monitoring adequacy of supply

Since serum iron accounts for less than 0.1% of total body iron, and moreover is affected by the acute-phase response, its measurement is rarely helpful in assessing iron status. Similarly, serum transferrin is affected by protein nutritional status and also by the acute-phase response, so changes are non-specific. In stable individuals, serum ferritin, originating from the RES, reflects total body iron stores. However, ferritin also responds as an acute-phase reactant in acute infection or chronic debilitating disease, and this limits the value of serum ferritin in stressed patients. Marrow concentration of stainable iron is therefore the most reliable test of the amount of iron stores.

Manganese

Metabolism

Although manganese is widely distributed in the body, with high concentrations especially in brain, kidney, pancreas and liver, its precise role is not well defined. It activates many enzymes in vitro, and it is believed to be particularly important for glycosyl transferase activity in mucopolysaccharide synthesis. It may also have a role in cholesterol and other steroid biosynthesis.

Manganese absorption from the diet is relatively low (less than 10%). Manganese is efficiently excreted in the bile, which maintains manganese homeostasis, little being excreted in urine.

Long-term deficiency syndromes

A manganese deficiency state involving an abnormality of cartilage, growth and sterility is well documented in animals. There are few well documented examples of manganese deficiency in man. Friedman et al (1987) have recently demonstrated that volunteers fed a manganese-deficient diet developed skin changes, anaemia and hypocholesterolaemia, which were reversible on supplementation with manganese. They also demonstrated that the obligatory manganese losses amounted to 1–4 μmol/day, whilst consuming an oral diet. There have not, however, been any definite cases of manganese deficiency during intravenous nutrition. This may result from the low dietary requirement for manganese, together with the inadvertent provision of manganese as a contaminant of intravenous nutrition infusions.

Provision of manganese

The recommended safe and adequate manganese intake orally is 46–91 μmol (2.5–5.0 μg) per day. Most but not all tube feeds provide this amount (Table 3). The AMA recommendation for intravenous provision is 3–15 μmol (0.15–0.8 mg), which is adequate to maintain serum manganese during long-term intravenous nutrition (Shenkin et al, 1986b). Manganese should be provided with caution in patients with cholestasis, since excretion is impaired.

Monitoring adequacy of supply

Serum manganese may not reflect tissue stores, but is nonetheless probably adequate to assess gross under- or overprovision. Careful attention to obtaining samples free of contamination is necessary if meaningful results are to be achieved (Versieck and Cornelis, 1980).

Selenium

Metabolism

The essential role of selenium in human nutrition has only recently been recognized. The selenoprotein glutathione peroxidase is found in most tissues and body fluids and is part of the cellular antioxidant system. Acting together with vitamin E, selenium protects cell mambranes and other structures from oxidative damage by peroxides and superoxides generated during metabolism.

Selenium is effectively absorbed in the upper small intestine as either selenite or selenomethionine, and is thereafter transported in the blood bound to serum proteins. Selenium homeostasis is maintained by urinary excretion, which therefore reflects the amount of dietary intake.

Long-term deficiency syndromes

The best evidence for the effects of selenium deficiency have come from patients receiving prolonged intravenous nutrition without selenium supplementation. There have now been several reports of patients developing fatal cardiomyopathy (e.g. Johnson et al, 1981) or reversible skeletal muscle myopathy (e.g. Mansell et al, 1987) after prolonged periods of intravenous nutrition during which severe selenium deficiency occurred. However, most patients receiving long-term intravenous nutrition develop biochemical depletion and it is not clear why only a small proportion of such cases develop clinical complications (Shenkin et al, 1986b). The cardiomyopathy resembles that found in Keshan disease, a cardiomyopathy endemic in some areas of China where dietary selenium is very low, and whose incidence has been dramatically lowered by intervention therapy with sodium selenite (Diplock, 1981). However, the seasonal variations in incidence of the disease suggest that other factors, e.g. viral infection, may contribute to the aetiology. Kaschin–Beck disease is an osteoarthropathy which occurs in some selenium-poor areas and which also appears, at least in part, to be due to selenium deficiency (Diplock, 1981).

Provision of selenium

Dietary intake is highly variable in different parts of the world but the recommended safe and adequate allowance is 50–200 µg/day in the USA. However, 30 µg/day orally appears adequate both in New Zealand (Thomson and Robinson, 1980) and in China in the prevention of Keshan disease (Chen et al, 1980). Levander (1984) has pointed out that since about half of the selenium excreted is in the faeces, only 25–30 µg/day should be necessary for long-term stable patients with reduced faecal losses. Not all tube feeds provide selenium, and indeed many do not quote analysed contents. Hence selenium intake may be inadequate during long-term tube feeding.

Selenium 30–200 µg/day has been given intravenously by different workers to stable adults. We have found that 30 µg/day (400 nmol/day) selenium, as sodium selenite, is adequate to maintain selenium status in most patients requiring intravenous nutrition. A higher daily intake may be necessary at first to correct the effects of prolonged selenium depletion. Considerable uncertainty still remains regarding the optimal dosage and chemical form of selenium during intravenous nutrition (Levander and Burk, 1986).

Monitoring adequacy of supply

Measurements of plasma or urine selenium provide suitable indices of recent intake, but where these are abnormal, measurement of red blood cell glutathione peroxidase or platelet glutathione peroxidase provides a more accurate index of whole-body selenium status (Levander, 1984).

Chromium

Metabolism

Although the mechanism is not clear, chromium is important in both carbohydrate and fat metabolism. In the form of glucose tolerance factor (a complex of chromium, nicotinic acid and amino acids) it promotes glucose uptake and metabolism, and also enhances lipogenesis and the proportion of cholesterol in high-density lipoproteins. The efficiency of absorption is poor, about 0.1%, although this may increase if chromium intake is low or if chromium is present in organic complexes in the diet. Excess chromium is excreted in the urine.

Effects of acute illness

The urinary excretion of chromium is increased after glucose infusions or in severe stress (Koslovsky et al, 1986). Moreover, trauma leads to excessive losses, due to the stress hyperglycaemia as well as to the infusion of chromium as contaminants of intravenous fluids used for resuscitation.

Long-term deficiency syndromes

Many individuals probably have marginal chromium status, leading to impaired glucose tolerance (Anderson, 1988). The best documented effects of chromium deficiency have occurred during long-term intravenous nutrition (Jeejeebhoy et al, 1977; Freund et al, 1979) in patients who developed glucose intolerance, weight loss and peripheral neuropathy.

Provision of chromium

The estimated safe and adequate chromium intake is 50–200 μg/day (Food and Nutrition Board, 1980). However, evidence to support this is limited. Despite there being no deliberate provision of chromium, patients receiving intravenous nutrition usually have high serum chromium as a result of contaminants of the intravenous solutions, especially of the amino acids (Shenkin et al, 1986b). The AMA recommended 0.3–0.4 μmol (15–20 μg) per day intravenously. A slight excess in provision is probably not important, provided renal function is satisfactory.

Monitoring adequacy of supply

The best test of adequate chromium provision probably is maintenance of glucose tolerance. Analytical methods are rarely sensitive enough to measure chromium at the lower limit of the reference range (Versieck and Cornelis, 1980) and collection of samples without chromium contamination requires special sampling techniques for both venepuncture and separation of serum.

Molybdenum

Metabolism

There are a number of molybdenum-dependent enzymes in man, including xanthine oxidase, sulphite oxidase and aldehyde oxidase. Molybdenum therefore plays an important role in nucleic acid and protein metabolism. Molybdenum is well absorbed from the oral diet, although there is some competition between copper and molybdenum for the absorption mechanism. Molybdenum is readily excreted in urine.

Long-term deficiency syndrome

Abumrad et al (1981) described a patient who developed severe intolerance to sulphur containing amino acids during long-term intravenous nutrition, associated with increased urinary sulphite, hypoxanthine and xanthine. Moreover, there were low serum and urine concentrations of uric acid. The patient had tachycardia, visual upsets and irritability, which were relieved by cessation of the infusion, and corrected by provision of ammonium molybdate.

Provision of molybdenum

The dietary requirement for molybdenum has been proposed to be 1.5–5 μmol (0.15–0.5 mg) per day when given orally, although intravenous requirements may be only about 0.2 μmol/day (Jacobson and Wester, 1977).

Monitoring adequacy of supply

Direct measurement of serum or urine molybdenum is technically difficult, and hence the best method of assessing adequacy of molybdenum is by measuring serum and urine uric acid, together with other urinary sulphur and purine metabolites.

Other essential elements

Many other elements have been suggested as essential in man, the evidence being strongest for arsenic, boron, nickel and silicon (Neilsen, 1984). At present, these elements appear to be of little practical significance. It is generally assumed, although there is little evidence to support it, that adequate amounts of such ultra-trace elements will be provided as contaminants of other infusions or dietary sources.

PRACTICAL PROVISION OF ESSENTIAL INORGANIC MICRONUTRIENTS

Most of the products intended for enteral use do contain stated amounts of many, but not all, the important essential elements (Table 3). There is considerable variation in the amount supplied compared with the dietary requirement. The actual content of elements found in a range of commercial preparations was significantly different from the stated content (Bunker and Clayton, 1983). This could lead to a serious undersupply of certain elements, particularly iron and copper.

During intravenous nutrition, the provision of a precise amount of inorganic nutrients is even more difficult. This is mainly due to uncertainty regarding the appropriate amount and chemical form of each element, together with the effect of the inevitable contamination of amino acid solutions and other intravenous nutrients with various elements. However, various commercial mixtures are available in the UK and these are listed in Table 4. The Expert Committee of the AMA recommended provision of each of the trace elements as a single-element ampoule in order to permit

Table 4. Additives used for trace element provision during intravenous nutrition.

	Units	Addamel[a] (1 vial)	Additrace[a] (1 vial)	Nutracel[b] (500 ml)	MTE-4[c] (1 dose)
Zinc	mg	1.3	6.5	2.6	2.9
	(μmol)	(20)	(100)	(40)	(45)
Copper	mg	0.3	1.3	—	1.3
	(μmol)	(5)	(20)	—	(21)
Manganese	mg	2.2	0.3	2.2	0.3
	(μmol)	(40)	(5)	(40)	(6)
Iron	mg	2.8	1.2	—	—
	(μmol)	(50)	(20)	—	—
Chromium	μg	—	10	—	12
	(nmol)	—	(200)	—	(230)
Selenium	μg	—	32	—	—
	(nmol)	—	(400)	—	—
Iodine	μg	131	131	—	—
	(μmol)	(1)	(1)	—	—
Fluoride	mg	0.95	0.95	—	—
	(μmol)	(50)	(50)	—	—
Molybdenum	μg	—	19.1	—	—
	(nmol)	—	(200)	—	—

[a]Kabi Vitrum, Stockholm. Addamel also has Ca (5 mmol) and Mg (1.5 mmol).
[b]Travenol Laboratories, UK.
[c]Lyphomed Inc., Illinois.

maximum flexibility of provision, but this is labour-intensive and might lead to error from multiple additions. At present, the best recommendations would seem to be to provide a reasonable intake of most elements, as suggested in Table 4, but also to have single elements available for provision to patients with increased requirements of, for example, zinc or selenium.

TOXICITY OF MICRONUTRIENTS

There is marked variation in the margin of safety associated with provision of micronutrients. Thus for the water-soluble vitamins, there is little concern regarding overdosage. On the other hand, overdosage of vitamins A and D are relatively common since there is little control of absorption or excretion. Similarly, for most of the trace elements, the normal homeostatic mechanisms will usually ensure adequate excretion of elements in bile or urine. However, in cases of liver disease, accumulation of copper or manganese may occur, and in renal disease there may be reduced excretion of chromium or selenium. One element of particular toxicological concern is selenium, because of the low margin between nutritional essentiality and toxicity. In cases of suspected overdosage of any of the micronutrients, measurement of plasma concentration is usually adequate to confirm or refute the diagnosis.

SUMMARY

An adequate provision of all micronutrients, vitamins and essential trace elements is necessary for maintenance of normal tissue function. In patients requiring nutritional support, these factors are essential for optimal utilization of the major nutrients and play a role in all aspects of intermediary metabolism.

In this chapter, some of the main features of the micronutrients have been described, together with suggestions regarding their provision enterally or parenterally. For most of these nutrients, diagnostic methods are not available to permit accurate assessment of status and hence the level of provision necessary for optimal results. However, there is now sufficient understanding of nutritional requirements such that few patients should now develop clinical or biochemical signs of under- or overprovision of micronutrients.

REFERENCES

Abumrad NN, Schneider AJ, Steel D & Rogers LS (1981) Amino acid intolerance reversed by molybdate therapy. *American Journal of Clinical Nutrition* **34:** 2551–2559.
Allwood MC (1984a) Compatability and stability of TPN mixtures in big bags. *Journal of Clinical and Hospital Pharmacy* **9:** 181–198.
Allwood MC (1984b) Factors affecting the stability of ascorbic acid in total parenteral nutrition infusions. *Journal of Clinical and Hospital Pharmacy* **9:** 75–85.
American Medical Association (1979) Guidelines for essential trace element preparations for parenteral use. *Journal of the American Medical Association* **241:** 2051–2054.
American Medical Association, Department of Food and Nutrition (1975) Multivitamin preparations for parenteral use: a statement by the Nutrition Advisory Group. *Journal of Parenteral and Enteral Nutrition* **3:** 258–265.
Anderson CE (1977) Vitamins. In Schneider HA, Anderson CE & Coursin DB (eds) *Nutritional Support of Medical Practice*, pp 24–56. Hagerstown, MD: Harper & Row.
Anderson RA (1988) Recent advances in the role of chromium in human health and disease. In Prasad AS (ed.) *Essential and Toxic Trace Elements in Human Health and Disease*, pp 189–197. New York: Alan R. Liss.
Ansell JE, Kumar R & Deykin D (1977) The spectrum of vitamin K deficiency. *Journal of the American Medical Association* **238:** 40–42.
Bach J-F, Plean J-M, Savino W et al (1988) The role of zinc in the biological activity of Thymulin, a thymic metallopeptide hormone. In Prasad AS (ed.) *Essential Trace Elements in Human Health and Disease*, pp 319–328. New York: Alan R. Liss.
Bayoumi RA & Rosalki SB (1976) Evaluation of methods of coenzyme activation of erythrocyte enzymes for detection of deficiency of vitamins B_1, B_2, and B_6. *Clinical Chemistry* **22:** 327–335.
Beard MEJ, Hatipov CS & Hamer JW (1980) Acute onset of folate deficiency in patients under intensive care. *Critical Care Medicine* **8:** 500–503.
Berthon G, Matuchansky C & May PM (1980) Computer simulation of metal ion equilibria in body fluids, 3. Trace metal supplementation in total parenteral nutrition. *Journal of Inorganic Chemistry* **13:** 63–73.
Bieri JG & Farrell PM (1976) Vitamin E. *Vitamins and Hormones* **34:** 31–75.
Bonjour JP (1977) Biotin in man's nutrition and therapy—a review. *International Journal of Vitamin Nutrition and Research* **47:** 107–118.
Brody T, Shane B & Stokstad ELR (1984) Folic acid. In Machlin LJ (ed.) *Handbook of Vitamins*, pp 459–496. New York: Marcel Dekker Inc.
Brubacher G (1982) Biochemical indicators which reflect the intake of vitamins. In Klaver W & Hautvast JGAJ (eds) *The Diet Factor in Epidemiological Research*, pp 125–135. The Netherlands: Ponsen & Looyen.
Bunker VW & Clayton BE (1983) Trace element content of commercial enteral feeds. *Lancet* **ii:** 426–428.
Burns JJ (1974) Water-soluble vitamins, ascorbic acid (vitamin C). In White PL, Nagy ME &

Fletcher DC (eds) *Total Parenteral Nutrition*, pp 1564–1569. Acton MA: Publishing Sciences Group.

Carr G & Wilkinson AW (1975) Zinc and copper urinary excretions in children with burns and scalds. *Clinica Chimica Acta* **61:** 199–204.

Chandra RK & Dayton DH (1982) Trace element regulation of immunity and infection. *Nutrition Research* **2:** 721–733.

Chen X, Yang G, Chen J, Chen X, Wen Z & Ge K (1980) Studies on the relations of selenium and Keshan Disease. *Biological Trace Element Research* **2:** 91–107.

Cook JD (1984) Parenteral trace elements: iron. *Bulletin of the New York Academy of Science* **60:** 156–162.

Cruickshank AM, Telfer ABM & Shenkin A (1988) Thiamine deficiency in the critically ill. *Intensive Care Medicine* **14:** 384–387.

Davies JWL & Fell GS (1974) Tissue catabolism in patients with burns. *Clinica Chimica Acta* **51:** 83–92.

Dempsey DT, Mullen JL, Rombeau JL et al (1987) Treatment effects of parenteral vitamins in total parenteral nutrition patients. *Journal of Parenteral and Enteral Nutrition* **11:** 229–237.

DHSS (1979) *Recommended daily amounts of food energy and nutrients for groups of people in the United Kingdom*. London: HMSO.

Diplock AT (1981) Metabolic and functional defects in selenium deficiency. *Philosophical Transactions of the Royal Society of London* **294:** 105–117.

Duhamel JF, Ricour C, Dufier JL et al (1979) Deficit en vitamine B_2 et nutrition parenterale exclusive. *Archive Francais Pédiatrique* **36:** 342–346.

Dunlap WM, James GW & Hume DM (1974) Anaemia and neutropenia caused by copper deficiency. *Annals of Internal Medicine* **80:** 470–476.

Editorial (1984) Vitamin D and the lymphomedullary system. *Lancet* **i:** 1105–1106.

Fleck A (1988) The acute phase response: Implications for nutrition and recovery. *Nutrition* **4:** 109–117.

Food and Nutrition Board, National Research Council (1980) *Recommended Dietary Allowances*, 9th edn. Washington DC: National Academy of Sciences.

Freund H, Atamian S & Fischer JE (1979) Chromium deficiency during total parenteral nutrition. *Journal of the American Medical Association* **241:** 496–498.

Frick PG, Riedler G & Brogli H (1967) Dose response and minimal daily requirements of vitamin K in man. *Journal of Applied Physiology* **23:** 387–389.

Friedman BJ, Freeland-Graves JH, Bales CW et al (1987) Manganese balance and clinical observations in young men fed a manganese deficient diet. *Journal of Nutrition* **117:** 133–143.

Gillis J, Jones G & Penchary P (1983) Delivery of vitamins A, D and E in total parenteral nutrition solutions. *Journal of Parenteral and Enteral Nutrition* **7:** 11–14.

Goldsmith GA (1977) Curative nutrition: Vitamins. In Schneider HA, Anderson CE & Coursin DB (eds) *Nutritional Support of Medical Practice*, pp 101–123. Hagerstown, MD: Harper and Row.

Goldsmith GC (1975) Vitamin B complex. *Progress in Food and Nutrition Sciences* **1:** 559–609.

Greene HL, Phillips BL, Franck L et al (1987) Persistently low blood retinol levels during and after parenteral feeding of very low birth weight infants: examination of losses into intravenous administration sets and a method of prevention by addition to a lipid emulsion. *Paediatrics* **79:** 894–900.

Horwitt MK (1974) Status of human requirements for vitamin E. *American Journal of Clinical Nutrition* **27:** 1182–1193.

Howard L, Chu R, Freman S, Mintz H, Oversen L & Wolf B (1980) Vitamin A deficiency from long-term parenteral nutrition. *Annals of Internal Medicine* **93:** 576–577.

Howard L, Oversen L, Satya-Marti S & Chu R (1982) Reversible neurological symptoms caused by vitamin E deficiency in a patient with short bowel syndrome. *American Journal of Clinical Nutrition* **36:** 1243–1249.

Innis SM & Allardyce DB (1983) Possible biotin deficiency in adults receiving long-term total parenteral nutrition. *American Journal of Clinical Nutrition* **37:** 185–187.

Jacobson S & Wester P-O (1977) Balance study of twenty trace elements during total parenteral nutrition in man. *British Journal of Nutrition* **37:** 107–126.

Jeejeebhoy KN, Chu RC, Marliss EB, Greenberg GR & Bruce A (1977) Chromium deficiency, glucose intolerance and neuropathy reversed by chromium supplementation in a patient receiving long-term parental nutrition. *American Journal of Clinical Nutrition* **30:** 531–538.

Jeppsson B & Gimmon Z (1983) Vitamins. In Fischer JE (ed.) *Surgical Nutrition*, pp 241–281. Boston: Little Brown & Co.

Johnson L, Schaffer D & Boggs TR (1974) The premature infant, vitamin E deficiency and retrolental fibroplasia. *American Journal of Clinical Nutrition* **27:** 1158–1173.

Johnson RA, Baker SS, Fallon JT et al (1981) An occidental case of cardiomyopathy and selenium deficiency. *New England Journal of Medicine* **304:** 1210–1212.

Kampschmidt RF (1980) Role of RES and leucocytic endogenous mediator in iron, zinc and copper metabolism. *Advances in Experimental Medicine and Biology* **121A:** 403–411.

Karpel JT & Peden VH (1972) Copper deficiency in long-term parenteral nutrition. *Journal of Pediatrics* **80:** 32–36.

Kay RG, Tasman-Jones C, Pybus J, Whitney R & Black H (1976) A syndrome of acute zinc deficiency during total parenteral alimentation in man. *Annals of Surgery* **183:** 331–340.

Klein GL, Targoff CM & Ament ME (1980) Bone disease associated with total parenteral nutrition. *Lancet* **2:** 1041–1044.

Konijn AM, Carmel N, Levy R & Hershko C (1981) Ferritin synthesis in inflammation. II. Mechanism of increased ferritin synthesis. *British Journal of Haematology* **49:** 361–370.

Koo WWD, Kaplan LA, Horn J, Tsang RC & Steichen JJ (1986) Aluminium in parenteral nutrition solution—sources and possible alternatives. *Journal of Parenteral and Enteral Nutrition* **10:** 591–595.

Koslovsky AS, Moser PB, Reiser S & Anderson RA (1986) Effects of diets high in simple sugars on urinary chromium losses. *Metabolism* **35:** 515–518.

La Selve P, Demolin P, Holzapfel L, Blanc PL, Teyssier G & Robert D. (1986) Shoshin beriberi: an unusual complication of prolonged parenteral nutrition. *Journal of Parenteral and Enteral Nutrition* **10:** 102–103.

Leape LL & Valae T (1976) Rickets in low birth weight infants receiving total parenteral nutrition. *Journal of Paediatric Surgery* **11:** 665–674.

Levander O (1984) The importance of selenium in total parenteral nutrition. *Bulletin of the New York Academy of Medicine* **60:** 144–155.

Levander OA & Burk RF (1986) Report on the 1986 ASPEN Research Workshop on Selenium in Clinical Nutrition. *Journal of Parenteral and Enteral Nutrition* **10:** 545–549.

Levander OA & Cheng L (1980) Micronutrient interactions; vitamins, minerals and hazardous elements. *Annals of the New York Academy of Sciences* **355:** 1–370.

Levine M (1986) New concepts in the biology and biochemistry of ascorbic acid. *New England Journal of Medicine* **314:** 892–902.

Main ANH, Mills PR, Russell RI et al (1983) Vitamin A deficiency in Crohn's Disease. *Gut* **24:** 1169–1175.

Manolagas SC, Provvedini M, Murray EJ, Tsouka CD & Deftos LJ (1986) The antiproliferative effect of calcitriol on human peripheral blood mononuclear cells. *Journal of Clinical Endocrinology and Metabolism* **63:** 394–400.

Mansell PI, Rawlings J, Allison SP et al (1987) Reversal of a skeletal myopathy with selenium supplementation in a patient on home parenteral nutrition. *Clinical Nutrition* **6:** 179–183.

Mock DM, Lorimer AA, Liebman WM, Sweetman K & Baker H (1981) Biotin deficiency: an unusual complication of parenteral nutrition. *New England Journal of Medicine* **304:** 820–823.

Moran JR & Greene HL (1979) The B vitamins and vitamin C in human nutrition. *American Journal of Disease of Children* **133:** 308.

Nadel AM & Burger PC (1976) Wernicke encephalopathy following prolonged intravenous therapy. *Journal of the American Medical Association* **235:** 2403–2405.

Neilsen FN (1984) Ultratrace elements in nutrition. *Annual Review of Nutrition* **4:** 21–41.

Norton JA, Peters ML, Westley R, Maher MM & Brennan MF (1983) Iron supplementation of total parenteral nutrition: a prospective study. *Journal of Parenteral and Enteral Nutrition* **9:** 457–461.

Prasad AS (1988) Clinical spectrum and diagnostic aspects of human zinc deficiency. In Prasad AS (ed.) *Essential and Toxic Elements in Human Health and Disease*, pp 3–53. New York: Alan R. Liss.

Ritchie JH, Fish MB, McMasters V et al (1968) Edema and hemolytic anemia in premature infants: a vitamin E deficiency syndrome. *New England Journal of Medicine* **279:** 1185–1190.

Robson JRK, Vanderveen T, Bennett K & Thomson T (1980) Ascorbic acid deficiency during TPN. *Journal of Parenteral and Enteral Nutrition* 4: 518.

Schepers GP, Dimitry AR, Eckhauser FE & Kirking DM (1988) Efficacy and safety of low dose intravenous versus intramuscular vitamin K in parenteral nutrition patients. *Journal of Parenteral and Enteral Nutrition* 12: 174–177.

Shearer MJ, Mallinson CN, Webster GR & Barkham P (1972) Clearance and excretion in urine, faeces, and bile of an intravenous dose of tritiated vitamin K_1 in man. *British Journal of Haematology* 22: 579–588.

Shearer MJ, McBurney A & Barkham P (1974) Studies on the absorption and metabolism of phylloquinone (vitamin K_1) in man. *Vitamins and Hormones* 32: 513–542.

Shearer MJ (1983) High-performance liquid chromatography of K vitamins and their antagonists. *Advances in Chromatography* 21: 243–301.

Shenkin A, Neuhauser M, Bergstrom J et al (1980) Biochemical changes associated with severe trauma. *American Journal of Clinical Nutrition* 33: 2119–2127.

Shenkin A, Richardson R & Garden OJ (1986a) Intestinal absorption of water soluble vitamins and essential trace elements. In Dietze G, Grunert A, Kleinberger G & Wolfram G (eds) *Clinical Nutrition and Metabolic Research*, pp 143–155. Basel: Kargerm.

Shenkin A, Fell GS, Halls DJ, Dunbar PM, Holbrook IB & Irving MH (1986b) Essential trace element provision to patients receiving home intravenous nutrition in the United Kingdom. *Clinical Nutrition* 5: 91–97.

Shenkin A, Fraser WD, McLelland AJD, Fell GS & Garden OJ (1987) Maintenance of vitamin and trace element status in intravenous nutrition using a complete nutritive mixture. *Journal of Parenteral and Enteral Nutrition* 11: 238–242.

Shike M, Harrison JE & Startridge WC (1980) Metabolic bone disease in patients receiving long-term parenteral nutrition. *Annals of Internal Medicine* 92: 343–350.

Shike M, Roulet M, Kurian R, Whitewell J, Stewart S & Jeejeebhoy KN (1981) Copper metabolism and requirements in total parenteral nutrition. *Gastroenterology* 81: 290–297.

Shils ME, Baker H & Frank O (1985) Blood vitamin levels of long-term adult home total parenteral nutrition patients: the efficacy of the AMA-FDA parenteral multivitamin formulation. *Journal of Parenteral and Enteral Nutrition* 9: 179–188.

Sokol RJ, Heubi JE, Iannaccone ST et al (1984) Vitamin E deficiency with normal serum vitamin E concentrations in children with chronic cholestasis. *New England Journal of Medicine* 310: 1209–1212.

Solomons NW (1986) Competitive interaction of iron and zinc in the diet. Consequence for human nutrition. *Journal of Nutrition* 116: 927–935.

Steinberg D (1972) Folic acid deficiency: Early onset of megaloblastosis. *Journal of the American Medical Association* 222: 490.

Stromberg P, Shenkin A, Campbell RA, Spooner RJ, Davidson JF & Sim AJW (1981) Vitamin status during total parenteral nutrition. *Journal of Parenteral and Enteral Nutrition* 5: 295–299.

Tennant GB, Smith RC, Leinster SJ, O'Donnell JE & Wardrop CAJ (1981) Amino acid infusion induced depression of serum folate after cholecystectomy. *Scandinavian Journal of Haematology* 27: 333–338.

Thomson CD & Robinson MD (1980) Selenium in human health and disease with emphasis on those aspects peculiar to New Zealand. *American Journal of Clinical Nutrition* 33: 303–323.

Versieck J & Cornelis R (1980) Normal levels of trace elements in human blood plasma or serum. *Analytica Chimica Acta* 116: 217–254.

Wardrop CA, Lewis MH, Tennant GB et al (1977) Acute folate deficiency associated with intravenous nutrition with amino acid–sorbitol–ethanol: Prophylaxis with intravenous folic acid. *British Journal of Haematology* 37: 521–526.

Weinberg ED (1978) Iron and infection. *Microbiology Review* 42: 45–66.

Wolman SL, Anderson GH, Marliss EB & Jeejeebhoy KN (1978) Zinc in total parenteral nutrition: requirements and metabolic effects. *Gastroenterology* 76: 458–467.

5

Vascular access for parenteral nutrition

A. J. W. SIM

One of the major advances in the techniques of intravenous feeding was the realization that in order to infuse hypertonic solutions for prolonged periods it was necessary to have a catheter whose tip lay in a large-calibre high-flow vein, the best being the superior vena cava. Percutaneous cannulation of the subclavian vein as described by Aubaniac (1952) was introduced for intravenous feeding by Dudrick in the late 1960s. Since then different approaches to central vein catheter insertion have been described and relative merits and disadvantages debated at length. The existence of so many different techniques for central vein cannulation is a reflection of the fact that no single technique is either complication-free or appropriate to any single individual's technical abilities. Before considering the techniques for central venous catheterization, it is important to discuss briefly the use of peripheral veins for intravenous feeding.

PERIPHERAL VEIN CANNULATION

The use of peripheral veins for intravenous feeding has a long history and some obvious attractions. Prior to the popularization of the subclavian route, most intravenous feeding was carried out via peripheral veins. The veins that were generally used were forearm veins and the long saphenous. An example of this is described by Griffiths (1963), who reported a patient who was fed intravenously for 2½ months through a cannula inserted into the 'main' saphenous vein. Because of concerns about the complicaton rate of central venous catheters, peripheral vein feeding has recently become more popular. In the hands of those dedicated to its use effective short-term nutrition can be achieved by a peripheral vein. Industry has responded by beginning to develop low-osmolality solutions appropriate for infusion into small-calibre veins.

The principal disadvantage of peripheral vein feeding is the development of thrombophlebitis. This condition is not only painful for the patient, but also, as the veins are slowly occluded, venous access becomes more difficult. Attempts to reduce the incidence of thrombophlebitis by the infusion of heparin (Tanner et al, 1980) and steriods (Isaacs et al, 1977) have been reported as being efficacious.

If a peripheral vein is to be used then special care in cannula insertion is necessary. It is not absolutely necessary to anaesthetize the overlying skin although this can make the insertion of a large cannula less unpleasant for the patient. A straight vein on the dorsal aspect of the forearm should be employed, and the surrounding skin should be shaved to allow easy removal of adhesive dressings. The cannula should be fixed to avoid mechanical trauma to the vein from unwanted movement. With a cannula in this position there should be no need to splint the arm, a practice which is inconvenient for the patient and which is usually ineffective in keeping a cannula in place. Ideally such catheters should be resited in the other forearm every 24 hours, although in practice it may only be feasible every 48 hours. The practice of only changing the cannula when 'necessary' should be deprecated; to allow a catheter to become unusable means that at the best the intravenous feeding will be interfered with in an uncontrolled fashion and at worst that the patient will develop a severe thrombophlebitis which can be extremely painful and will damage the vein so that it cannot be used in the future.

The future of peripheral vein feeding will depend on the development of better solutions and perhaps on the introduction of agents which will improve the utilization of infused nutrients and thus reduce the quantity of nutrients required for effective feeding.

CENTRAL VEIN CANNULATION

Before describing specific techniques it is necesary to consider some general principles.

Catheter type

Specially designed catheters for intravenous feeding are available and should be used. They are usually made of silicone rubber or polyurethane. Catheters with integral hub systems are generally safest although those with detachable hubs are easier to tunnel and the compression-type junction between hub and catheter is usually strong enough.

Recently there has been interest in the use of catheters with more than one lumen, and although at first sight this seems to contradict the dictum that the intravenous catheter should be sacrosanct, experience has shown that as long as both lumens are cared for in a meticulous fashion the catheter sepsis rate is not substantially increased. The second (or third) lumen can be used to infuse other intravenous fluids, intravenous antibiotics and other drugs. In addition, it can be used for blood sampling.

Our initial study (Patterson-Brown et al, 1987), when experience with 36 single and 32 double lumen catheters was described, reported that the catheter sepsis rates (the definition of catheter sepsis employed is described in detail in the relevant section below) were similar, and the recommendation was made that a double lumen catheter should be considered in all surgical patients. Since then the policy of using a double lumen catheter on most occasions has been pursued and a further 104 double lumen catheters have been inserted; of these, complete data necessary to define catheter sepsis is available in 66, and 8 episodes of catheter sepsis occurred. The catheter sepsis rate of approximately 12% is high. It is certainly possible that the second lumen contributes to this but it is important to weigh the benefits of the second lumen in overall patient care against the risk of catheter sepsis, bearing in mind that with proper vigilance catheter sepsis can be recognized early and effective measures taken to control it.

There is an increasing interest in the use of catheters with a subcutaneous injection port (Rich, 1986). These catheters can be inserted by most of the techniques used to insert the standard 'open-ended' catheter. Because the whole of the catheter is subcutaneous, the patient does not have the concerns relating to a foreign body protruding through the skin; in those requiring long-term venous access, this improves the patient's body image and will allow more flexibility in activities which could compromise a catheter whose distal end was outside the body. The subcutaneous port is punctured through a diaphragm with a specially designed needle. It is claimed that this diaphragm can be punctured as many as 2000 times without damage. The subcutaneous injection port is placed in a 'pouch' under the skin on the anterior chest wall. Recommendations about siting the incision for this to denervate the overlying skin have been made but the author's experience is that this is far from reliable and it is necessary to accept that a disadvantage of this form of venous access is the discomfort associated with repeated needle puncture. The diagnosis of an infected port can be difficult but if it is cared for with appropriate care and attention the sepsis rate should be low.

Catheter insertion technique

The techniques described can be carried out under either local or general anaesthesia. Catheters should always be inserted in an operating theatre, where the controlled environment is capable of sustaining aseptic principles. A quiet, disciplined attitude, with the knowledge that all facilities are readily available if a problem arises, promotes confidence in both patient and doctor. Although catheter insertion in the operating theatre may seem time-consuming and inconvenient, it should be borne in mind that the catheter, once inserted, may have to remain in place for months, and time expended on a careful insertion at this juncture will be rewarded in the future. The central venous catheter should be accorded the importance it deserves and not relegated to a quick procedure in an open ward.

Failure to cannulate a vein is particularly likely to happen with a blind percutaneous technique and occurs because of unrecognized abnormal venous anatomy and thrombosed or collapsed veins. The latter may occur in the fluid-depleted patient, and intravenous infusion of suitable intravascular expanding fluid should be considered prior to catheter insertion. A direct-exposure technique will go part of the way to solving the problem of cannulation failure.

Before infusing intravenous nutrients the position of the catheter must be checked, and although techniques involving ECG tracings have been described, the gold standard should be documentation by X-ray. Ideally, the position of the catheter should be checked at the time of insertion by use of X-ray image intensification. It is both inefficient and inconvenient to both patient and theatre staff to have to return to the operating theatre after an X-ray, taken on the ward or in the radiology department, has shown the catheter to be in the wrong position. X-rays are especially important when techniques in which a blind percutaneous approach close to the root of the neck is used. In these circumstances a good-quality radiograph, rather than image intensification, is required to exclude a pneumothorax; this is particularly so when an attempt has failed on one side and a further attempt to cannulate a vein on the other side could meet with disaster if a second pneumothorax was induced. Pneumothorax is more common after an unsuccessful cannulation attempt.

Most would consider it routine to tunnel the catheter subcutaneously away from the vein entry site so that the skin exit site is on a flat area of skin, usually the anterior chest wall. One study has demonstrated a reduction in catheter sepsis rates with this manoeuvre (Garden and Sim, 1983) but others (von Meyenfeldt et al, 1980; Keohane et al, 1983) have failed to demonstrate such an effect. Despite this, the increased ease of dressing and comfort for the patient have become established as potent reasons to recommend tunnelling of all intravenous feeding catheters, whatever insertion technique is used.

Most patients will be anxious about having a central venous catheter inserted, and if this is to be done under local anaesthesia, irrespective of which approach is employed, the patient should be reassured and sedation given prior to the commencement of the procedure.

TECHNIQUES OF CENTRAL VENOUS CATHETER INSERTION

Arm vein cannulation with advancement of a long catheter to the superior vena cava

For a time this was considered acceptable by some, and long catheters, such as the drum catheter, were frequently used. Experience, however, demonstrated that thrombophlebitis often developed and the catheter had to be removed. The principal veins used are the cephalic and the median basilic, the better of the two being the median basilic vein because of its more direct route to the superior vena cava. Further disadvantages are the immobility of the arm, which inconveniences patients, and the difficulties in keeping a skin entry site in the antecubital fossa reliably clean. Those who are inexperienced in the insertion of central venous catheters will continue to use this route, and while it may be valuable in the short term, long-term intravenous feeding still requires specific expertise in inserting proper catheters. This will only come when individuals recognize that intravenous feeding is a specific therapy which requires training, practice and experience.

Blind percutaneous cannulation of a major vein

The fundamental principle underlying this method of catheter insertion relies on a sound knowledge of surface anatomy and a tacit belief that anatomical variations are sufficiently infrequent not to create major difficulties. It is also important that potential alterations in venous anatomy associated with disease are considered; amongst these are smaller calibre veins because of decreased intravascular volume and the effect of previous surgery or trauma in the vicinity of the vein to be cannulated. Because of this it may be wise to use a fine needle to identify the vein before insertion of a larger bore cannula. Insertion of a Seldinger wire to define the course of the cannulated vein can be used prior to dilatation of the puncture site to introduce a wider bore catheter over the wire.

As with any invasive technique the individual inserting a catheter must be prepared for the complications that could arise as a result. This implies that the individual himself should be able to cope or have ready access to the facilities and personnel who can. Pneumothorax, air embolus and arterial and venous laceration are serious complications which, if not managed expeditiously, can prove fatal; fortunately, in experienced hands these complications are rare, but care must be exercised to avoid complacency.

In all percutaneous techniques where it is necessary to thread a catheter through an introducing needle, the potential for air embolus exists, and therefore specific measures have to be taken to ensure that this potentially fatal event does not occur. In order to raise the venous pressure to a level higher than right atrial pressure a head-down tilt should be employed. At the times when there is an 'open' system, conscious patients should be instructed to perform a Valsalva manoeuvre.

One of the main arguments advanced for the use of the percutaneous techniques is the speed with which a catheter can be inserted. However, before accepting this as a valid reason, it is worth considering whether the time factor is one which should determine the technique of catheter insertion. As previously stated, catheters may have to remain in situ for many months and the saving of a few minutes on catheter insertion would appear inappropriate in the circumstance where other techniques without the complication rates, and which can often be carried out by individuals with less experience, are available.

Excellent descriptions of the techniques for percutaneous insertion of catheters mentioned in this section are to be found in Rosen et al (1981).

Internal jugular vein

The internal jugular vein lies along with the carotid artery and vagus nerve within the carotid sheath. As it passes down the neck its position changes from being behind the artery to being in front and to the side. The principal landmarks used in determining the site of skin entry to cannulate the internal jugular vein are the sternomastoid muscle and the carotid artery. The confluence of the sternal and clavicular heads of the sternomastoid at the level of the cricoid cartilage separate the approaches into high and low.

The right internal jugular vein is, in the first instance, the vein of choice, as the success rate for correct catheter tip placement is greater than with the left (Rosen et al, 1981). Complication rates vary between series but are usually low. The commonest, carotid artery puncture, occurs in approximately 2% of cases. In a review of the literature by Rosen et al (1981) no fatal complications occurred in over 2700 cases.

High approach. In experienced hands this technique is safe and straight-forward. The vein can be approached centrally (though the sternomastoid) or from either the medial or lateral border of the sternomastoid above the level of the cricoid cartilage. The principal advantage of this technique is that the vein is entered above the upper extension of the dome of the pleura and therefore pneumothorax should be avoided. Care must be taken to avoid damage to the carotid artery.

Low approach. This technique is advocated by some because the vein is more superficial and the cannulation failure rate is reported as being lower than with any other percutaneous approach to the internal jugular vein. It does, however, carry a greater risk of pneumothorax and trauma to sur-rounding structures; furthermore, difficulty may be encountered in advanc-ing the catheter because the vein is entered at a virtual right angle.

The vein can be approached centrally through the middle of the triangle made by the two heads of sternomastoid and the clavicle or laterally from the posterior edge of the clavicular head.

Subclavian vein

The subclavian vein commences at the lower border of the first rib and is a direct continuation of the axillary vein; it lies in front of and slightly below the subclavian artery, with the dome of the pleura rising above and behind the arch of the subclavian artery. The external jugular vein joins the sub-clavian from above, near to the midpoint of the clavicle. The phrenic nerve lies between the vein and artery behind the sternoclavicular joint. On the left side the thoracic duct enters the subclavian vein from above and behind, just before its confluence with the internal jugular vein.

Supraclavicular approach. Because of the potential hazards of pneumo-thorax and the unsatisfactory skin exit site, this technique of catheter insertion is only rarely used for intravenous feeding. Its main attractions are the close proximity of the vein to the skin and the reported ease of getting satisfactory catheter tip position (Haapaniemi and Slatis, 1974).

Both a high approach (Haapaniemi and Slatis, 1974), where the catheter is inserted from a point 2–3 cm above the clavicle just behind the posterior border of the sternomastoid muscle, and a low approach (Yoffa, 1965; James and Myers, 1973), where the catheter is inserted into the angle between the posterior border of the sternomastoid and the clavicle, have been described. Reports of complication rates vary from 0% (Yoffa, 1965) to 11% (James and Myers, 1973).

Infraclavicular approach. For intravenous feeding the infraclavicular approach to the subclavian vein is the most popular method of inserting central venous catheters. It was initially introduced by Dudrick et al (1969) and has remained popular ever since. The technique employed by Dudrick was that originally described by Aubaniac in 1952. Despite its popularity, it is a technique fraught with complications, although, as demonstrated by Bernard and Stahl (1971), complications are rare with those experienced in this technique of insertion. The principal complications are pneumothorax and subclavian artery puncture or laceration. Dudrick et al (1969) reported no complications in 400 insertions, but James and Myers (1973) described an overall complication rate of 15% in 511 insertions; 7% were major, 3% being pneumothoraxes. It is the fear of rates such as the latter that deters some medical practitioners from using this approach, and in the absence of knowledge about other routes of venous access leads them to deprive their patients of valuable intravenous nutrition.

The catheter is introduced from a point below the midpoint of the clavicle and advanced under the clavicle in the direction of the jugular notch until the vein is entered.

Direct exposure and cannulation

These techniques require that the vein to be cannulated is dissected and the catheter inserted under direct vision, allowing control of haemorrhage from the site of insertion and ensuring that inadvertent damage to surrounding structures is avoided. Although this can be categorized as a surgical procedure (and therefore comes into the remit of a trained surgeon), 'cut downs' to permit rapid venous access are used by other medical practitioners in emergencies. The simpler of the direct-exposure techniques should not be beyond the wit of any competent medically qualified individual, especially if they have a particular interest in intravenous feeding and will be inserting catheters on a regular basis.

According to the situation and the state of the patient, either local or general anaesthesia can be employed, but if local anaesthetic is to be used then the patient should be sedated.

Tributary vein

The advantage of these veins is that they are relatively superficial and thus easily accessible. The cephalic and the external jugular are in 'safe' anatomical sites distant from any major structure. Because they are relatively small they can be readily mobilized and ligated distal to the catheter entry point.

Their size, however, can be a disadvantage, as on occasions the vein may be too small to accept a catheter, but in experienced hands this is rare. Sometimes it may be difficult to advance the catheter past the venous valves. Dilatation of the vein with a rapid instillation of saline can overcome this. Because the route to the superior vena cava is not direct, greater care in checking the position of the tip is required to avoid malposition.

With appropriate care and attention the direct exposure of a tributary vein can be the easiest and safest of all techniques. Unfortunately the cannulation success rate can be low and it is therefore necessary for the individual to be able to use another technique when circumstances dictate.

Cephalic

The cephalic vein arises at the wrist, and passes up the lateral aspect of the forearm and across the front of the antecubital fossa, where it communicates with the median basilic vein. It then lies on the surface of the biceps and passes through the groove between the deltoid and pectoralis major muscles before passing deep to the pectoralis major through the clavipectoral fascia to join the axillary vein. Its anatomy can be variable and it may be absent in as many as 10% of individuals.

The technique of insertion was described by Ellis and Fielding in 1977. A short (2–4 cm) transverse or longitudinal incision overlying the delto-pectoral groove usually gives good access. The scar produced can sometimes be wide and unsightly but tunnelling from this site has the advantage that the catheter does not have to cross the clavicle, which in a thin patient can be both unsightly and uncomfortable.

In an unreported consecutive series of 68 cephalic vein catheter insertion attempts carried out by nine different individuals (inserting between 1 and 30 catheters each) in the Royal Infirmary, Glasgow, there were two failed insertions, one because of an absent cephalic vein and one because the vein was too small; in three other cases the cephalic vein was not identified but an adjacent vein (one supraclavicular and two the venae comitantes of the lateral thoracic artery) was used; one cephalic vein was aberrant, lying over the middle of the deltoid muscle; malposition of the catheter tip occurred on four occasions—in three the catheter was repositioned and in one the catheter was removed and a new one inserted at the same site. Thus 58 (85%) of cephalic vein insertions were uncomplicated. The mean time taken was 38 min (range 15–90).

External jugular

The external jugular vein is formed from the confluence of the posterior facial and posterior auricular veins. It passes down the neck, crossing the anterior aspect of the sternomastoid muscle to enter the subclavian vein. It is variable in both size and position.

Percutaneous cannulation is possible but the direct-exposure technique with a short incision in the root of the neck overlying a previously marked vein is more reliable; our small experience with 26 insertions, 4 left and 22 right, has been complication-free.

Major vein

Internal jugular. Exposure of the internal jugular vein can be achieved with a small incision across the lower part of the triangle formed between the two heads of the sternomastoid muscle. The technique has been described by Benotti et al (1977). Although the internal jugular vein is important for venous drainage of the brain, it can, particularly in young children, be ligated, as long as other venous channels are patent. The catheter can be inserted under local anaesthetic and in all but the very obese the dissection is straightforward. The scar left from this approach is small and rapidly becomes inconspicuous, being the least of all the scars resulting from direct-exposure techniques.

In our experience of 244 internal jugular cannulations, 194 were inserted into the right and 50 into the left. Complications at the time of insertion were encountered in 7.4%. Malposition was the commonest, 4.5% (five (10%) occurring on the left and six (3%) on the right), followed by excessive, but controllable, bleeding in 2%. Air was noted to enter the catheter on one occasion without clinical effect, one patient developed a transient hemiparesis, one a venous tear requiring suture and one patient with pneumonia died within an hour of insertion—post mortem examination failed to demonstrate a cause of death related to catheter insertion.

Subclavian. The vein is approached through an incision under the mid-portion of the clavicle as described by Oosterlee and Dudley (1980). Technically this is more exacting than the internal jugular and should be reserved for those patients in whom other approaches are inappropriate. It is a particularly difficult approach in the obese patient. The scar is often long and can be unsightly.

Of 43 subclavian cannulations, the right subclavian vein was used on 35 occasions and the left on 8. Complications occurred in five patients (15%), malposition on three occasions, bleeding on one and the only pneumothorax, with a concomitant 'hydrothorax', of our series of 341 cannulations by direct exposure, occurred after insertion of a right subclavian catheter.

COMPLICATIONS OF CENTRAL VENOUS CATHETERS

Catheter sepsis

As with any foreign material introduced into the body, avoidance of bacterial contamination of the catheter is essential. Once infected the catheter may act as a focus for systemic sepsis, and removal is the only reliable way of ensuring eradication of this source of infection. Catheter sepsis remains the single most common complication of intravenous nutrition performed through a catheter inserted into a central vein. The incidence varies between 0% (Jacobs et al, 1984) and 40% (Sitges Serra et al, 1984). Catheter sepsis can produce a response which may be as insignificant as a low-grade pyrexia without other systemic effect or as serious as overt septic shock.

Catheter sepsis is difficult to define accurately and no definition will encompass all of its manifestations. A widely used definition (Garden and Sim, 1984) employs the combination of the clinical syndrome of a pyrexia which resolves on catheter removal (clinical catheter sepsis) and positive bacterial cultures of the same organism from two or more of the three cultures obtained from peripheral blood, drawback through the catheter and the catheter tip (bacteriological sepsis—this implies that the catheter was infected but not necessarily the primary cause of systemic sepsis). This definition allows the identification of not only those patients with catheter sepsis but also those who have clinical or bacteriological catheter sepsis, either of which might be a manifestation of 'true' catheter sepsis.

Using this definition the diagnosis of catheter sepsis is retrospective to the removal of the catheter. The identification of infected catheters in situ would allow timely removal and avoid the removal of non-infected catheters. A high index of suspicion of catheter sepsis should be entertained when the patient is pyrexial and a drawback culture grows Gram-positive organisms (Ponting et al, 1985). The development of readily available quantitative blood culture techniques may be of use in identifying in situ infected catheters (Meguid et al, 1987). Catheter sepsis is highly likely when quantitative cultures reveal a colony count five or more times greater in blood withdrawn through the catheter than in blood withdrawn simultaneously from a peripheral vein.

At present the principal organisms in catheter sepsis are the staphylococci, *Staphylococcus epidermidis* being the most common. Gram-negative gut-derived organisms are only rarely implicated. Before the late 1970s *S. epidermidis* was only rarely reported in this context and *Candida albicans* was the principal infecting agent. There are certain characteristics of *S. epidermidis*, production of slime substance and its ability to etch into silicone catheters, which make it well suited to infect catheters, and staphylococcus may be considered the opportunistic infecting organism of intravenous nutrition. There is no doubt that it is pathogenic and should not be considered merely as a skin commensal. It is a difficult organism to type, and identification of the source of origin in a case of catheter sepsis is not usually possible.

Apart from direct seeding of a catheter with organisms from an endogenous septic focus related to the primary disease, transmission of bacteria to the catheter may be from the patient's skin or the person looking after the catheter. Data on the origin of infecting organisms conflict; Sitges Serra et al (1984) failed to demonstrate any relationship between the organisms cultured from the patient's skin and that responsible for catheter sepsis, whereas Snydman et al (1982) reported that the presence of an organism on the skin had a positive predictive value of 61% and the absence of any organism had a negative predictive value of 98%.

An observation that some patients have multiple catheter infections has been reported by Faubion et al (1986). Most of the patients with multiple infected catheters had severe intra-abdominal sepsis, their long and complex management making strict adherence to catheter care protocols more difficult. It may therefore be reasonable to designate such patients as being at greater risk of developing catheter sepsis.

Although catheters inserted for intravenous feeding should be sacrosanct and not used for any other purpose, there is a role for multi-lumen catheters.

If one is to be used, then one lumen should be used exclusively for intravenous nutrition and the other(s) used for additional fluid replacement, drug infusion, central venous pressure monitoring or blood sampling, All lumens must be cared for with rigid adherence to aseptic technique.

Once inserted, the catheter should be cared for by specifically designated or specially trained nursing staff. The nursing staff who care for catheters vary from institution to institution. In some, specially employed nursing teams are responsible for all catheter care (Hamoui, 1987), in others, special units exist for intravenous feeding, and in yet others, there may be an individual who oversees catheter care; commonly, though, it is the nurses who staff a particular ward who carry out the day to day care of central venous catheters (Sim et al, 1984). There is ample information demonstrating that specialist nurses produce low catheter sepsis rates (Keohane et al, 1983; Haddock et al, 1985; Faubion et al, 1986). It is necessary, however, to consider why this is so, as the expense involved in providing specialist teams to care for catheters and intravenous nutrition is often more than can be borne by a hospital budget.

The fundamental of any catheter care system is a protocol. The fact that there is no universally accepted protocol relates to differing nursing practices, differing interpretation of published data and the different experience of individuals involved. Wherever possible the protocol must be simple to learn and carry out, it must make use of commonly used materials and it should not differ radically from other similar practices.

A protocol may include such things as hair removal, skin defatting, topical antibiotics, frequent dressing changes, special types of dressing, in line filters etc. All or none of these may be considered of value. Controlled studies to demonstrate their efficacy in reducing catheter sepsis are few and the results often fail to prove that a single aspect of catheter care is important (Murphy and Lipman, 1987). Despite this, if they are part of a defined protocol which produces the desired outcome they should be retained; it is the whole protocol and not an individual component which will determine efficacy. Breaches in defined protocols are often identified as being responsible for individual incidences of catheter sepsis.

Based on the findings of Sitges Serra et al (1984) that contamination of the junction between the giving set and the catheter was an important cause of catheter sepsis, we instituted a policy of junctional care in which particular attention is paid to the catheter–giving set junction (Stotter et al, 1987). This policy change reduced catheter sepsis rates dramatically.

Prevention of catheter sepsis is a complex undertaking which involves consideration not only of the details of catheter management such as insertion, nutrient solutions and catheter care but also of the intellectual environment in which it is carried out. Without an analytical approach which fosters informed discussion and permits rational change, the exercise of catheter care becomes mechanistic and rigid without opportunity for improvement. One aspect of this is to keep accurate records of each catheter inserted, and a system of catheter audit should be established. Without this the catheter sepsis rate will be unknown and knowledge will not be available to judge whether present practices are achieving the required standards. This information must be analysed regularly and the results communicated to all personnel involved in catheter care. This can alert them to the possibility that sepsis rates are increasing and that a cause must be sought. Of equal importance is the fact that it can reinforce the assumption that techniques are adequate and that catheter sepsis is under control.

The general approach to catheter care must include aseptic technique which pays attention to care of the catheter skin exit site and the junction between the catheter and the giving set. If a catheter care protocol has been demonstrated to be effective then continued meticulous attention to its details will ensure the maintenance of good results.

Central vein thrombosis

High incidences (up to 30%) of radiologically demonstrated thrombus formation in central veins have been reported, but fortunately in most intravenous feeding this does not often produce clinically evident problems. In long-term (home) parenteral nutrition, it is a cause for concern. Reduction of thrombosis by addition of heparin to the nutrient solution has not been proven but many clinicians include it in their regimen. Catheters made of materials such as silastic or polyurethane, which are less thrombogenic, should be used. Insertion techniques should avoid venous endothelial damage. Phlebitis, which may lead to thrombosis, is associated with infusion of irritant hypertonic solutions and may be avoided by ensuring that the solution is rapidly diluted in a large vein with a high blood flow. Routine echocardiography may be employed in home parenteral nutrition patients to detect clot associated with the catheter tip.

Embolism

Air embolism

This potentially fatal complication is rare. Because catheter tips are positioned in a part of the venous system where negative pressures occur during inspiration, specific measures must be taken at the time of giving set changes to avoid air being 'sucked' into the bloodstream. The measures that should be considered are placing the patient in the Trendelenberg position, Valsalva manoeuvre and catheter clamping or switching off. To avoid accidental disconnection, giving set–catheter connections should be protected by a Luer lock or firmly taped. Care must be taken to avoid catheter breakage.

Catheter embolism

With the decrease in use of 'catheter through a needle' insertion techniques, catheter embolism at the time of insertion is now rare. Improperly secured or completely broken catheters can migrate into the bloodstream. Catheters can be secured by suture of the catheter or hub to the skin or by subcutaneous implantation of a Dacron cuff incorporated onto the outside of the catheter.

Catheter blockage

This occurs because blood, allowed to flow retrogradely into the catheter, clots, or a complex solid material forms within the catheter lumen. The former can be prevented by ensuring continuous infusion of solutions, and although most people would endorse the use of positive pressure pumping systems to ensure this, continuous flow can be maintained with accurate flow control devices (Isoflux). The formation of complex solids in the lumen has been reported with lipid-containing mixtures which have been infused for prolonged periods. Precautions to avoid this include: not infusing fat-containing mixtures every day; providing fat separately; using wider internal diameter catheters; and regular daily flushing of catheters with heparin-containing solutions. Once it is blocked, attempts to clear the catheter may be made with lytic agents (urokinase, alcohol etc.); often they are unsuccessful and the catheter will require replacement.

Catheter breakage

Silastic catheters are soft and can be broken by careless handling, an example of which is the application of metal clamps during giving set change. This can be avoided by using soft clamps or employing a catheter with an integral clamping or switching device. Damage to the catheter hub can occur with faulty hub design or overzealous tightening of the Luer lock. Silastic catheters can be repaired with the special kits that are available. In catheters with detachable hubs, a broken hub can be replaced, but in catheters with an integral hub, the catheter hub has to be cut off and a new one attached or a new catheter has to be inserted.

Catheter removal

Accidental

Catheters may be prematurely pulled out by agitated patients or inadvertent pulling on giving sets. Suture to the skin or use of a catheter with a Dacron cuff with propitious taping of the giving set or extension tube will prevent this and thwart all but the most determined patient.

Elective

Haemorrhage after catheter removal is uncommon, and firm pressure over the venotomy site at the time of removal should prevent this. Catheters with integral Dacron cuffs can be removed by simple traction but on occasions the cuff comes off the catheter and remains in the subcutaneous tissues; in the thin patient this may require surgical removal. Formal dissection of the cuff under local anaesthetic at the time of removal will obviate this problem.

CONCLUSION

The central venous catheter is an essential component of effective intravenous feeding but its insertion and subsequent care are not without problems. The responsibility of the medical practitioner involved in intravenous nutrition is to ensure that he or his staff are capable of guaranteeing that the central venous catheter is a reliable means of providing an essential therapy. To this end all involved must be ready to take on new techniques or adapt old ones if evidence is made available that this will improve their standard of care.

REFERENCES

Aubaniac R (1952) L'injection intraveineuse sous-claviculaire; avantages et technique. *Presse Médicale* **60:** 1456.
Benotti PN, Bothe A, Miller JDB & Blackburn GL (1977) Safe cannulation of the internal jugular vein for long term hyperalimentation. *Surgery, Gynecology and Obstetrics* **144:** 574–576.
Bernard RW & Stahl WM (1971) Subclavian vein catheterisations: A prospective study. 1. Non-infectious complications. *Annals of Surgery* **173:** 184–190.
Dolin BJ, Davis PD, Hollard TA & Turner JA (1987) Contamination rates of 3 in 1 total parenteral nutrition in a clincial setting. *Journal of Parenteral and Enteral Nutrition* **11:** 403–405.
Dudrick SJD, Wilmore DW, Vars HM & Rhoads JE (1969) Can intravenous feeding as the sole means of nutrition support growth in the child and restore weight loss in the adult? *Annals of Surgery* **169:** 974.
Faubion WC, Wesley JR, Khalidi N & Silva J (1986) Total parenteral nutrition catheter sepsis: Impact of the team approach. *Journal of Parenteral and Enteral Nutrition* **10:** 642–645.
Garden OJ & Sim AJW (1983) A comparison of tunnelled and non-tunnelled subclavian vein catheters: a prospective study of complications during parenteral feeding. *Clinical Nutrition* **2:** 51–54.
Griffiths JD (1963) Uses of intravenous fat and protein in intestinal surgery. In *Parenteral Nutrition Colloquium*, p 35. London: Lowe and Brydon.
Haapeniemi L & Slatis P (1974) Supraclavicular catheterisation of the superior vena cava. *Acta Anaesthesiologica Scandinavica* **18:** 12.
Haddock G, Barr J, Burns HJG & Garden OJ (1985) Reduction of central venous catheter complications. *British Journal of Parenteral Therapy* **6:** 124–128.
Hamoui E (1987) Assessing the nutritional support team. *Journal of Parenteral and Enteral Nutrition* **11:** 412–421.
Isaacs JW, Millikan WJ, Stackhouse J, Hersh T & Radman D (1977) Parenteral nutrition of adults with a 900 mOsm solution via peripheral veins. *American Journal of Clinical Nutrition* **30:** 552–559.
Jacobs DO, Melnik G & Forlaw L (1984) Impact of a nutritional support service on VA surgical patients. *Journal of American College Nutrition* **3:** 311–315.
James PM & Myers RT (1973) Central venous pressure monitoring: complications and a new technique. *American Surgeon* **39:** 75.
Keohane PP, Jones BJM, Attrill H et al (1983) Effect of catheter tunnelling and a nutrition nurse on catheter sepsis during parenteral nutrition. *Lancet* **ii:** 1388–1390.
Meguid MM, Mosca R, Curtas S & Forbes B (1987) Use of isolator cultures to manage suspected catheter sepsis. *Clinical Nutrition* **6** (special supplement): 94.
Mershon J, Nogami W, Williams JM, Yoder C, Eitzen HE & Lemons JA (1986) Bacterial/ fungal growth in combined parenteral nutrition solution. *Journal of Parenteral and Enteral Nutrition* **10:** 498–502.
von Meyenfeldt MM, Stapert J, deJong PC, Soeters PB, Wesdorp RIC & Greep JM (1980) TPN catheter sepsis: lack of effect of subcutaneous tunnelling of PVC catheters on sepsis rate. *Journal of Parenteral and Enteral Nutrition* **4:** 514–517.
Murphy LM & Lipman TO (1987) Central venous catheter care in parenteral nutrition: A review. *Journal of Parenteral and Enteral Nutrition* **11:** 190–201.

Oosterlee J & Dudley HAF (1980) Central catheter placement by puncture of the exposed subclavian vein. *Lancet* **1**: 19–20.

Patterson-Brown S, Parry BR & Sim AJW (1987) The role of double lumen catheters in intravenous nutrition. *Intensive Therapy and Clinical Monitoring* **8**: 54–56.

Ponting GA, Stotter A, Waterfield AH & Sim AJW (1985) Drawback and peripheral cultures in the diagnosis of catheter sepsis. *Clinical Nutrition* **4** (special supplement): 103A.

Rich AJ (1986) An implantable reservoir for long term venous access. *British Journal of Parenteral Therapy* **7**: 64–68.

Rosen M, Latto IP & Ng WS (1981) *Handbook of Percutaneous Venous Catheterisation.* London, Philadelphia, Toronto: WB Saunders Co. Ltd.

Segura Badia M, Alia Aponte C, Torres Rodriguez JM, Gil Egea J & Sitges Serra A (1987) 'In vitro' bacteriological study of a new hub model for intravascular catheters and infusion equipment. *Clinical Nutrition* **6** (special supplement): 99.

Sim AJW, Guest J, Carr K, Urwin J, Mundell C & Shenkin A (1984) Nutritional support—the role of a surgical nutritional advisory group. *British Journal of Parenteral Therapy* **5**: 5–7.

Sitges Serra A, Puig P & Linares J (1984) Hub colonisation as the initial step in an outbreak of catheter related sepsis due to coagulase −ve staphylococci. *Journal of Parenteral and Enteral Nutrition* **8**: 668–672.

Snydman DR, Gorbea HF, Pober BR, Majka JA, Murray SA & Perry LK (1982) Predictive value of surveillance skin cultures in total-parenteral-nutrition-related infection. *Lancet* **ii**: 1385–1388.

Stotter AT, Ward H, Waterfield AH, Hilton J & Sim AJW (1987) Junctional care: the key to prevention of catheter sepsis in intravenous feeding. *Journal of Parenteral and Enteral Nutrition* **11**: 159–162.

Tanner WA, Delaney PV & Hennessay TP (1980) The influence of heparin on intravenous infusions: a prospective study. *British Journal of Surgery* **67**: 311–312.

Yakoun M, Armynot du Chatelet AM & Simeon de Buochberg M (1987) Reduction of catheter related sepsis in long term parenteral nutrition using subcutaneous infusion ports. A prospective study on 44 patients. *Clinical Nutrition* **6** (special supplement): 96.

Yoffa D (1965) Supraclavicular subclavian venepuncture and catheterisation. *Lancet* **2**: 614.

6

Enteral nutrition: background, indications and management

JASON PAYNE-JAMES
DAVID SILK

Progress in enteral nutrition has to some extent been overshadowed by the developments and advances in total parenteral nutrition (TPN) that originated from Dudrick's work reported in 1968. Although enteral feeding techniques had been used spasmodically, particularly in the United States, for at least 50 years (Stengel and Ravdin, 1939; Boles and Zollinger, 1952; Pareira et al, 1954; Smith and Lee, 1956), it was not until the latter half of the 1970s that formal re-evaluation of enteral nutrition led to it being recognized as a valuable therapeutic tool, Enteral nutrition is considerably cheaper, more physiological and has fewer complications than total parenteral nutrition (Heymsfield et al, 1979; Shanbhogue et al, 1987). Undoubtedly there may be situations in which TPN alone is indicated, but it is equally clear that many patients who would benefit from enteral nutrition, are inappropriately prescribed TPN. For the purposes of this chapter enteral nutrition will be considered to refer to nutrition administered artificially to the gastrointestinal tract of patients who are unable or unwilling to consume an adequate diet by mouth. Oral nutritional supplementation will be considered elsewhere in this volume. Before considering the indications for, and management of enteral nutrition it is necessary to review present knowledge about digestion and absorption of protein, carbohydrate and fat, in order to put into perspective the necessity for administering particular dietary formulas. The techniques by which these diets should be administered will then be reviewed.

DIGESTION AND ABSORPTION OF PROTEINS, LIPIDS AND CARBOHYDRATES

Protein digestion

The two sources of protein available for intestinal luminal digestion are dietary protein (about 70–100 g per day in a normal western diet) and endogenous protein originating from gastric, biliary, pancreatic and related secretions composed of digestive enzymes and secretory proteins. It has been demonstrated that in man, exogenous dietary protein is the major source of free amino acides and peptides in intraluminal contents (Adibi and Mercer, 1973). Most exogenous protein appears to be absorbed in the upper jejunum (Nixon and Mawer, 1970a; 1970b; Johansson, 1975; Silk & Dawson, 1979), although there is still some present in the ileum where absorption may also take place (Adibi and Mercer, 1973; Chung et al, 1979). Recent studies on patients with established ileostomies (Russell and Evans, 1987) support this. Animal studies suggest the colon as the primary site of endogenous protein assimilation (Curtis et al, 1978). Protein is denatured in the stomach by substrate specific pepsins, allowing large polypeptides to enter the duodenum where they are further hydrolysed by pancreatic proteolytic enzymes. A small proportion of free amino acids is released in the stomach. In addition to the pancreatic proteolytic enzymes, solubilized intestinal brush border and cytoplasmic mucosal amino-oligopeptidases are present in intestinal contents (Josefsson and Lindberg, 1967; Silk et al, 1976a; 1976b). These luminal peptidases are probably functionally more important in the ileum than in the jejunum. Free amino acids and small peptides with chain lengths of 2 to 6 amino acid residues are the products of luminal proteolysis (Chen et al, 1962; Nixon and Mawer, 1970a; 1970b; Adibi and Mercer, 1973).

Amino acid absorption

It is thought that absorption of free amino acids is dependent on a sodium gradient across the brush border membrane of intestinal epithelial cells (Schultz and Curran, 1970), but confirmation of dependency has not been clearly demonstrated in man (Silk and Dawson, 1979). Animal studies have suggested the existence of four main group-specific active transport systems (Wellner and Meister, 1979; Matthews and Payne, 1980; Matthews and Burston, 1984):

1. monoamino monocarboxylic (neutral amino acids)
2. dibasic amino acids (e.g. ornithine)
3. glycine, proline, hydroxyproline
4. dicarboxylic (acidic amino acids)

The first two mechanisms have been confirmed in man (Matthews, 1975; Matthews and Adibi 1976; Silk and Dawson, 1979).

Peptide absorption

Recent research has shown that complete digestion of protein to free amino acids is not necessary for absorption. Craft et al (1968) showed that when glycine was administered orally in the form of di- and tri-peptides it was absorbed faster than when given in the free form. This work resulted in much more detailed study of the uptake of peptides from the intestinal lumen. Intestinal absorption studies of patients with Hartnup disease (a defect in neutral amino acid absorption) and cystinuria (a defect in dibasic amino acid absorption) showed that normal or near normal uptake of the affected amino acids occurred if they were presented to the mucosa as dipeptides (Asatoor et al, 1970; Nawab and Asatoor, 1970; Asatoor et al, 1972; Hellier et al, 1972; Silk et al, 1975). If the dipeptides had undergone hydrolysis within the bulk phase in the gut lumen, or by brush border peptidases, then uptake would not have taken place. Work supporting this evidence of intact dipeptide uptake has shown that competition between free amino acids for mucosal uptake is lessened when solutions of dipeptides instead of the equivalent free amino acids are presented to the gut (Hellier et al, 1972; Silk et al, 1973; Silk, 1974). Other studies have demonstrated intact dipeptides in plasma samples during in vivo intestinal perfusions (Adibi, 1971) and during oral feeding (Hueckel and Rogers, 1970). The mechanism of dipeptide uptake is dependent on a carrier-mediated transport mechanism, as has been shown by the competitive inhibition of two dipeptides (Adibi and Soleimanpoor, 1974), and the mechanism can be saturated by increasing solute concentration (Adibi, 1971; Silk, 1977). The possibility of more than one transport mechanism has been postulated but not confirmed (Lane et al, 1975; Fairclough et al, 1977; Chung et al, 1979). It is however considered that a dual hypothesis for dipeptide uptake is valid (Silk, 1986a). Peptides with a high affinity for brush border peptidases are hydrolysed to their component amino acids, whilst a second group of peptides with a lower affinity for those peptidases are absorbed intact and hydrolysed by cytoplasmic peptidases. Studies on tripeptide uptake and absorption also demonstrate an enhanced uptake when compared with the equivalent free amino acid solution (Silk et al, 1974; Adibi et al, 1975). Again it is likely that a dual uptake mechanism is operating. Nicholson and Peters (1977a; 1977b) have demonstrated tripeptidases in both brush border and soluble fractions in a series of subfractionation studies which suggests that hydrolysis to dipeptides and free amino acid takes place in significant amounts. Tobey et al (1985) confirmed the existence of dipeptidases and tripeptidases in the human brush border and also commenced biochemical characterization of these enzymes. Few tetrapeptides have been studied, and the conclusions about mechanisms of uptake of these and longer chain peptides are conflicting (Smithson and Gray, 1977; Chung et al, 1979). As a means of study of the possible nutritional advantages of peptide versus amino acid transport, in vivo intestinal perfusion studies have been performed comparing uptake of amino acid residues from partial enzymic hydrolysates of whole protein and from equivalent free amino acid mixtures. Results have consistently demonstrated improved uptake of α-amino nitrogen from partial enzymic hydrolysates of protein compared to their equivalent free amino acid mixtures (Silk et al, 1980). The pattern of absorption of amino acid residues from the different protein hydrolysate studies has been variable. Further studies have shown that the amino acid composition of the starter protein as well as the techniques of hydrolysis influence nitrogen uptake (Keohane et al, 1981). Perfusion studies examining the effect of peptide chain length have demonstrated that a small increase in peptide chain length from 2–3 to 3–5 has a clear deleterious effect on α-amino N absorption (Keohane et al, 1982a; Rees et al, 1984).

Relevance of protein digestion and absorption to enteral nutrition

Clinical studies have clearly shown that the optimal form of nitrogen source in normal subjects with intact functioning gut is whole protein (Jones et al, 1983; Moriarty et al, 1985). The studies outlined in the previous section have demonstrated a theoretical advantage for amino acids or peptides as nitrogen sources in those patients with severely impaired gastrointestinal function where luminal hydrolysis is rate limiting, e.g. short bowel syndrome. A recent double-blind crossover study comparing the effect of a whole protein versus an oligopeptide diet on the nutritional parameters of patients with *moderately* severe impairment of gastrointestinal function highlighted the similarities in nitrogen utilization (Rees et al, 1988). Stein-hardt et al (1986) showed no significant difference in nitrogen balance or plasma amino acid profiles when comparing utilization of a predigested and a polymeric diet in patients after total pancreatectomy. A study of patients with high jejunostomies after bowel resection showed no consistent difference in nitrogen absorption between either peptide-based or poly-meric diets (McIntyre et al, 1986). Unfortunately, all these studies compare diets with different amino acid compositions. The answer to the question 'What is the optimal form of nitrogen to present to the gut?' requires a study comparing nitrogen uptake using diets of identical amino acid composition.

At the present state of knowledge the following guidelines are appro-priate. Patients with a normal functioning gastrointestinal tract should receive whole protein as the nitrogen source in enteral diets. Patients with moderately severe impairment of gastrointestinal function may in many cases be capable of handling a polymeric diet, but in a minority of cases may require a predigested protein nitrogen source. In those patients where luminal hydrolysis is rate limiting with regard to determining absorption (e.g. short bowel syndrome and severe exocrine pancreatic insufficiency) then predigested protein should be administered. However other factors also influence choice of diet and these will be discussed later in the chapter.

DIGESTION AND ABSORPTION OF LIPID

The major dietary lipids are triglycerides, cholesterol and the fat soluble vitamins. Triglycerides are triesters of glycerol and the majority are water insoluble, consisting of fatty acids with 16–18 carbon atoms – the long chain triglycerides (LCT) – and the more soluble medium chain triglycerides (MCT) containing fatty acids with 6–12 carbon atoms. Digestion and absorption of lipids requires hydrolysis of ester lipids by lipases and ester-ases, and micellar solubilization of the products of the lipolysis. Emulsifi-cation of dietary lipid occurs in the stomach by mechanical action and the emulsion is mixed with bile and pancreatic secretions after passage into the duodenum. Lipolysis of triglyceride in the stomach by pharyngeal lipase (Hamosh et al, 1975), producing diglycerides and fatty acids, promotes further emulsification. This cycle continues in duodenal and jejunal lumens, with the aid of pancreatic lipase, which produces free fatty acids and a 2-monoglyceride resulting in eventual micellar solubilization. Other lipases may be present but their significance is as yet undetermined. Cholesterol ester is hydrolysed by pancreatic cholesterol esterase to produce free cholesterol.

Absorption of products of lipid digestion

Monoglycerides, free cholesterol and fatty acids (the products of luminal lipid hydrolysis) are poorly soluble in the gut lumen water, and require solubilization for adequate absorption. The pH (6–7) of intraluminal jejunal contents results in a high degree of ionization. Bile salts are soluble in this mileu. Above the Critical Micellar Concentration, pure bile salt micelles are formed. Fatty acids, monoglycerides and phospholipids are incorporated in the centres of these micelles forming mixed mixcelles. The mixed micelles then diffuse across the unstirred water layer, allowing lipolysis products to reach the surface of microvilli. As the products of lipolysis are predominantly absorbed in the proximal small intestine and bile salts in the distal ileum, it is necessary for micellar dissociation to take place prior to absorption. The dissociation is assisted by local acidity resulting from mucosal cell hydrogen secretion deep to the unstirred water layer. Mucosal uptake of long chain fatty acids occurs as a result of binding to specific microvillous binding proteins, possibly as a result of a carrier-mediated transport mechanism. Having entered the cytoplasm, the long chain fatty acids bind to fatty acid binding protein, which direct the fatty acids to the smooth endoplasmic reticulum where triglyceride is synthesized (Stremmel et al, 1985). The re-esterified triglycerides then transfer along the cholesterol, phospholipids and fat soluble vitamins to the Golgi apparatus.

Chlyomicrons are formed and the Golgi vesicles discharge these into the intercellular space from where they progress to the lacteal and then lymphatic system. The absorption of short and medium chain fatty acids differs as they are more water soluble and are rapidly hydrolysed by lingual and pancreatic lipase. Bile salt micelles are not required for their absorption. In contrast to long chain fatty acids, short and medium chain fatty acids are generally not re-esterified and incorporated into chylomicrons. After release from the mucosal cell these free fatty acids bind to albumin and enter the portal circulation (Silk, 1986a).

Relevance of lipid digestion and absorption to enteral nutrition

It is clear that normal lipid digestion and absorption is dependent on an adequate supply of pancreatic lipase and bile acids along with adequate absorptive area. There is a group of patients in whom these factors are defective and therefore diets containing large amounts of long chain triglycerides (LCT) should be avoided, as assimilation will be impaired and essential fatty acid deficiency (Dodge and Yassa, 1980) and vitamin depletion may occur. These patients include those with severe exocrine pancreatic insufficiency (chronic pancreatitics and cystic fibrotics), severe intestinal mucosal abnormalities (untreated coeliac disease), or extensive small bowel resections. An alternative that has been suggested are medium chain triglycerides (MCT), which are composed of triglycerides of 6–12 carbon atoms, but predominantly 8–10. They do not contain the essential fatty acid linoleic acid, and risk promoting essential fatty acid deficiency for this reason. They may be beneficial, because they are more water soluble than LCT, and intraluminal hydrolysis of MCTs is more efficient than hydrolysis of LCTs (MacBurney and Young, 1984). There is some debate as to how efficiently MCTs are utilized (Hashim, 1967; MacBurney and Young, 1984; Silk, 1984) the proponents suggesting that they should be used for all disorders of fat absorption or lymph drainage of the intestine. Despite these controversies it is known that MCTs are assimilated more efficiently than LCTs in patients with reduced luminal lipase activity, and in these circumstances enteral diets using MCT as the predominant lipid energy source would be preferable (Silk, 1986a). In addition, exogenous pancreatic supplements will enhance utilization of MCTs and reduce steatorrhoea in cases of exocrine pancreatic insufficiency and small intestinal resection (Forstner et al, 1980).

CARBOHYDRATE DIGESTION AND ABSORPTION

In the western world the average adult ingests more than 300 g of carbohydrate daily, providing at least 50% of total caloric intake. The majority is in the form of starch (64%) or sucrose (26%) with a smaller amount of lactose (6.5%) and fructose (3%). α-Amylase secreted by the pancreas and salivary glands cleaves α1–4 glycosidic linkages of starch. The digestion of amylose, a linear component of starch, yields maltotriose and maltose. The α1–6 linkages of amylopectin, the other, highly-branched component of starch, are not cleaved by α-amylase so that the products consist of α-limit dextrins (oligo 1–6 glucosides comprising $\geq$ 4 glucose units). Thus luminal digestion of starch yields a mixture of α-limit dextrins, maltotriose and maltose. Sucrose and lactose are not hydrolysed by α-amylase (Silk, 1986a). The end stage of digestion of these groups of substances is cellular processes from which monosaccharides are formed. The enzymes responsible are located at the microvillus membrane fraction of intestinal mucosa. Several maltases have been characterized and in vivo intestinal perfusion experiments have demonstrated that the α1–4 glucosidase isolated by Kelly and Alpers (1973) is one of the most functionally important. Sucrase-isomaltase is the enzyme responsible for cleavage of the α1–2 linkage of sucrose and the α1–6 linkage of α-limit dextrins. Lactose is hydrolysed by a β-galactosidase which has a high substrate specificity for lactose and is located in the brush border fraction of small intestinal mucosa. In summary, for a person consuming an average western diet, the dietary carbohydrates starch, sucrose and lactose are hydrolysed to monosaccharides in the proportions, glucose 80%, fructose 15% and galactose 5%.

Absorption of carbohydrate digestion products

Monosaccharides

Glucose absorption is considered an active mechanism dependent, at least in part, on a sodium gradient across the brush border membrane and this has been supported by the studies of Biederdoft et al (1975) and of Debnam and Levin (1975). It had been considered that galactose shared the same glucose transport system but other work suggests that multiple carrier systems exist (Debnam and Levin, 1976). Fructose absorption is almost certainly via a carrier-mediated mechanism that may use a transmembrane sodium gradient (Gracey et al, 1972; Millar et al, 1977).

Intestinal assimilation of glucose polymer mixtures

In vivo intestinal perfusion experiments have clearly shown that monosaccharide uptake from the disaccharide sucrose occurred as rapidly as when the constituent monosaccharides themselves were presented for absorption. In the case of maltose and maltotriose, glucose uptake has been shown to occur faster than from the free form (Cook, 1973; Sandle et al, 1977; Jones et al, 1987). This provoked further studies of the intestinal handling of glucose polymers. The composition of the carbohydrate sources used in enteral diets have been submitted to gel-permeation chromatography, and approximately 50% of the total glucose component was present as polymers consisting of greater than 10 glucose molecules (high molecular weight polymers) and 50% was present as polymers consisting of less than 10 glucose molecules (low molecular weight polymers) (Jones, 1984; Jones et al, 1984). In vivo intestinal perfusion studies in man showed a different handling of the high and low molecular weight fractions. In the absence of luminal α-amylase activity a purified low molecular weight fraction exerted a kinetic advantage on glucose uptake. It was also shown that glucose uptake from maltose, maltotriose and the highly purified fraction containing 5–8 glucose molecules occurs faster than from pure glucose (Jones et al, 1981).

Relevance of carbohydrate digestion and absorption to enteral nutrition

In conditions when there is severe impairment of gastrointestinal function consideration should therefore be given to using purified low molecular weight glucose polymer as the carbohydrate source. In other situations where gastrointestinal function is not compromised, considerable savings in diet osmolality could be achieved if purified high molecular weight glucose polymers are used. As mentioned earlier, fructose is absorbed by a separate transport mechanism from glucose. Recent intestinal perfusions have demonstrated that sugar absorption can be enhanced if sucrose is added to a glucose polymer mixture, as fructose will continue to be absorbed despite saturation of the glucose transport mechanism (Spiller et al, 1987).

Lactase deficiency may have an incidence as high as 100% in some ethnic and racial groups (Neale, 1968). This problem has been cited as evidence for one of the causes of diarrhoea in enteral feeding. It may be that lactase deficiency by itself, does not always *have* to result in enteral feeding related diarrhoea. A study (O'Keefe et al, 1984) has demonstrated that bolus feeding of lactose-containing enteral diets will result in diarrhoea. Haverberg et al (1980) and Kwon et al (1980), however, showed no different incidence of gastrointestinal side-effects when administering milk or lactose-free milk to patients with lactose malabsorption. The explanation lies in the pathology of the disease. β-galactosidase is a brush border hydrolase whose specific activity is reduced but not absent in lactose malabsorbers. Thus 'intolerance' is dependent on the load of lactose presented to the brush border. As 'load' is a product of 'concentration' and 'rate', continuous infusion of a lactose-containing diet over 24 hours will have a low load administered per unit time whereas in O'Keefe's study a high load was presented when the diet was administered by bolus techniques. In the most recent study from that unit they question the clinical necessity of administering lactose-free diets to adults with confirmed lactose intolerance (O'Keefe et al, 1988). In practice however, most commercial enteral diets are essentially lactose free.

WATER AND ELECTROLYTE ABSORPTION

Water

The approximate quantities of water and electrolytes handled by the normal adult gut are summarized in Table 1.

There are no specific active transport processes for water absorption, as the intestinal mucosa acts as a semi-permeable membrane with water flowing in either direction in response to changes in osmotic pressure. Intestinal luminal digestion creates a hypertonic bulk phase, resulting in movement of water into the gut lumen. With gradual absorption of luminal

Table 1. Water and electrolyte handling by the gut in 24 hours.

	Water (ml)	Sodium (mmol)	Chloride (mmol)	Potassium (mmol)
Input				
Diet (exogenous)	1500	150	150	80
Gut secretions (endogenous)	7500	1000	750	40
Total	9000	1150	900	120
Uptake				
Small intestine	7500	950	800	110
Colon	1350	195	97	−3
Output				
Faeces	150	5	3	12

contents hypotonicity occurs and water is absorbed along with the solutes. In such a way near isotonicity is maintained.

The jejunal mucosa is more freely permeable than the ileum which in turn is more permeable than the colon. Water absorption in the upper small intestine is determined by absorption of nutrients. In contrast, water absorption in the ileum and dehydration of colonic contents is primarily related mainly to the absorption of salt.

Electrolytes

Over 100 mmol of sodium chloride enters the upper small intestine every 24 hours. As is seen from Table 1, conservation is extremely efficient with about 5 mmol being excreted in stool. In the upper small intestine sodium and chloride diffuse down a concentration gradient resulting in luminal concentration similar to plasma levels. Glucose, amino acids, di- and tripeptides and bicarbonate ions within the gut lumen all stimulate sodium uptake. Sodium-linked, carrier-mediated uptake mechanisms are utilized in these situations. Bicarbonate reacts with actively secreted hydrogen ions and is removed as CO_2. The hydrogen ions are secreted by exchange with absorbed sodium on a specific cation-exchange carrier. Sodium and chloride ions are also considered to move in response to the movement of water that occurs via the intercellular spaces. As yet the quantitative significance of 'solvent drag' is unclear. Sodium and chloride absorption by means of ion exchange takes place in the ileum, and because the ileal mucosa is less permeable to ions than the jejunum, therefore less back diffusion occurs. The colon absorbs a considerable quantity of water in 24 hours (see Table 1), but can absorb up to three or four times this load before the absorptive capacity becomes insufficient and diarrhoea results. Absorption of sodium, chloride and short chain fatty acids determines the degree of water absorption (Spiller and Silk, 1988).

Relevance of water and electrolyte absorption in short bowel syndrome

Following massive resection of intestine for whatever reason, one of the early problems is the massive fluid and electrolyte loss either per rectum or per stoma. Often these patients are treated with a combination of both TPN and enteral nutrition, allowing maintenance of nutritional state, whilst at the same time promoting gut adaptation. Recent work has demonstrated that the administration of a diet with a sodium concentration of less than 70–90 mmol/l will result in a sodium flux from mucosa to lumen with associated water movement, thereby aggravating the underlying problem. Unfortunately many enteral diets may have a low concentration of sodium. A sodium concentration greater than 90 mmol/l should be ensured in all enteral diets administered to this group of patients (Spiller et al, 1987; Jones, 1987).

TYPES OF DIET

Prior to 1981 the proportion of hospitals using commercial feeds was just under 50%, the great majority using 'home-brew' diets prepared in hospital kitchens (Tredger et al, 1981). Problems with microbial contamination of these feeds (Bastow et al, 1982) and the time required for preparation have been partly responsible for the great increase in the proportion of commercial enteral diets now used in hospitals, from 47% in 1981 to 96% in 1987 (Green et al, 1987). In the last 10 years as enteral nutrition has expanded, many different commercial enteral diets have been developed. Heimburger and Weinsier (1985) examined a variety of diets and suggested parameters of relative importance by which clinicians could evaluate new and current enteral feeding products. A recent review of diets available in the UK emphasizes the range available (at least 30 different diets) and the difficulties in deciding the most appropriate product for a given patient (Drugs and Therapeutics Bulletin, 1986). The types of diet available can be considered in four main groups (Table 2), of which the first two can be considered the most important.

Table 2. Categories of enteral diet.

Polymeric
Predigested chemically defined or elemental diets
Disease specific formulations
Modular diets

Polymeric diets

Polymeric diets contain whole protein as a nitrogen source and are appropriate diets for all patients with a normal or near normal functioning gastrointestinal tract. Most of these diets have an energy density of 1 kcal/ml and a nitrogen concentration of 5–7 g/litre. Although the non-nitrogen calorie:nitrogen ratio of these diets ranges from 150:1 to 200:1 there is little evidence to suggest whether the low or high figure is more appropriate for the majority of non-catabolic patients. A lower ratio providing a greater proportion of nitrogen for a given energy intake is required to maintain nitrogen balance in heavily catabolic patients such as those with burns or sepsis.

Recently a few nitrogen dense and/or energy dense diets have become available. The nitrogen dense diets contain up to 9 g nitrogen/litre and may find a wider application in the future particularly in non-catabolic patients as recent studies have highlighted the benefits of such a diet in terms of nitrogen balance (Twyman et al, 1985; Rees et al, 1986a). Bunker and Clayton (1983) have shown that the majority of commercial feeds contain adequate trace elements, vitamins and essential fatty acids to prevent deficiency in patients requiring feeding for just a few weeks. It must be noted however that quoted values for Recommended Daily Allowances are derived from requirements of normal subjects and may not be sufficient in patients with pre-existing deficiencies or for some disease states.

Predigested 'chemically defined' or elemental diets

When first produced, these diets, consisting of a nitrogen source of synthetic L-amino acids or predigested protein providing oligopeptides and amino acids, were purported to be indicated for the majority of patients with impaired gastrointestinal function and for those patients where minimum residue was required. In practice the majority of polymeric diets are themselves low residue, and those studies examining absorption from polymeric and elemental diets show little or no difference between the two groups (Andersson et al, 1984; McIntyre et al, 1986; Russell and Evans, 1987). Many of the studies outlined in the first section above have clearly indicated that except in severely impaired gastrointestinal digestive and absorptive function, the theoretical advantages of these diets when compared with a polymeric diet are not borne out in clinical practice (Fick et al, 1986). Clearly this is significant when it is realized that there may be a threefold price difference when supplying the same amount of calories or nitrogen. The increased osmolality of the majority of predigested elemental diets may also increase the incidence of side-effects such as abdominal cramps and bloating, although a recent study has once again emphasized the concept of 'osmoles administered per unit time' being clinically more relevant than 'osmoles per unit volume of feed' (Bastow et al, 1985). The main indications for a predigested or elemental diet include exocrine pancreatic insufficiency, the nutritionally inadequate short bowel syndrome and possibly as primary therapy in Crohn's disease.

Disease specific enteral diets

Early in the history of nutritional support it became clear that there were certain groups of patients in whom 'standard nutritional support' may not be appropriate, or may be potentially disadvantageous. Much work has been undertaken to improve the clinical condition of patients by manipulation of aspects of their nutritional support, particularly directed at the underlying pathological process. Diets have been designed and manufactured specifically for liver disease, renal disease, respiratory disease and states of marked metabolic stress such as trauma or sepsis.

Patients with *advanced cirrhosis* are often malnourished and in many of these ingestion of protein may precipitate or worsen hepatic encephalopathy. Those patients with hepatic disease who are malnourished but without impairment of mental state may be treated with standard diets (Silk, 1986b). Fischer and Balderssarini (1971) were the first to suggest that encephalopathy might be improved by attempting to correct existing abnormalities of the plasma amino acid profile. A number of controlled clinical trials performed in patients with cirrhosis and portosystemic encephalopathy have now examined the efficacy of diets containing a modified free amino acid nitrogen source enriched with branched chain amino acids (BCAAs) and containing low concentrations of aromatic amino acids and methionine. Results are conflicting and until more data become available it must be concluded that there are no clear indications for using these diets (Silk, 1988).

Patients with acute *renal failure* have been shown to have improved survival and recovery when administered intravenous solutions rich in essential amino acids (Dudrick et al, 1970; Abel et al, 1973). No prospective randomized trial has yet been undertaken with the specially formulated renal enteral diets, which are rich in essential amino acids, therefore the diets that are available are as yet of unproven value, and not appropriate for every type of renal failure (Steffee and Anderson 1984).

A detailed of study of the respiratory, cardiovascular and metabolic effects of enteral nutrition has been reported (Heymsfield et al, 1984). It shows clearly that when an increasing amount of energy was infused into patients on continuous enteral feeding, their CO_2 production, minute ventilation and heat production increased. This concurred with earlier studies which had identified refeeding as the cause of respiratory problems in patients receiving high carbohydrate loads (Askanasi et al, 1980; Covelli et al, 1981). Heymsfield's study (1984) confirmed that these changes were less marked when fat was used as a calorie source. An enteral diet with a reduced amount of carbohydrate and an increased amount of fat is available for patients in respiratory failure. It is our current practice to use this diet for patients with respiratory failure or when patients are being weaned from ventilators in the Intensive Therapy Unit.

Severely metabolically stressed patients, such as those with multiple trauma, burns or sepsis, are extremely catabolic with a resulting markedly negative nitrogen balance. There is considerable interest in using BCAAs in the stressed patient. Although potential benefits with regard to metabolic parameters have been seen in humans and animals with sepsis or after injury, we are unaware of any significant *clinical* advantage having been demonstrated using BCAAs as the nitrogen source (Freund et al, 1979; Cerra et al, 1984; Iapichino et al, 1985). Currently the problem of reducing post-trauma catabolism and improving nitrogen balance is being approached in another way by using the ornithine salt of the Kreb's cycle intermediate, alpha-ketoglutarate. Ornithine alpha-ketoglutarate (OαKG) was developed and used originally for the treatment of encephalopathy (Michel et al, 1971). A series of studies have suggested that OαKG as a supplement to both enteral nutrition or total parenteral nutrition may reduce protein catabolism after injury and result in better postoperative nitrogen economy (Cynober et al, 1984; Leander et al, 1985). These results appear to be supported in clinical studies of nitrogen balance and protein synthesis in skeletal muscle of postoperative patients (Wernerman et al, 1987), and in a study of nitrogen balance in septic and polytraumatized patients (Mertes et al, 1987). Further studies to confirm these results, and to clarify the mode of action of OαKG, are being undertaken in our unit at the present time.

Modular diets

Despite the large number of commercially available complete enteral diets there are some patients who may be deficient in one particular group of nutrients. For these patients specific nutrients, particularly carbohydrate, protein, medium chain triglycerides and vitamins are available to be administered separately and can be used to correct the overall dietary intake.

INDICATIONS FOR ENTERAL FEEDING

It is over 10 years since the classic studies of Bistrian and colleagues (1974; 1976), and of Hill et al (1977) demonstrated the high incidence of nutritional deficiencies in patients admitted to both medical and surgical wards. It was to be hoped that the information obtained from these studies might have led to a general improvement in the nutritional status in hospitalized patients by increasing the use of nutritional support. A recent study (Neithercut et al, 1987) comparing different nutritional parameters showed a prevalence of malnutrition on a general surgical ward of between 16 and 35% depending on the parameter used. It is clear that malnutrition in hospitalized patients remains a major problem. However the indications for instigating nutritional support remain controversial and difficult to define.

In general terms our current indications for nutritional support include first, those patients with severe malnutrition as manifest by marked weight loss, an albumin level of less than 30 g/l, obvious muscle wasting and/or peripheral oedema. We will also consider providing nutritional support to patients whom we consider to be only moderately malnourished. In these patients nutritional parameters may be suggestive of malnutrition but a dietary history shows an impaired nutrient intake for the preceding two to four weeks. Finally, in our experience there exists a significant group of patients who, on initial assessment, have normal or near-normal nutritional status. These patients however may have an underlying pathology (medical or surgical) which is likely to result in malnutrition if nutritional support is withheld. Our indications for *enteral* rather than parenteral nutritional support can be summarized as:

Enteral nutrition should be considered for all patients in the above groups with a functioning, accessible gastrointestinal tract.

These will include patients with an enormous range of differing pathologies (see Table 3), some of which will be discussed in further detail. The means of obtaining access to the gut will be reviewed later in the chapter. There are very few contraindications to enteral nutrition. Indeed many situations requiring nutritional support originally considered to be the sole province of TPN, such as fistulas, have now been shown to be successfully treated by enteral nutrition (Esteve et al, 1987). In some conditions, such as short bowel syndrome, the two techniques may be used concurrently. However three main contraindications to enteral nutrition remain, paralytic ileus, bowel obstruction and major intra-abdominal sepsis.

Table 3. Categories of patients suitable for enteral nutrition. (References indicate detailed reviews of the literature).

Patient group	Disease state
Medical	Inflammatory bowel disease
	Hepatic failure
	Renal failure
	Respiratory failure
Neurological	Cerebrovascular accidents
	Motor neurone disease
Surgical	Preoperative
	Postoperative
	Fistula
	Burns
	Sepsis
Orthopaedic	Trauma
Psychiatric	Anorexia nervosa
Paediatric	Cystic fibrosis
	(Courtney Moore et al, 1986)
Miscellaneous	Intensive care patients
	Cancer
	Short bowel (Jones, 1987)

Enteral feeding and specific disease states

Inflammatory bowel disease

Enteral feeding was used in the late 1960s and early 1970s by some workers, as a means of maintaining or improving nutritional status in inflammatory bowel disease, whilst standard medical management controlled the disease or the patient was prepared for surgical intervention. The idea of enteral diet having a therapeutic role was proposed by O'Morain et al whose work (1980; 1984) suggested that an elemental enteral diet might be an appropriate primary therapy. Further studies investigating this are currently in progress. A recent study (Rao et al, 1987) has demonstrated that nutritional support via the enteral route using a polymeric diet is an effective method of improving nutritional status in patients with severe Crohn's colitis or ulcerative colitis, whilst remission is induced by standard medical means. In a prospective randomized study Gonzalez-Huix and colleagues (1987) compared a polymeric diet with TPN in the treatment of Crohn's disease and ulcerative colitis. Nutritional indices remained similar for the two groups but the enteral diet group had a significant improvement in disease activity indices.

Neurological

Many patients admitted to hospital acutely with cerebrovascular accidents will eventually be fit enough to return home. In many cases at admission the patient is in a state of altered consciousness, or has a temporarily suppressed gag reflex or swallowing mechanism that may preclude adequate oral intake of nutrients. Common practice has been to treat these patients with a dextrose/saline drip until a spontaneous improvement occurs. It would seem logical to commence enteral feeding from day 1 in the majority of these patients so that the circle of anorexia, apathy and malnutrition (Allison, 1986) does not become established, with a resultant delay in recovery and an increased risk of the development of decubitus ulcers and infection. The advisability of commencing or continuing nutritional support in this difficult group of patients, some with extremely poor prognosis, requires close liaison between the supervising clinician and the nutrition team.

Surgical

Surgical patients are a group who until recent years have traditionally received nutritional support via the parenteral route. Undoubtedly there are many theoretical reasons why nutritional support may be beneficial to the surgical patient. Studley's classical paper (1937) on surgical risks in patients with chronic peptic ulcer, first alerted surgeons to the dangers of weight loss in patients. Subsequent studies have confirmed this, and recent elegant studies by Haydock and Hill (1986) have demonstrated an abnormality in the wound healing response in malnourished patients. The same two workers have recently demonstrated an improvement in this response after only one week of intravenous nutrition (Haydock and Hill, 1987). Although the majority of these studies relate to intravenous nutrition, recent work has concentrated on comparing parenteral with enteral nutrition. A prospective study by Fletcher and Little (1986), of patients who had undergone aortic aneurysm surgery concluded that 'postoperative nutritional support after major surgery can be given as effectively by the enteral route as by TPN'. Preoperative regimens for colorectal surgery often include two or three days of clear fluids by mouth, in a patient who may already be malnourished. A recent study comparing a conventional preoperative regimen with one where clear fluids were replaced by a low residue enteral diet, demonstrated a significantly earlier return of intestinal function with a trend towards shorter hospitalization in the patients prepared with an enteral diet (Rumley et al, 1987). Conventional wisdom dictates that there is a period of 'ileus' post-laparotomy and that fluid and food should not be ingested until the presence of bowel sounds and the passage of flatus indicate that the ileus has resolved. However small bowel function returns to normal within a few hours of a laparotomy, whilst the stomach and colon may take 48 and up to 96 hours respectively to revert to normal function (Shoemaker and Wright, 1970; Nachlas et al, 1972). Many investigators have now demonstrated the efficacy and safety of immediate or early postoperative feeding into the jejunum (Sagar et al, 1979; Hoover et al, 1980; Moss, 1984; Schattenkerk, 1984) and others have confirmed the safety of delivering the diet *proximal* to a bowel anastomosis (Merkle et al, 1984; Pasurka et al, 1984; Takala et al, 1985). This is a practice not readily accepted by all surgeons but on theoretical grounds it could be beneficial, as gut with luminal contents has an increased blood supply which should promote anastomotic healing, and a proportion of the energy required for normal gut function derives from intraluminal contents. Indeed, 'bowel rest' which may be achieved by withholding food or by creating a diverting colostomy, can promote colonic atrophy which may affect healing adversely (Blomquist et al, 1984; 1985). Studies by Rolandelli et al (1986a; 1986b) on rats suggest that perfusing the newly anastomosed colon with a diet containing the fibre pectin, or its fermentation products, short chain fatty acids, promotes colonic healing and produces a stronger anastomosis.

Fistulas

The treatment of *bowel fistulas* by enteral nutrition is still controversial and in a review Rombeau and Rolandelli (1987) emphasized the importance of careful patient selection. They also emphasized that mortality and spontaneous closure rates were comparable to those patients treated with TPN, and that elemental diets offered no clear advantage over polymeric diets. Enteral nutrition would seem to be indicated for oesophageal, gastric and high small bowel fistulas if distal access is possible, and otherwise for low output ileal and colocutaneous fistulas.

Intensive therapy units

Patients on intensive therapy units (ITU) who require nutritional support often require artificial ventilation. In our experience the majority of these patients will tolerate enteral feeding. In our unit the underlying pathological process determines whether enteral or total parenteral nutrition is initially prescribed. In general, total parenteral nutrition is prescribed after extensive gastrointestinal surgery or in the presence of major abdominal sepsis. The absence of bowel sounds in ITU patients is not a contraindication to enteral feeding (Shelley and Church, 1987). Enteral nutrition *is* however contraindicated in the presence of gross abdominal distension, or if there are more than 400 ml of gastric aspirate in 24 hours (Payne-James et al, 1987a). If abdominal distension or a high volume gastric aspirate is not present and the patient is unlikely to be able to feed normally for a minimum of 72 hours, then enteral nutrition should be commenced as early as possible. For the first 24 hours 2-hourly gastric aspiration is undertaken and if the volume of feed aspirated back is more than 100 ml then the rate of infusion is decreased or stopped temporarily. If there is clearly little residual volume of feed after 24 hours regular aspiration then the 2-hourly aspiration can be abandoned.

MANAGEMENT OF ENTERAL FEEDING

Administration techniques

Despite the theoretical reasons for using particular diets in particular circumstances, none of this theory is appropriate if the administration of the diet into the patient's gut fails for some technical reason. Techniques of administration are vitally important as studies have indicated that as much as one third of the prescribed diet may not be administered to the patient because of technical problems (Keohane et al, 1983a; Rees et al, 1986b). A number of factors account for this. Table 4 lists some of the factors that may affect nutritional intake and which should therefore be considered for each patient's particular circumstances prior to commencing enteral nutrition.

Table 4. Factors to be considered prior to commencing enteral nutrition.

Factor	What options?

Route	Pernasal (fine-bore tube) — nasogastric
	                                 — nasoduodenal
	                                 — nasojejunal
	Pharyngostomy
	Oesophagostomy
	Gastrostomy — percutaneous endoscopic
	                           — surgical
	Jejunostomy — needle catheter
	                           — surgical

Reservoir & Giving sets	Bag? Bottle? Volume?
Infusion v. bolus	Continuous? Intermittent? Pump?
Starter regimens	Yes? No?

Route

Nasoenteral tubes

The wide variety of techniques now available for gaining access to the gastrointestinal tract, mean that there are very few patients, with normal or near-normal gastrointestinal function, in whom enteral feeding is impossible. The use of fine-bore nasoenteral tubes was pioneered in the United Kingdom by McMichael (Brown, 1979). Many of the complications associated with the use of larger bore Ryle's type tube, such as rhinitis, pharyngitis, oesophagitis, oesophageal strictures, gastritis and upper gastrointestinal haemorrhage are no longer seen. A prospective study of 340 debilitated patients intubated pernasally at the bedside showed an incidence of malposition into the airways in 2.4% of subjects with other complications in 7.6% of patients, including three episodes of massive pulmonary aspiration of feed (Ghahremani and Gould, 1986). The presence of a stylet to stiffen the tube has resulted in sporadic reports of pneumothorax after tube insertion (Eldar and Meguid, 1984) and oesophageal perforation (James, 1978). Guidelines to avoid these complications have been suggested, including the use of fine-bore tubes where the stylet cannot exit proximally through a side port, tube insertion to be undertaken by staff trained in the technique, and confirmatory X-rays to be obtained after insertion in conscious and alert patients if either auscultation or aspiration of gastric contents through the tube is impossible. In patients with altered consciousness, an altered cough or gag reflex or who are on a ventilator, then X-ray is mandatory (Payne-James et al, 1987b). One of the major problems with nasoenteral tubes is unplanned or non-elective extubations which occur with distressing frequency, in up to 62% of patients in some series (Keohane et al, 1983a; Keohane et al, 1986; Rees et al, 1986c; Meer, 1987). The major reason, accounting for between 50% and 90% of non-elective extubations is accidental or deliberate removal by the patient. Many different techniques for retaining tubes have been suggested including the 'bridle' described by Armstrong et al (1980). The most effective technique is regular patient surveillance (Payne-James JJ, Rees RG, Doherty J and Silk DBA – personal observation). Some workers have advocated the use of tubes with a weight incorporated at the distal end, but recent studies do not support the theory that addition of a weight prolongs length of tube usage (Keohane et al, 1986; Payne-James et al, 1988a). As the ability to aspirate through the nasoenteral tube is desirable, studies were undertaken to compare a standard polyvinylchloride tube with a newly designed tube constructed of polyurethane coated with water-activated lubricant and with a modified outflow port at the distal end (Corpak Co., Wheeling, Illinois, USA). In a prospective randomized controlled trial it was shown that aspiration of gastric luminal contents was achieved in a significantly higher percentage of occasions with the new outflow port, and in addition the new tube remained in position significantly longer than the standard tube (Rees et al, 1986c).

Nasogastric versus nasoduodenal/jejunal feeding

In the majority of patients nasogastric delivery of nutrients is the route of choice. In some patients however, nasogastric feeding is relatively contraindicated, e.g. in those with gastric atony or gastroparesis. Neurosurgical patients, diabetic patients (with neuropathy), severely hypothyroid patients, ventilated patients, postoperative patients are all examples where nasoduodenal or nasojejunal feeding might be indicated to reduce the risk of regurgitation and pulmonary aspiration of feed (Kiver et al, 1984). Many authors have described techniques for achieving intubation of the duodenum/jejunum pernasally, and these include fluoroscopic placement (Hatfield and Beck, 1981), endoscopic placement (Keohane et al, 1982b), using metoclopramide (Whatley et al, 1984; Kittinger et al, 1987), and a manipulative technique at the bedside (Thurlow, 1986). These techniques have met with variable success, generally more successful in the authors' hands than in others. It had been observed that some tubes of adequate length would pass spontaneously into the duodenum/jejunum after a time, and clearly a suitable tube would simplify the technique of post-pyloric feeding. Three specially lengthened tubes of the type described earlier (Rees et al, 1986c) were entered into a prospective randomized controlled trial to attempt to find the design most suitable for spontaneous transpyloric passage. Two had weights incorporated into the distal end. The unweighted tube performed better than the two weighted tubes when considering length of time in situ, but varying the tip design did not alter the incidence of spontaneous transpyloric passage of the tube tip (Payne-James et al, 1988a).

Endoscopic placement of the fine-bore tube ensures correct positioning for the patient in whom spontaneous transpyloric passage fails to occur.

Cervical pharyngostomy and oesophagostomy

These techniques have been used for almost 40 years. Klopp (1951) developed oesophagostomy as a technique for feeding patients with oropharyngeal cancer, and this technique was then adapted for patients with neurological disease, trauma and after extensive facial surgery. In general the technique has been performed under general anaesthetic, but Bucklin and Gilsdorf (1985) described a technique to be undertaken at the bedside under local anaesthetic, for patients requiring long-term or indefinite nutritional support. This technique allowed a fine-bore tube to be passed percutaneously into the pharynx and down into the stomach with a minimum of discomfort. Indications for this technique are now limited as the percutaneous endoscopic gastrostomy described below is probably more appropriate for long-term feeding.

Gastrostomy

Gastrostomies may be fashioned surgically at the time of a concurrent surgical procedure to allow temporary access to the gastrointestinal tract for drainage or feeding. In other cases they may be formed specifically to allow permanent access to the gastrointestinal tract for patients with chronic disease such as multiple sclerosis or stroke, who require long-term feeding. Until recently this procedure required a laparotomy and a general anaesthetic. In 1980 Gauderer et al described a new technique of gastrostomy in which the gastrostomy tube was inserted under local anaesthesia under endoscopic control. This procedure – percutaneous endoscopic gastrostomy (PEG) – has now become well established with a number of different technical variations, and represents a great advance in the care of patients requiring long-term feeding. A gastroscope is passed into the stomach which is then inflated with air. The gastroscope is directed anteriorly and a cannula is introduced under direct vision through the anterior abdominal wall into the stomach, at a point where the endoscope light can be seen. The two commonly used techniques differ at this point, in that either a strong suture is pushed through the cannula into the stomach, the suture being withdrawn through the mouth by the endoscope, or a guide wire is pushed through the cannula into the stomach, the guide wire again being grasped by the endoscope and being withdrawn through the mouth. The gastrostomy tube is either attached to the thread and *pulled* through the oesophagus, into the stomach and out through the abdominal wall and fixed by a flange, or *pushed* into place over the guidewire. In a prospective randomized study (Hogan et al, 1986) of the two techniques, the insertion time was similar, with a mean of 15 minutes. Complications included an episode of aspiration during one procedure, and a death from pulmonary aspiration of gastric contents several days later. Other complications were minor and compare favourably with a surgically placed gastrostomy. Two complications that may be specifically related to this technique are pneumoperitoneum (Plumser et al, 1984), probably arising after failure to correctly fix the gastrostomy tube securely, and necrotizing fasciitis of the anterior abdominal wall (Greif et al, 1986). The cases of necrotizing fasciitis emphasize the importance of the routine use of prophylactic antibiotics during the procedure. A further study (Larson et al, 1987) concluded that this procedure 'is safe and has a low mortality even in patients who are medically debilitated'. Undoubtedly this technique is the procedure of choice for gaining access to the gastrointestinal tract in any patient likely to require long-term or permanent feeding.

Jejunostomy

Jejunostomies may be created at laparotomy as a separate surgical procedure or concurrently with other abdominal surgery. Delaney et al (1973) first described the technique of needle catheter jeunostomy (NCJ). Using this technique a fine catheter is inserted into the jejunum and brought through the anterior abdominal wound wall, away from the laparotomy wound, in order to facilitate postoperative enteral feeding. The technique has a low morbidity with a major complication rate of less than 2% (Page, 1981). The procedure is generally performed in association with major surgery of the gastrointestinal tract to provide access for enteral feeding if there are postoperative problems, or a prolonged convalescence is anticipated. Ryan and Page (1984) in a review of the subject consider that NCJ should be recommended for patients who are malnourished at the time of laparotomy, or who are undergoing major upper gastrointestinal surgery, or who may receive adjuvant radiotherapy or chemotherapy after surgery and for those patients subject to laparotomy after major trauma. Heberer et al (1987) suggest one further group in whom a NCJ is indicated. They recommend inserting the NCJ in patients who *might* require enteral feeding. The decision can then be delayed, but access is available if required. They cite the low incidence of complications as the reason for this practice, and the availability of this route means that total parenteral nutrition with its attendant risks may be avoided. This reason is unlikely to be widely adopted as an indication for insertion of an NCJ.

Reservoirs and giving sets

500 ml glass bottles were originally used for diet administration, but now much larger bags or containers with capacities of up to 3 litres are available for enteral nutrition. Controlled clinical trials comparing containers of different sizes (varying from 500 ml to 2 litres) demonstrated that as little as 70% of *prescribed* diet was administered to the patient using the smaller volume containers, as compared with 85% using the 2 litre pouches (Keohane et al, 1983b; Rees et al, 1986b). The potential dangers of bacterial contamination of these larger containers hanging at room temperature proved unfounded as long as aseptic techniques were used for preparation, although significant microbial contamination of enteral diets is not uncommon (Bastow et al, 1982; De Vries et al, 1983; Keohane et al, 1983b). Giving

sets should be changed every 24 hours to reduce the risk of infective complications, as apart from exogenous contamination, ascending contamination by proximal migration along the feeding tube from the gut has been reported (Van Alsenoy et al, 1985).

Bolus versus infusion (continuous or intermittent)

Although bolus feeding of enteral diet was the accepted technique of administration of feed for many years, in the majority of centres it has been superseded by a continuous infusion, maintained either by gravity or a mechanical pump. In this way feeds are not omitted, and considerable nursing time is saved (Allison et al, 1979). Despite the arguments that bolus feeding is more physiological, it has a greater incidence of side-effects, such as regurgitation and diarrhoea. Two studies directly comparing intermittent and continuous infusion of enteral diet both support the technique of continuous infusion (Parker et al, 1981; Hiebert et al, 1981). For patients who are immobile or who are confined to bed, a continuous infusion of approximately 2 litres of diet over 24 hours is appropriate. Our practice is to have the head of the patient's bed elevated to 20 or 30° to prevent regurgitation and aspiration. Bastow et al (1985) have demonstrated the practicalities of overnight tube feeding in certain groups of patients, and a further study (Pinchovsky–Devin and Kaminski, 1985) has shown improved nutritional parameters in patients fed continuously for 16 hours and then fasted for 8 hours. This may well be the ideal technique for the majority of mobile in-patients requiring enteral nutrition, as they can be disconnected from the pump and their tube spigotted for a substantial part of the day. The main practical problem with overnight or interrupted feeding is the increased frequency of micturition related to the fluid load.

Starter regimens

The technique of using small volume, diluted enteral diets when commencing enteral feeding, in order to reduce the incidence of gastrointestinal side-effects is still utilized although not for any valid reasons. Two studies have conclusively demonstrated that the only measurable effect of starter regimens over the first three or four days of enteral feeding is to reduce nutrient intake and adversely affect nitrogen balance (Keohane et al, 1984; Rees et al, 1986d). At present, enteral feeding is commenced in the majority of patients in this unit by administering 2 litres of full strength feed in the first 24 hours.

Monitoring

Diet charts

It is essential that an accurate record of enteral feed administered to a patient is recorded. For the many reasons discussed earlier, prescribed diet does not necessarily equate to administered diet. A standardized diet administration form is extremely useful in following a patient's progress. In addition, a patient's oral intake must be assessed so that an appropriate time for cessation of enteral feeding can be decided.

Weight

Regular weighing of the patient is probably the single most useful test of the adequacy of enteral nutrition. Maintenance of a steady weight, or in the case of the severely malnourished, a gradual increase in weight being the object of the therapy.

Anthropometric and dynamometric measurements

These techniques have been used generally as research tools. However they can, over a period of weeks and months, demonstrate very effectively responses to therapy. In the short term, in most clinical situations, their value is limited. Dynamometry has been shown to be a useful predictor for malnutrition that may predispose to serious postoperative morbidity (Klidjian et al, 1980).

Biochemical measurements

In the initial stages of enteral nutritional support careful watch should be kept for manifestations of hyperglycaemia. Twelve-hourly BM Stix or Dextrostix provide adequate information. The plasma electrolytes should be estimated at least twice weekly, and in severely malnourished patients who are being refed, these and calcium and phosphate should be measured daily for at least a week, or until the patient is stable. Acute hypophosphataemia after refeeding in the severely malnourished has long been recognized as a cause of respiratory failure or sudden death in patients being parenterally fed. It is now clear that this abnormality may also become manifest with potentially fatal consequences after refeeding by the enteral route (Payne-James et al, 1988b). Plasma zinc and magnesium levels should be estimated at the outset and corrected if abnormal. Urinary electrolytes and 24 hour urinary urea excretion are valuable, particularly for estimating nitrogen balance. The plasma proteins, albumin, transferrin and thyroid binding pre-albumin (TBPA) are good biochemical markers for response to feeding (Church and Hill, 1987; Fletcher et al, 1987). Transferrin and TBPA are useful in the short term and albumin, because of its longer half-life, over a period of three weeks or more. Trace elements such as selenium and other assays such as vitamin E levels are not undertaken unless clinically indicated.

Urinary urea can be used to calculate the estimated nitrogen excretion, and thus determine nitrogen balance. Direct urinary nitrogen measurement is the most accurate way of determining nitrogen loss, and has been demonstrated to correlate poorly in some patient groups with the estimates achieved indirectly using the urinary urea measurements (Steinhorn and Radmer, 1986; Grimble et al, 1988). Other losses, such as from fistulae or drain sites must also be considered, as considerable nitrogen loss may occur from these sites.

PREVENTION AND TREATMENT OF COMPLICATIONS

Complications of enteral feeding can be divided into three main groups (see Table 5).

Table 5. Complications of enteral nutrition.

1. Tube related	malposition
	unwanted removal
	blockage
2. Diet related	diarrhoea
	bloating
	abdominal distension
	nausea
	cramps
	regurgitation
	pulmonary aspiration
	drug interactions
	vitamin, mineral, trace element, essential fatty acid deficiencies
3. Metabolic/biochemical	see text

Tube related

No matter what type of tube is used for access to the gastrointestinal tract, all have the ability to fall out, become displaced or blocked, necessitating replacement. In some cases, such as needle catheter jejunostomies, replacement is impossible without a further laparotomy. Meticulous care is therefore required in the use of all these feeding tubes, particularly with regard to both fixation and maintaining patency. All unused tubes should be flushed at regular intervals during the day to prevent occlusion. Malposition of tubes at insertion will be avoided by attention to correct technique, and in the case of the pernasally inserted nasoenteral tubes, by following the guidelines mentioned earlier and always confirming the position with an X-ray if in doubt.

Diet related

If the techniques of administration of diet outlined above are adhered to, the classical diet-related symptoms of diarrhoea, abdominal cramps, bloating, abdominal distension and nausea should be avoided. Although the generally accepted causes for enteral feed related diarrhoea are osmolality and lactose intolerance, the most significant relationship between diarrhoea and enteral feeding is in those patients on concurrent antibiotic therapy (Keohane et al, 1984). If diarrhoea is a persistent problem and/or if antibiotic therapy cannot be stopped, then symptomatic relief can be obtained using loperamide or codeine phosphate. The most dangerous and potentially fatal complications of enteral feeding are undoubtedly regurgitation and pulmonary aspiration of feed. These are avoided by feeding post-pylorically in patients at risk of gastric atony or paresis, or in those patients with altered consciousness or a suppressed gag reflex. Elevating the head of the bed by 20 or 30° when diet infusion is in progress is considered useful. In cases where gastric stasis or pooling is suspected, 2-hourly aspiration is appropriate. If there is more than 100 ml of aspirate the feed rate should be decreased or stopped. Once the aspirate has reduced to less than 400 ml in 24 hours, no further aspiration is required. In some cases metoclopramide is beneficial by promoting gastric emptying. It is common practice to administer drugs, in crushed tablet or liquid form with enteral diets. Two recent reports (Watson et al, 1984; Holtz et al, 1987) have shown the dangers of adding particular drugs – theophylline, digoxin, methyldopa and warfarin – to enteral diets. The lesson is to have a high index of suspicion about drug interactions with enteral diets if a patient fails to respond to a particular medication.

Metabolic complications

In a study of 100 patients undergoing tube feeding, Vanlandingham et al (1981) found a surprisingly wide range of biochemical abnormalities in a high proportion of patients. These include hyperkalaemia in 40%, hypophosphataemia in 30% and hyperglycaemia in 29%. Other abnormalities recorded included hypokalaemia, hyperphosphataemia, hypomagnesaemia and hypozincaemia. Nearly 50% of the subjects studied had previously been in the Intensive Care Unit. Their recommendations included regular monitoring along similar lines to those described earlier. Certainly it is important to look for these abnormalities and review regularly until the patient is completely stable.

Enteral nutrition team

Undoubtedly awareness of potential complications allows anticipation and prevention, but the idea of an enteral nutritional support team well versed in the practice and management of enteral feeding techniques has rarely formally been considered. The benefits of a Total Parenteral Nutrition Team are well documented (Nehme, 1980; Dalton et al, 1984). Brown et al (1987) report a prospective study comparing team versus non-team management of enterally fed patients. The conclusion reached was that team management reduces associated morbidity and optimizes nutrient delivery in patients receiving enteral nutrition. Considering that up to 80% of patients requiring nutritional support will require enteral rather than total parenteral nutrition, it would seem appropriate to encourage the development of such specialized teams.

SUMMARY

Enteral nutrition is only part of the wider field of clinical nutrition in which great advances in both theory and practice have been made over the last decade. We have attempted to summarize what we consider to be the advances that have most relevance to the clinical practice of enteral nutrition. This chapter reviews our present understanding of the processes of digestion and absorption of protein, carbohydrate and fats, and examines how this theoretical understanding can be applied to patients in the clinical situation. A broad classification of the different enteral diets is undertaken, and the reasons for the development of particular diets are discussed. The clinical value of these diets is assessed. The wide variety of indications for enteral (as opposed to parenteral) nutrition are discussed and the specific benefits of enteral nutrition for the patient are highlighted. Techniques of administration of enteral nutrition are reviewed in detail, and the methods by which enteral nutrition should be monitored are outlined. Finally, complications of enteral nutrition are summarized and advice given on how to prevent or treat them.

REFERENCES

Abel RM, Beck CH, Abbot WM et al (1973) Improved survival from renal failure after treatment with intravenous essential L-amino acids and glucose. *New England Journal of Medicine* **288:** 695–699.

Adibi SA (1971) Intestinal transport of dipeptides in man: relative importance of hydrolysis and intact absorption. *Journal of Clinical Investigation* **50:** 2266–2275.

Adibi SA & Mercer DW (1973) Protein digestion in human intestine as reflected in luminal mucosal and plasma amino acid concentrations after meals. *Journal of Clinical Investigation* **53:** 1586–1594.

Adibi SA & Soleimanpoor MR (1974) Functional characterization of depeptide transport system in human jejunum. *Journal of Clinical Investigation* **53:** 1368–1374.

Adibi SA, Morse EL, Masilamani S & Amin P (1975) Evidence for two different modes of tripeptide disappearance in human intestine, uptake by peptide carrier systems and hydrolases. *Journal of Clinical Investigation* **56:** 1355–1363.

Allison SP (1986). Some psychological and physiological aspects of enteral nutrition. *Gut* **27 (supplement 1):** 18–24.

Allison SP, Walford S, Todorovic V & Elliott ET (1979) Practical aspects of nutritional support. *Research and Clinical Forums* **1:** 49–57.

Andersson H, Hulten L, Magnusson O & Sandstrom B (1984) Energy and mineral utilization from a peptide-based elemental diet and a polymeric enteral diet given to ileostomists in the early postoperative course. *Journal of Parenteral and Enteral Nutrition* **8:** 497–500.

Armstrong C, Luther W & Sykes T (1980) A technique for preventing extubation of feeding tubes. 'The bridle'. *Journal of Parenteral and Enteral Nutrition* **4:** 603.

Asatoor AM, Cheng B, Edwards KDG et al (1970) Intestinal absorption of two dipeptides in Hartnup disease, *Gut* **11:** 380–387.

Asatoor AM, Harrison BDW, Milne MD & Prosser DI (1972) Intestinal absorption of an arginine containing peptide in cystinuria. *Gut* **13:** 95–98.

Askanasi J, Rosenbaum SH, Hyman AI et al (1980) Respiratory changes induced by the large glucose loads of parenteral nutrition. *Journal of the American Medical Association* **243:** 1444–1447.

Bastow MD, Allison SP & Greaves P (1982) Microbial contamination of nasogastric feeds. *Human Nutrition and Applied Nutrition* **36A:** 213–217.

Bastow D, Rawlings J & Allison SP (1985) Overnight nasogastric tube feeding. *Clinical Nutrition* **4:** 7–11.

Biederdoft FA, Morawski S & Fordtran JS (1975) Effect of sodium, mannitol and magnesium on glucose, galactose, 3–0 methylglucose and fructose absorption in the human ileum. *Gastroenterology* **68:** 58–66.

Bistrian BR, Blackburn GL, Hallowell E & Heddle R (1974) Protein status of general surgical patients. *Journal of the American Medical Association* **230:** 858.

Bistrian BR, Blackburn GL, Vitale J et al (1976) Prevalence of malnutrition in general medical patients. *Journal of the American Medical Association* **235:** 1597.

Blomquist P, Jiborn H & Zederfeldt B (1984) The effect of relative bowel rest on collagen metabolism and suture holding capacity in the colonic wall. *Research and Experimental Medicine* **184:** 221–226.

Blomquist P, Jiborn H & Zederfeldt B (1985) Effect of diverting colostomy on breaking strength of anastomoses after resection of the left side of the colon. *American Journal of Surgery* **149:** 712–715.

Boles T Jr & Zollinger RM (1952) Critical evaluation of jejunostomy. *Archives of Surgery* **65:** 358–366.

Brown JM (1979) Narrow bore naso-gastric feeding. *Anaesthesia* **34:** 368–369.

Brown RO, Carlson SD, Cowan GSM, Powers DA & Luther RW (1987) Enteral nutritional support management in a university teaching hospital: team vs nonteam. *Journal of Parenteral and Enteral Nutrition* **11:** 52–56.

Bucklin DL & Gilsdorf RB (1985) Percutaneous needle pharyngostomy. *Journal of Parenteral and Enteral Nutrition* **9:** 68–70.

Bunker VW & Clayton BE (1983) Trace element content of commercial enteral feeds. *Lancet* **ii:** 426–428.

Cerra F, Mayusky J, Chute E et al (1984) Branched chain metabolic support: a prospective randomised double-blind trial in surgical stress. *Annals of Surgery* **3:** 286–290.

Chen ML, Rogers QR & Harper AG (1962) Observations on protein digestion in vivo: IV further observations on the gastrointestinal contents of rats fed different dietary proteins. *Journal of Nutrition* **76:** 235–241.

Chung YC, Kim YS, Shadchehr A, Garrido A, MacGregor IL & Sleisenger MH (1979) Protein digestion and absorption in human small intestine. *Gastroenterology* **76:** 1415–1421.

Church JM & Hill GL (1987) Assessing the efficacy of intravenous nutrition in general surgical patients: dynamic nutritional assessment with plasma proteins. *Journal of Parenteral and Enteral Nutrition* **11:** 135–139.

Cook GC (1973) Comparison of absorption rates of glucose and maltose in man in vivo. *Clinical Science* **44:** 425–428.

Courtney Moore M, Greene HL, Donald WD & Dunn GD (1986) Enteral tube feeding as adjunct therapy in malnourished patients with cystic fibrosis: clinical studies and literature review. *American Journal of Clinical Nutrition* **44:** 33–41.

Covelli HD, Black JW, Oslen MS & Beekman JF (1981) Respiratory failure precipitated by high carbohydrate loads. *Annals of Internal Medicine* **95:** 579–591.

Craft IL, Geddes D, Hyde CW, Wise IJ & Matthews DM (1968) Absorption and malabsorption of glycine and glycine peptides in man. *Gut* **9:** 425–437.

Curtis KJ, Kim YC, Perdonna JM, Silk DBA & Whitehead JS (1978) Protein absorption and digestion in the rat. *Journal of Physiology* **274:** 409–419.

Cynober L, Saizy R, Dinh FD, Lioret N & Giboudeau I (1984) Effect of enterally administered ornithine alpha-ketoglutarate on plasma and urinary amino acid levels after burn injury. *Journal of Trauma* **24:** 590–596.

Dalton MJ, Schepers G, Gee JP et al (1984) Consultative total parenteral nutrition teams. The effect on the incidence of total parenteral nutrition related complications. *Journal of Parenteral and Enteral Nutrition* **8:** 146–152.

Debnam ES & Levin RJ (1975) An experimental method of identifying and quantifying the active transfer electrogenic component from the diffusional component during sugar absorption measured in vivo. *Journal of Physiology* **246:** 181–196.

Debnam ES & Levin RJ (1976) Influence of specific dietary sugars on the jejunal mechanisms for glucose, galactose and methylglucoside absorption: evidence of multiple sugar carriers. *Gut* **17:** 92–99.

Delaney HM, Carnevale NJ & Garvey JW (1973) Jejunostomy by a needle catheter technique. *Surgery* **73:** 786–790.

De Vries EG, Mulder NH, Houwen B et al (1983) Enteral nutrition by nasogastric tube in adult patients treated with intensive chemotherapy for acute leukaemia. *American Journal of Clinical Nutrition* **35:** 1490–1496.

Dodge JA & Yassa JG (1980) Essential fatty acid deficiency after prolonged treatment with elemental diet. *Lancet* **ii:** 1256–1257.

Drugs and Therapeutics Bulletin (1986) *Enteral feeds for adults: an update* **24:** 61–64.

Dudrick SJ, Wilmore DW, Vars HM & Rhoads JE (1968) Long-term total parenteral nutrition with growth, development, and positive nitrogen balance, *Surgery* **64:** 134–142.

Dudrick SJ, Steiger E & Long JM (1970) Renal failure in surgical patients, treatment with intravenous essential amino acids and hypertonic glucose. *Surgery* **68:** 180–186.

Eldar S & Meguid MM (1984) Pneumothorax following attempted nasogastric intubation for nutritional support. *Journal of Parenteral and Enteral Nutrition* **8:** 450–452.

Esteve M, Fernandez-Banares F, Cabre E et al (1987) The effect of total enteral nutrition as the unique nutritional support in patients with gastrointestinal fistulas. *Clinical Nutrition* **6 (supplement) P78:** 93.

Fairclough PD, Silk DBA, Webb JPW, Clark ML & Dawson AM (1977) A reappraisal of osmotic evidence for intact peptide absorption. *Clinical Science and Molecular Medicine* **53:** 241–248.

Fick TE, van Rooyen W, Schattenkerk ME et al (1986) A nonelemental versus an elemental diet for early postoperative enteral feeding by needle catheter jejunostomy. *Clinical Nutrition* **5:** 105–107.

Fischer JE & Baldessarini RJ (1971) False neurotransmitters and hepatic failure. *Lancet* **ii:** 75–79.

Fletcher JP & Little JM (1986) A comparison of parenteral nutrition and early postoperative enteral feeding on the nitrogen balance after major surgery. *Surgery* **100:** 21–24.

Fletcher JP, Little JM & Guest PK (1987) A comparison of serum transferrin and serum prealbumin as nutritional parameters. *Journal of Parenteral and Enteral Nutrition* **11:** 144–147.

Forstner G, Gall G, Corey M et al (1980) *Proceedings of the 8th International Congress of Cystic Fibrosis*, pp 137–138. Toronto: Canadian Cystic Fibrosis Foundation.

Freund HR, Yoshimura N & Fischer JE (1979) Infusion of the branched chain amino acids in post-operative patients. *Annals of Surgery* **190:** 18–22.

Gauderer MWL, Ponsky JL & Izant RJ (1980) Gastrostomy without laparotomy: a percutaneous endoscopic technique. *Journal of Pediatric Surgery* **15:** 872–875.

Ghahremani GG & Gould RJ (1986) Nasoenteric feeding tubes: radiographic detection of complications. *Digestive Diseases and Sciences* **31:** 574–585.

Gonzales-Huix F, Abad-Lacruz A, Esteve M et al (1987) TPN vs TEN in the management of acute attacks of inflammatory bowel disease: a prospective, randomised study. *Clinical Nutrition* **6 (supplement) P32:** 70.

Gracey M, Burke V & Oshin A (1972) Transport of fructose by the intestine. In Burland WL & Samuel PD (eds) *Transport Across the Intestine* pp 99–104. Edinburgh: Churchill Livingstone.

Green C, Tredger J & Dickerson (1987) Enteral feeding: a survey to investigate current practices and attitudes of dietitians. *Human Nutrition: Applied Nutrition* **41A:** 360–363.

Greif JM, Ragland JJ, Ochsner MG & Riding R (1986) Fatal necrotizing fasciitis complicating percutaneous endoscopic gastrostomy. *Gastrointestinal Endoscopy* **32:** 292–296.

Grimble GK, West MFE, Acuti ABC et al (1988) Assessment of an automated chemiluminescence nitrogen analyzer for routine use in clinical nutrition. *Journal of Parenteral and Enteral Nutrition* **12:** 100–106.

Hamosh M, Klaeveman HL, Wolf RD & Scow RD (1975) Pharyngeal lipase and digestion of dietary triglyceride in man. *Journal of Clinical Investigation* **55:** 908–913.

Hashim SA (1967). Medium chain triglycerides: clinical and metabolic aspects. *Journal of the American Dietetics Association* **57:** 221–227.

Hatfield DR & Beck JL (1981) An improved technique for feeding tube placement. *Radiology* **141:** 823.

Haverberg L, Kwon PH & Scrimshaw NS (1980) Comparative tolerance of adolescents of differing ethnic backgrounds to lactose-containing and lactose-free dairy drinks. Initial experience with a double-blind procedure. *American Journal of Clinical Nutrition* **33:** 17–21.

Haydock DA & Hill GL (1986) Impaired wound healing in surgical patients with varying degrees of malnutrition. *Journal of Parenteral and Enteral Nutrition* **10**: 550–554.

Haydock DA & Hill GL (1987) Improved wound healing response in surgical patients receiving intravenous nutrition. *British Journal of Surgery* **74**: 320–323.

Heberer M, Bodoky A, Iwatschenko P & Harder F (1987) Indications for needle catheter jejunostomy in elective abdominal surgery. *American Journal of Surgery* **153**: 545–552.

Heimburger DC & Weinsier RL (1985) Guidelines for evaluating and categorizing enteral feeding formulas according to therapeutic equivalence. *Journal of Parenteral and Enteral Nutrition* **9**: 61–67.

Hellier, MD, Holdsworth CD, McColl I & Perrett D (1972) Dipetide absorption in man. *Gut* **13**: 965–969.

Heymsfield SB, Bethel RA, Ansley JD, Nixon DW & Rudman D (1979) Enteral hyperalimentation: an alternative to central venous hyperalimentation. *Annals of Internal Medicine* **90**: 63–71.

Heymsfield SB, Head CA, McManus CB et al (1984) Respiratory, cardiovascular, and metabolic effects of enteral hyperalimentation: influence of formula dose and composition. *American Journal of Clinical Nutrition* **40**: 116–130.

Hiebert JM, Brown A, Anderson RG et al (1981) Comparison of continuous versus intermittent tube feeding in adult burn patients. *Journal of Parenteral and Enteral Nutrition* **5**: 73–75.

Hill GL, Pickford I, Young GA et al (1977) Malnutrition in surgical patients. *Lancet* i: 689–692.

Hogan RB, DeMarco DC, Hamilton JK, Walker CO & Polter DE (1986) Percutaneous endoscopic gastrostomy – to push or pull. *Gastrointestinal Endoscopy* **32**: 253–259.

Holtz L, Milton J & Sturex JK (1987) Compatibility of medications with enteral feedings. *Journal of Parenteral and Enteral Nutrition* **11**: 183–186.

Hoover HC, Ryan JA, Anderson EJ & Fischer JE (1980) Nutritional benefits of immediate postoperative jejunal feeding of an elemental diet. *American Journal of Surgery* **139**: 153–159.

Hueckel HJ & Rodgers QR (1970) Urinary excretion of hydroxyproline-containing peptides in man, rat, hamster, dog, and monkey after feeding gelatin. *Comparative Biochemistry and Physiology* **32**: 7–16.

Iapichino G, Radazzani D, Bonetti G et al (1985) Parenteral nutrition of injured patients: effect of manipulation of amino acid infusion (increasing branched chain while decreasing aromatic and sulphated amino acids) *Clinical Nutrition* **4**: 121–123.

James RH (1978) An unusual complication of passing a narrow bore nasogastric tube. *Anaesthesia* **33**: 76.

Johansson C (1975) Characteristics of the absorption pattern of sugar, fat and protein from composite meals in man: a quantitative study. *Scandinavian Journal of Endocrinology* **10**: 33–42.

Jones BJM (1984) *Glucose-polymer-saline absorption from the human jejunum*, MD thesis, University of London.

Jones BJM (1987) Nutritional management of short bowel syndrome. *Journal of Clinical Nutrition and Gastroenterology* **2**: 99–103.

Jones BJM, Brown BE, Spiller RC & Silk DBA (1981) Energy dense enteral feeds – the use of high molecular weight glucose polymers. *Journal of Parenteral and Enteral Nutrition* **5**: 567.

Jones BJM, Lees R, Andrews J, Frost P & Silk DBA (1983) Comparison of an elemental and polymeric enteral diet in patients with normal gastrointestinal function. *Gut* **24**: 78–84.

Jones BJM, Brown BE, Loran JS et al (1984) Glucose absorption from starch hydrolysates in the human jejunum. *Gut* **24**: 1152–1160.

Jones BJM, Higgins BE & Silk DBA (1987) Glucose absorption from maltotriose and glucose oligomers in the human jejunum. *Clinical Science* **72**: 409–414.

Josefsson L & Lindberg T (1967) Intestinal dipeptidases IX. Studies on dipeptidases of human intestinal mucosa. *Acta Chemica Scandinavica* **21**: 1965–1966.

Kelly JJ & Alpers DH (1973) Properties of human intestinal gluco-amylase. *Biochemica et Biophysica Acta* **315**: 113–120.

Keohane PP, Brown BE, Grimble GK & Silk DBA (1981) The peptide nitrogen source of elemental diets: comparisons of absorptive properties of five partial enzymic hydrolysates of whole protein. *Journal of Parenteral and Enteral Nutrition* **5**: A61 568.

Keohane PP, Grimble GK, Brown BE, Kaminski MV & Silk DBA (1982a) Influence of peptide chain length on absorption from protein hydrolysates in man. *Journal of Parenteral and Enteral Nutrition* **6:** A28 578.

Keohane PP, Attrill H & Silk DBA (1982b) Endoscopic placement of fine bore nasogastric and nasoenteric feeding tubes. *Clinical Nutrition* **1:** 245–247.

Keohane PP, Attrill H, Jones BJM & Silk DBA (1983a) Limitations and drawbacks of 'fine bore' nasogastric feeding tubes. *Clinical Nutrition* **2:** 85–86.

Keohane PP, Attrill H, Love M, Frost P & Silk DBA (1983b) A controlled trial of aseptic enteral diet preparation – significant effects on bacterial contamination and nitrogen balance. *Clinical Nutrition* **2:** 119–122.

Keohane PP, Attrill H, Love M, Frost P & Silk DBA (1984) Relation between osmolality of diet and gastrointestinal side effects in enteral nutrition. *British Medical Journal* **228:** 678–680.

Keohane PP, Attrill H & Silk DBA (1986) Clinical effectiveness of weighted and unweighted 'fine-bore' nasogastric feeding tubes in enteral nutrition: a controlled clinical trial. *Journal of Clinical Nutrition and Gastroenterology* **1:** 189–193.

Kittinger JW, Sandler RS & Heizer WD (1987) Efficacy of metoclopramide as an adjunct to duodenal placement of small-bore feeding tubes: a randomized, placebo-controlled double-blind study. *Journal of Parenteral and Enteral Nutrition* **11:** 33–37.

Kiver KF, Hayes DP, Fortin DF, Main BS (1984) Pre- and post-pyloric enteral feeding: analysis of safety and complications. *Journal of Parenteral and Enteral Nutrition* **8:** 95.

Klidjian AM, Foster KJ, Kammerling RM, Cooper A & Karran SJ (1980) Relation of anthropometric and dynamometric variables to serious postoperative complications. *British Medical Journal* **281:** 899–901.

Klopp CT (1951) Cervical esophagostomy. *Journal of Cardiovascular Surgery* **21:** 490.

Kwon PH, Rorick MH & Scrimshaw NS (1980) Comparative tolerance of adolescents of differing ethnic backgrounds to lactose-containing and lactose-free dairy drinks II. Improvement of a double blind test. *American Journal of Clinical Nutrition* **33:** 22–26.

Lane AE, Silk DBA & Clark ML (1975) Absorption of two proline-containing peptides by rat small intestine in vivo. *Journal of Physiology* **248:** 143–149.

Larson DE, Burton DD, Schroeder KW & DiMagno EP (1987) Percutaneous endoscopic gastrostomy: indications, success, complications and mortality in 314 consecutive patients. *Gastroenterology* **93:** 48–52.

Leander U, Furst P, Vesterberg K & Vinnars E (1985) Nitrogen sparing effect of Ornicetil in the immediate postoperative state: clinical biochemistry and nitrogen balance. *Clinical Nutrition* **4:** 43–51.

MacBurney MM & Young LS (1984) Formulas. In Rombeau JL & Caldwell MD (eds) *Enteral and Tube Feeding*, pp 171–198. Philadelphia: WB Saunders Company.

McIntyre PB, Fitchew M & Lennard-Jones JE (1986) Patients with a high jejunostomy do not need a special diet. *Gastroenterology* **91:** 25–33.

Matthews DM (1975) Intestinal absorption of peptides. *Physiological Reviews* **55:** 537–608.

Matthews DM & Adibi SA (1976) Peptide absorption. *Gastroenterology* **71:** 151–161.

Matthews DM & Burston D (1984) Uptake of a series of neutral dipeptides including L-alanyl-L-alanine, glycylglycine and glycylsarcosine by hamster jejunum in vitro. *Clinical Science* **67:** 541–549.

Matthews DM & Payne JW (1980) Transmembrane transport of small peptides. *Current Topics In Membranes and Transport* **14:** 331–425.

Meer JA (1987) Inadvertent dislodgement of nasoenteral feeding tubes: incidence and prevention. *Journal of Parenteral and Enteral Nutrition* **11:** 187–189.

Merkle NM, Wiedeck H, Herfarth Ch & Grunert A (1984). Die unmittelbare postoperative enterale Sondenernahrung nach Dickdarmresektion. *Chirurg* **55:** 267–274.

Mertes N, Puchstein C, Zander J, Mangold J & Furst P (1987) Ornithine alpha-ketoglutarate improves nitrogen balance in septic or polytraumatized patients. *Clinical Nutrition* **6:** (supplement) P85: 97.

Michel H, Oge P & Bertrand L (1971) Action de l'alpha ketoglutarate d'ornithine sur l'hyper-ammoniemic du cirrhotique. *Presse Médecine* **79:** 867–868.

Millar PJ, Oyesiku JEJ, Muller DPR & Harries JT (1977) Fructose absorption and the effects of other monosaccharides on its absorption in the rat jejunum in vitro. *Gut* **18:** A425.

Moriarty KJ, Hegarty JE, Fairclough PD et al (1985) Relative nutritional value of whole protein, hydrolysed protein and free amino acids in man. *Gut* **26:** 694–699.

Moss G (1984) Efficient gastroduodenal decompression with simultaneous full enteral nutrition: a new gastrostomy catheter technique. *Journal of Parenteral and Enteral Nutrition* **8:** 203–208.

Nachlas MM, Younis MT, Roda CP et al (1972) Gastrointestinal studies as a guide to postoperative management. *Annals of Surgery* **175:** 510–522.

Nawab F & Asatoor AM (1970) Studies on intestinal absorption of amino acids and a dipeptide in a case of Hartnup disease. *Gut* **11:** 373–379.

Neale G (1968) The diagnosis, incidence and significance of disaccharidase deficiency in adults. *Proceedings of the Royal Society of Medicine* **61:** 1099–1117.

Nehme AE (1980) Nutritional support of the hospitalized patient; the team concept. *Journal of the American Medical Association* **24:** 1906–1908.

Neithercut WD, Smith ADS, McAllister JM & La Ferla GA (1987) Nutritional survey of patients in a general surgical ward: is there an effective predictor of malnutrition? *Journal of Clinical Pathology* **40:** 803–807.

Nicholson JA & Peters TJ (1977a) Subcellular distribution of di- and tri-peptide activity in human jejunum. *Clinical Science and Molecular Medicine* **52:** 16.

Nicholson JA & Peters TJ (1977b) Subcellular distribution of di-, tri-, tetra- and pentapeptidase in human digestion *Gut* **18:** A969-A961.

Nixon SE & Mawer GE (1970a) The digestion and absorption of proteins in man 1. The site of absorption. *British Journal of Nutrition* **24:** 227–240.

Nixon SE & Mawer GE (1970b) The digestion and absorption of protein in man 2. The form in which digested protein is absorbed. *British Journal of Nutrition* **24:** 241–258.

O'Keefe SJD, Adam JK, Cakata E & Epstein S (1984). Nutritional support of malnourished lactose intolerant African patients. *Gut* **25:** 942–947.

O'Keefe SJD, Young GD & Rund J (1988) Lactose intolerance and the malnourished African. *Journal of Parenteral and Enteral Nutrition* **12:** supplement A57.

O'Morain C, Segal AW & Levi AJ (1980) Elemental diets in treatment of acute Crohn's disease. *British Medical Journal* **281:** 1173–1175.

O'Morain C, Segal AW & Levi AJ (1984) Elemental diets in treatment of acute Crohn's disease; a controlled trial. *British Medical Journal* **288:** 1859–1862.

Page CP (1981) Needle catheter jejunostomy. *Contemporary Surgery* **19:** 29–47.

Pareira MD, Conrad EJ, Hicks W & Elman R (1954) Therapeutic nutrition with tube feeding. *Journal of the American Medical Association* **156:** 810–816.

Parker P, Stroop S & Green H (1981) A controlled comparison of continuous versus intermittent enteral feeding in the treatment of infants with intestinal disease. *Journal of Pediatrics* **99:** 360–364.

Pasurka B, Filler D & Kahle M (1984) Enterale Ernährung nach Colonresektionen. *Chirurg* **55:** 275–279.

Payne-James JJ, Rees RG & Silk DBA (1987a) Bowel sounds. *Anaesthesia* **42:** 893–894.

Payne-James JJ, Rees RG & Silk DBA (1987b) Dangers of placement of narrow bore nasogastric feeding tubes. *Annals of the Royal College of Surgeons of England* **69:** 251.

Payne-James JJ, Rees RG, King C & Silk DBA (1988a) Enteral tube design and its effect on spontaneous transpyloric passage and duration of tube usage. *Journal of Parenteral and Enteral Nutrition* **12 (supplement) P111.**

Payne-James JJ, Rees RG, Newton M & Silk DBA (1988b). Respiratory failure with acute hypophosphataemia after enteral refeeding in anorexia nervosa. *Journal of Clinical Nutrition and Gastroenterology* (in press).

Pinchovsky-Devin GD & Kaminski MV (1985). Visceral protein increase associated with interrupted versus continuous enteral hyperalimentation. *Journal of Parenteral and Enteral nutrition* **9:** 474–476.

Plumser AB, Gottfried EB & Clair MR (1984) Pneumoperitoneum after percutaneous endoscopic gastrostomy. *American Journal of Gastroenterology* **79:** 440–441.

Rao SSC, Holdworth CD & Forrest ARW (1987) Small intestinal absorption and tolerance of enteral nutrition in acute colitis. *British Medical Journal* **295:** 698.

Rees RG, Grimble GK, Keohane PP et al (1984) Peptide chain length of protein hydrolysates influences jejunal nitrogen absorption. *Gut* **25:** 547.

Rees RG, Cooper TM, Frost PG & Silk DBA (1986a) Influence of energy and nitrogen contents of enteral diets on nitrogen balance: a double blind prospective controlled clinical trial. *Gut* 27: (10) A1274.

Rees RG, Springford J, Attrill H & Silk DBA (1986b) Superiority of 2 l prepackaged delivery system compared with 1 l containers in enteral nutrition. *Clinical Nutrition* 5 (supplement) P18: 105.

Rees RG, Attrill H, Quinn D & Silk DVA (1986c) Improved design of nasogastric feeding tubes. *Clinical Nutrition* 5: 203–207.

Rees RG, Keohane PP, Grimble GK et al (1986d) Elemental diet administered nasogastrically without starter regimens to patients with inflammatory bowel disease. *Journal of Parenteral and Enteral Nutrition* 10: 258–262.

Rees RG, Payne-James JJ, Cooper T & Silk DBA (1988). Requirements of peptides versus whole protein in patients with moderately impaired gastrointestinal function: a double-blind controlled crossover study. *Journal of Parenteral and Enteral Nutrition* 12 (supplement) P58: 12.

Rolandelli RH, Koruda MJ, Settle RJ & Rombeau JL (1986a) The effect of enteral feedings supplemented with pectin on the healing of colonic anastomoses in the rat. *Surgery* 99: 703–707.

Rolandelli RH, Koruda MJ, Settle RG & Rombeau JL (1986b) Effects of intraluminal infusion of short chain fatty acids on the healing of colonic anastomoses in the rat. *Surgery* 100: 198–203.

Rombeau JL & Rolandelli RH (1987) Enteral and parenteral nutrition in patients with enteric fistulas and short bowel syndrome. *Surgical Clinics of North America* 67: 551–571.

Rumley TO, Lineaweaver WC & Davis JM (1987) Low residue nutritional supplementation as an adjunct to mechanical preparation for surgical treatment of the colon. *Surgery, Gynecology and Obstetrics* 164: 345–350.

Russell CA & Evans SJ (1987) A comparison of the absorption from a 'chemically defined elemental' and a 'whole protein' enteral feed by the human small bowel. *Clinical Nutrition* 6: 127–130.

Ryan JA & Page CP (1984) Intrajejunal feeding: development and current status. *Journal of Parenteral and Enteral Nutrition* 8: 187–198.

Sagar S, Harland P & Shields R (1979) Early post-operative feeding with elemental diet. *British Medical Journal* 1: 293–295.

Sandie GI, Lobley RW & Holmes R (1977) Effect of maltose on the absorption of glucose in the jejunum in man. *Gut* 18: A944–A945.

Schattenkerk ME, Obertop H, Bruining HA, van Rooyen Wm & van Houten H (1984) Early postoperative enteral feeding by a needle catheter jejunostomy after 100 oesophageal resections and reconstructions for cancer. *Clinical Nutrition* 3: 47–49.

Shultz SG & Curran PF (1970) Coupled transport of sodium and organic solutes. *Physiological Reviews* 50: 637–672.

Shanbhogue LKR, Bistrain BR & Blackburn GL (1987) Trends in enteral nutrition in the surgical patient. *Journal of the Royal College of Surgeons of Edinburgh* 31(5): 267–273.

Shelly MP & Church JJ (1987) Enteral feeding and bowel sounds. *Anaesthesia* 42: 207–209.

Shoemaker CP & Wright HK (1970) Rate of water and sodium absorption from the jejunum after abdominal surgery in man. *American Journal of Surgery* 119: 62–63.

Silk DBA (1974) Peptide absorption in man – progress report. *Gut* 15: 494–501.

Silk DBA (1977) Amino acid and peptide absorption in man. In *Peptide transport and hydrolysis. CIBA Foundation Sympsoium 50* (New series) pp 15–36. Amsterdam: North Holland/Elsevier/Excerpta Medica.

Silk DBA (1984) Future directions in supplemented nutrition. In Lawson D (ed) *Cystic Fibrosis Horizons* pp 99–114. Chichester: John Wiley and Sons.

Silk DBA (1986a) Digestion and absorption of carbohydrate, protein and fat. In Woolfson AMJ (ed) *Biochemistry of Hospital Nutrition*, pp 7–40. London: Churchill Livingstone.

Silk DBA (1986b) Branched chain amino acids in liver disease: fact or fantasy? *Gut* 27 (supplement 1): 103–110.

Silk DBA (1988) Use of modified amino acid based enteral diets in the nutritional support of patients with portosystemic encephalopathy: a rethink. Editorial. *Nutrition* (in press).

Silk DBA & Dawson AM (1979) Intestinal absorption of carbohydrate and protein in man. In Crane RK (ed) *International Review of Physiology (III Gastrointestinal Physiology)* 15: 151–204, Baltimore: University Park Press.

Silk DBA, Perrett D & Clark ML (1973). Intestinal transport of two dipeptides containing the same two neutral amino acids in man. *Clinical Science and Molecular Medicine* **49:** 523–526.

Silk DBA, Perrett D, Webb JPW & Clark ML (1974) Absorption of two tripeptides by the human small intestine: a study using a perfusion technique. *Clinical Science & Molecular Medicine* **46:** 393–402.

Silk DBA, Perrett D & Clark ML (1975) Jejunal and ileal absorption of dibasic amino acids and an arginine containing dipeptide in cystinuria. *Gastroenterology* **68:** 1426–1432.

Silk DBA, Nicholson JA & Kim YS (1976a) Hydrolysis of peptides within the lumen of small intestine. *American Journal of Physiology* **231:** 1322–1329.

Silk DBA, Nicholson JA, & Kim YS (1976b) Release of peptide hydrolase during incubation of intact intestinal segment in vitro. *Journal of Physiology* **258:** 489–497.

Silk DBA, Fairclough PD, Clark ML et al (1980) Use of a peptide rather than free amino acid nitrogen source in chemically defined 'elemental diets'. *Journal of Parenteral and Enteral Nutrition* **4:** 548–553.

Smith DW & Lee RM (1956) Nutritional management of duodenal fistula. *Surgery, Gynecology and Obstetrics* **103:** 666–672.

Smithson KW & Gray GM (1977) Intestinal assimilation of the tetrapeptide in the rat. Obligate function of brush border amino peptidase. *Journal of Clinical Investigation* **60:** 665–674.

Spiller RC & Silk DBA (1988) The small intestine. In Hardy JD & Kyle J (eds) *Scientific Foundations of Surgery* London: Heinemann Medical. (in press).

Spiller RC & Jones BJM & Silk DBA (1987) Jejunal water and electrolyte absorption from two proprietary enteral feeds in man – importance of sodium content. *Gut* **28:** 681–687.

Steffee WP & Anderson CF (1984) Enteral nutrition and renal disease. In Rombeau JL & Caldwell MD (eds) *Clinical Nutrition Vol 1, Enteral and Tube Feeding*, pp 362–375. Philadelphia, WB Saunders Company.

Steinhardt HJ, Wolf A, Jakober B et al (1986) Efficiency of nitrogen absorption from whole vs. hydrolysed protein after total pancreatectomy in man. *Clinical Nutrition* **5 (supplement) P23:** 108.

Steinhorn D & Radmer W (1986) Urea synthesis is not consistent throughout the acute phase of stress. *Journal of Parenteral and Enteral Nutrition* **10 (supplement) A 49.**

Stengel A Jr & Ravdin IS (1939) The maintenance of nutrition in surgical patients with a description of the orojejunal method of feeding. *Surgery* **6:** 511–519.

Stremmel W, Lotz G, Strohmeyer G & Berk PD (1985) Identification isolation and partial characterisation of a fatty acid binding protein from rat jejunal microvillus membranes. *Journal of Clinical Investigation* **75:** 1068.

Studley HO (1937) Percentage of weight loss; a basic indicator of surgical risk in patients with chronic peptic ulcer. *Journal of the American Medical Association* **106:** 458–460.

Takala J, Havia T, Heinonen R & Renvall S (1985) Immediate enteral feeding after abdominal surgery. *Acta Chirurgica Scandinavica* **151:** 143–145.

Thurlow PM (1986) Bedside enteral feeding tube placement into duodenum and jejunum. *Journal of Parenteral and Enteral Nutrition* **10:** 104–105.

Tobey N, Heizer W, Yeh R, Huang T-I & Hoffner C (1985) Human intestinal brush border peptidases. *Gastroenterology* **88:** 913–926.

Tredger J, Bazin C & Dickerson JWT (1981) Nasogastric tube feeding – a survey to investigate current practices and attitudes of dietitians. *Journal of Human Nutrition* **35:** 188–122.

Twyman D, Young AB, Ott L, Norton JA & Bivins BA (1985) High protein enteral feedings: a means of achieving positive nitrogen balance in head injured patients. *Journal of Parenteral and Enteral Nutrition* **9:** 679–684.

Van Alsenoy L, De Leeuw I, Delvigne C & Van De Woude (1985) Ascending contamination of a jejunostomy feeding reservoir. *Clinical Nutrition* **4:** 95–98.

Vanlandingham S, Simpson S, Daniel P & Newmark SR (1981) Metabolic abnormalities in patients supported with enteral tube feeding. *Journal of Parenteral and Enteral Nutrition* **5:** 322–324.

Watson AJM, Pegg M & Green JRB (1984) Enteral feeds may antagonise warfarin. *British Medical Journal* **288:** 557.

Wellner D & Meister A (1979) A survey of inborn errors of amino acid metabolism and transport in man. *Annual Review of Biochemistry* **50:** 911–968.

Wernerman J, Hammarqvist F, von der Decken A & Vinnars E (1987) Ornithine-αketoglutarate improves skeletal muscle protein synthesis as assessed by ribosome analysis and nitrogen use after surgery. *Annals of Surgery* **206:** 674–678.

Whatley K, Turner WW, Dey M et al (1984). When does metoclopramide facilitate transpyloric intubation? *Journal of Parenteral and Enteral Nutrition* **8:** 679–681.

7

The metabolic and nutritional effects of injury and sepsis

H. J. G. BURNS

Previous chapters have outlined the basis for the development and identification of malnutrition in patients who have disordered gastrointestinal tract function. That such malnourished states are common in everyday clinical practice is well recognized. Similarly, it is widely accepted that injury or the development of sepsis will exacerbate many of the harmful effects of malnutrition. Other chapters describe specific therapeutic approaches to many of the most important nutritional problems seen clinically. In this chapter, the mechanisms by which injury can modify and worsen the effects of malnutrition will be examined.

THE CHARACTER OF THE METABOLIC RESPONSE TO INJURY

The modern concept of a generalized response to injury has evolved from the work of the military surgeons who worked with the armed forces of Europe in the seventeenth and eighteenth centuries. They recognized that many of their patients suffered injuries which were apparently trivial and yet produced an inexorable collapse of the vital processes. Cooper (1836) noted that many battle casualties died without serious loss of blood or evidence of severe injury at post mortem examination. During this time venesection was recommended in cases of injury where bleeding had not already occurred. Macleod, who was an army surgeon in the Crimea, advised venesection and debridement for the management of compound fractures of the femur (Wangensteen and Wangensteen, 1978). Since the venesection was carried out in the upright position and proceeded until the patient became limp, it is likely that sufficient relaxation was obtained to allow reduction of the fracture! Not surprisingly, death was usually inevitable in these circumstances.

The first suggestion that the response to injury could be beneficial to the patient was made by the Scots surgeon John Hunter in 1796. While endorsing, albeit unenthusiastically, the notion of bleeding for gunshot wounds, he suggested that it would be likely that injury would produce in the body changes which would provide the means and disposition for cure of the injuries.

Only with the advances in experimental physiology made in the nineteenth century, together with the stimulus to injury research of a world war, could Hunter's suggestion begin to be examined. Bernard (1877) noted that haemorrhage caused a rise in blood sugar, and shortly after this Crile (1899) published an experimental study of shock. For the first time, arterial vasoconstriction with reduced tissue perfusion was identified as a common feature of injury. Evidence to link the circulatory abnormality with a metabolic lesion was produced by Cannon and Bayliss (1919), who used the Van Slyke apparatus to show that fixed acids (such as lactic acid) accumulated in the blood of injured soldiers with low blood pressure. They suggested impaired oxygen transport as the cause. At the same time, Dale and Richards (1918) were studying the effects of tourniquet removal from injured limbs. They noted improved survival if amputation was carried out before the tourniquet was removed. They suggested that a major factor in injury was the release of toxic materials into the systemic circulation from the wound.

The relationship between injury and nutritional state became obvious when Sir David Cuthbertson first described an apparently co-ordinated and consistent series of biochemical changes in young men following fracture of a long bone (Cuthbertson, 1930). Similar responses to infection with typhoid fever had been described earlier by Shaffer and Coleman (1909). Elevated energy expenditure and release of nitrogen and minerals into the urine suggested that injured patients required more energy and protein. In addition, these two contributions indicated for the first time that the response to sepsis and injury was likely to be identical. Since then research has been directed towards three major questions. Firstly, a clearer understanding of the type and quantity of energy required by stressed individuals was necessary. Secondly, the abnormal protein metabolism seen after injury required elucidation. What was its purpose, could it be manipulated or even should we manipulate it? Thirdly, identification of the mediators which control the response was seen to be important. Consideration of these three areas forms the basis for the rest of this chapter.

ENERGY METABOLISM

Consideration of energy metabolism in injured patients is often complicated by failure to clarify the terms by which it is defined. For example, 'metabolic rate' can be measured in either the basal or the resting state. Measurement of the basal metabolic rate requires many conditions relating to activity, nutritional intake and ambient temperature to be met (Little, 1985). These conditions are often clinically impractical and therefore the resting metabolic rate or resting energy expenditure (REE) is usually measured (Elwyn et al, 1980). The REE represents the sum of basal energy expenditure together with the energy expended on maintenance of body functions in the resting state. At room temperature, for example, the body expends energy to maintain the temperature difference between itself and its environment.

Oxygen consumption and heat production are two terms which also give rise to some confusion. Oxygen consumption is measured by indirect calorimetry and reflects total amount of oxygen consumed by chemical reactions in the body. Since energy is produced by oxidation of substrate, oxygen consumption is a good approximation of energy expenditure. In the short term, however, heat production differs from oxygen consumption, since the amount of heat produced per unit of oxygen consumed depends on the substrate being oxidized. Most clinical studies of energy expenditure in trauma have used indirect calorimetry to measure oxygen consumption and in most cases it is the resting rather than the basal state which has been assessed.

Little and Stoner (1981) showed that body temperature falls after severe injury and Little et al (1981) found some evidence for a reduction in oxygen consumption at the same time. The significance of these observations is not clear, since not all patients had a low oxygen consumption and it did not appear to correlate with severity of injury. These patients were studied before resuscitation, and the low oxygen consumption might be a reflection of reduced tissue perfusion. After fluid replacement and restoration of a satisfactory level of delivery of oxygen to the tissues, an increase in oxygen consumption is observed.

The magnitude of the increase in REE is related to the severity of the injury. Elective hip replacement surgery may only increase REE by 5% (Michelsen et al, 1979). Where bony injury is accidental and associated with pain, blood loss and muscle injury, the increase in REE is greater. Roe and Kinney (1965) found an elevation of between 10% and 20% in such cases. The most severe injuries in metabolic terms appear to be large-area, full-thickness burns which can produce increases in REE of up to 100% above predicted values (Davies, 1982). At least some of the increase in REE observed in burns patients is due to the necessity to generate energy to maintain body temperature in the light of evaporative water losses from the burned area (Davies, 1982). Wilmore has argued, however, that the main cause of the increased REE in burned patients is an alteration in the control of body temperature by the hypothalamus (Wilmore, 1977). An alternative explanation for the raised REE in stressed patients has been advanced by Wolfe et al (1987). They measured rates of conversion of glucose to glucose 6-phosphate and the rate of simultaneous breakdown and synthesis of stored triglyceride in severely burned patients. These metabolic pathways involve opposing reactions which are catalysed by different enzymes. Shuttling carbon round these cycles involves the expenditure of energy for no apparent gain in stored fat or glucose. Hence, they have been called 'futile cycles'. It is now thought that they play a role in determining the response of biochemical pathways to controlling influences such as hormones (Newsholme and Crabtree, 1976). In burned patients, it was shown that these substrate cycles were turning at greatly increased rates. The triglyceride–fatty acid cycle was restored to near normal by infusion of propranolol, confirming the stimulatory influence of catecholamines in post-injury metabolism.

Cycling of glucose was not affected by adrenergic blockade, confirming the suggestion that glucagon is the main stimulator of glucose turnover after injury (Jahoor et al, 1986).

The energy expended in fuelling these cycles in burned patients could be calculated to account for 15% of the increase in energy expenditure seen following injury. There are several other possible futile cycles which may be accelerated in stressed individuals and they may provide an explanation for a significant proportion of the thermogenic effects of injury.

While the mechanism which causes the increase in REE in injured patients is not completely understood, it should be noted that the extent of the increase is often not great. Ill patients are confined to bed and often sedated. They may have lost weight due to longstanding illness, and recent food intake may be negligible. These factors result in a reduction in REE, and therefore while the percentage increase in REE may be great, it may only serve to produce a small absolute increase in energy requirements compared to the patient's normal demands. Very few patients require more than 3000 kcal/day (Askanazi et al, 1980a).

GLUCOSE METABOLISM

The observation by Bernard of hyperglycaemia after haemorrhage has already been mentioned. Elevation of glucose level in the plasma could occur as a result of either increased release or decreased removal of glucose into the circulation. There has been much controversy as to the predominant influence on plasma glucose level. At present it seems likely that there is an increased release of glucose into the plasma, and most authorities would also accept evidence for decreased glucose oxidation in stressed patients.

Glucose release into the plasma

Glucose entering the plasma is derived from two sources. It can either come from glycogen stored in liver or it can be synthesized from precursor molecules. The glucose entering the plasma in fasting humans will initially come from stored glycogen, and there is evidence that the initial hyper-glycaemia of injury is the result of depletion of glycogen stores (Stoner, 1958). Glycogenolysis mediated by adrenaline release together with a transient inhibition of insulin release are the initial causes of the elevated blood glucose (Shuck et al, 1977; Stoner et al, 1979). Plasma adrenaline increases within a few minutes of injury, and the extent of the rise observed is related to severity of injury (Davies et al, 1984). Adrenaline level declines fairly rapidly and has often returned to near-normal levels in the first 24 hours. Glucagon levels rise in the plasma within a few hours of injury and reach a peak between 12 hours and 48 hours (Meguid et al, 1974). The possibility that glucagon is the prime determinant of the rate of glucose production in the later phase of injury has already been mentioned (Jahoor et al, 1986). Both these hormones contribute to the elevation in plasma glucose and their effects are potentiated by elevation in blood cortisol (Shamoon et al, 1981). Within 24 hours, glycogen stores will be exhausted and the hyperglycaemic effects of adrenaline will lessen.

When the injury receives appropriate treatment, plasma glucose falls slowly over the next few days to normal levels (Frayn et al, 1984). Effective anaesthesia can attenuate or even abolish these changes in elective surgery (Traynor and Hall, 1981). Continued stress arising from an unexcised burn wound or unresolved sepsis will provide a reason for continued metabolic derangement.

Any glucose entering the plasma at this stage will be newly synthesized under the influence of glucagon. The principal source of the new glucose entering the plasma will be conversion of three-carbon precursor molecules into glucose by the process of gluconeogenesis. Glycerol, lactate and alanine derived from protein breakdown are the major sources of carbon for glucose production. Wolfe (1979) has demonstrated that an elevated glucose production is related to the rate of protein breakdown seen in burned patients. Recent work has shown that somatostatin infusion in burned patients can, by reducing glucagon output from the pancreas, reduce hepatic synthesis of glucose (Jahoor et al, 1986). A combination of increased substrate availability and an appropriate hormonal environment probably accounts for the increased glucose production.

Glucose removal from the plasma

In the uninjured state, gluconeogenesis is suppressed by glucose infusion. This effect is probably mediated by an elevation in insulin levels, which determine the rate of disappearance of glucose from the plasma (Exton et al, 1970). Injured patients are unable to respond normally to infusions of glucose and this is because insulin appears to be less efficient in enhancing the rate of clearance of glucose from the plasma (Allsop et al, 1978). After a transient fall, plasma insulin levels begin to rise soon after injury and are consistently elevated within a few days (Stoner et al, 1979). The plasma insulin level at that time is usually inappropriately high for the plasma glucose concentration, and it appears that a degree of resistance to the effects of insulin exists (Wolfe et al, 1979; Frayn et al, 1984). The concept of 'insulin resistance' has been evolved to explain the failure to suppress glucose production. In addition, the role of cortisol in sustaining hyperglycaemia has been emphasized by Bessey et al (1984), who found that infusion of cortisol, in association with glucagon and adrenaline, significantly increased plasma glucose and caused apparent insulin resistance in normal volunteers. An elevation in plasma cortisol after injury has been recognized for many years (Moore, 1957). Other workers have suggested that the major factor in the production of insulin resistance is elevation in catecholamine levels (Alberti et al, 1980). This suggests that insulin resistance is probably a reflection of the balance of hormones released following injury, with adrenaline and cortisol antagonizing the effect of insulin on glucose clearance.

Another factor which apparently reduces clearance of glucose from the plasma is its fate within the cell. In general, oxidation of glucose is directly proportional to its availability, and while circulating glucose is increased, the amount which is actually available within the cell is reduced by the effect of insulin resistance. Some attempt must be made, therefore, to express glucose oxidation as a percentage of available glucose. When the problem is looked at in these terms, a substantial weight of evidence exists to suggest that glucose oxidation is reduced after injury (Heath and Corney, 1973; Wolfe et al, 1976; Shaw et al, 1985a,b).

However, Frayn et al (1984) have studied young patients with long bone fractures and concluded that glucose oxidation is elevated in absolute terms in these patients. They concluded also that oxidation of glucose relative to plasma concentrations of insulin and glucose was also increased. Long (1983) has also suggested that burned and septic patients have elevated glucose oxidation rates, but the Manchester group has recently examined the glucose utilization rate in septic patients and concluded that it is decreased (White et al, 1987). In a review of this subject, Long (1987) has argued strongly that methodological considerations make much of the existing data unreliable and that inconsistencies in the present published work require further studies to resolve them. Until further work clarifies the situation, it seems reasonable to hold the view that glucose removal from the plasma is reduced both by resistance to the effects of insulin and reduced intracellular oxidation, possibly due to inhibition of intracellular pathways (Vary et al, 1986).

FAT METABOLISM

It is generally agreed that any stress resulting in a release of adrenaline and glucagon will result in lipolysis with a rise in plasma free fatty acid (FFA) concentrations (Herndon and Riseborough, 1978; Stoner et al, 1979). Cortisol also has a lipolytic influence but its effect is thought to be less important than that of the other two hormones (Fain, 1979). Uncertainty as to the effects of trauma on fat metabolism arose because different injuries have different effects on the degree of mobilization of FFAs, since any injury which results in hypovolaemia will inevitably reduce perfusion of adipose tissue. In addition, lactic acid stimulates re-esterification of triglycerides in the adipocyte, and in the shocked patient, acidosis will tend to reduce availability of FFAs (Miller et al, 1964). A further factor to be considered in chronic illness is the reduced serum albumin commonly seen in these patients which will reduce transport capacity of the blood for FFAs (Wannemacher et al, 1979). A variable elevation in plasma FFAs can therefore be expected immediately after injury. Restoration of perfusion of adipose tissue following adequate resuscitation will allow the lipolytic hormones to proceed with mobilization of FFAs.

Oxidation of FFAs is normally proportional to plasma FFA levels, and elevated FFA oxidation has been confirmed in septic and injured patients (Nordenstrom et al, 1983). Measurement of respiratory quotient (R/Q) in patients oxidizing fat gives a value of 0.7. As the amount of carbohydrate oxidized increases, the R/Q increases to 1.0. Measurement of R/Q in septic patients confirms that FFA oxidation is increased (Stoner et al, 1979). Shaw and Wolfe (1987) have used stable isotope-labelled fatty acid to show that not only is the rate of FFA oxidation elevated in absolute terms, but also, even allowing for the rise in plasma levels, the proportion of circulating FFAs that is oxidized is increased. A further interesting observation is that the elevated FFA oxidation rate is not inhibited by glucose infusion, implying a loss of the normal inhibiting effects on fat mobilization of insulin (Carpentier et al, 1979). The mechanism by which elevated FFA oxidation is produced is not clear. Elevated plasma insulin would normally be expected to inhibit lipolysis, and the relatively unrestrained fat mobilization in stressed patients suggests that adipocytes participate in the insulin resistance phenomenon. Elevated FFA oxidation is also detectable in cancer-bearing patients (Hansell et al, 1986). Using oxygen consumption figures, it is possible to calculate that weight-losing cancer patients had a significantly greater fat oxidation rate than weight-stable cancer patients. This effect appeared to be related to the extent of tumour. The more widespread the tumour, the greater the effect on fat metabolism. Further studies in cancer patients have indicated that fatty acid turnover is as sensitive to glucose infusion in cancer-bearing patients as it is in normal individuals. The major difference between the two groups appears to be that the cancer patients have higher basal levels of fatty acid turnover than control patients (Selberg et al, 1988).

Triglyceride metabolism is poorly understood in injury. Elevation in the rate of production of triglyceride has been postulated (Wolfe et al, 1985) and it appears that triglyceride concentration may be increased in the plasma for this reason. Others have suggested that severe sepsis results in reduced triglyceride clearance and that this is the explanation for lipaemic serum observed occasionally in critically ill patients (Cerra et al, 1979a; Lindholm and Rossner, 1983). Lipoprotein lipase is also thought to be inhibited at this stage (Robin et al, 1981). With progressive sepsis, R/Q rises, indicating that lipogenesis is taking place. The triglyceride–FFA futile cycle is becoming more active at this stage and the rising R/Q may be an indicator of poor prognosis.

Plasma ketones are markedly reduced in trauma and sepsis (Rich and Wright, 1979). A possible explanation for this observation is the high circulating insulin level, since this failure of ketogenesis is not seen in diabetic rats maintained on a constant insulin infusion (Neufeld et al, 1980).

At present, therefore, it seems that injured patients break down adipose tissue and oxidize fatty acid in preference to glucose. This conclusion has obvious implications for the provision of energy for the injured or septic patient.

PROTEIN METABOLISM

The negative nitrogen balance seen after injury and first described by Cuthbertson (1930) is indicative of a net body protein loss. If prolonged, protein loss can seriously compromise recovery. The existence of well organized trauma centres and intensive care units, however, now allows prolonged survival of patients with severe protein catabolism after injury, and some consideration of the mechanisms responsible for protein depletion in these patients is necessary.

Since proteins are being synthesized continually, a net protein loss may be due to decreased synthesis or increased breakdown. The factors responsible for control of muscle protein synthesis and breakdown are discussed in Chapter 11.

Whole-body protein synthesis and breakdown have been extensively studied in injured humans, and the whole-body figure obtained by isotope infusion studies obviously includes visceral protein turnover as well as the contribution from muscle. A balance between the muscle compartment and the visceral compartment is maintained in health. Injury upsets this balance, and muscle and viscera respond to injury in different ways. Overall, whole-body protein turnover is said to increase after injury (Cuthbertson and Tilstone, 1977; Birkahn et al, 1980), sepsis (Hasselgren et al, 1986b) and burns (Kien et al, 1978a). In the case of serious injury, the elevation in turnover is due to increases in both synthesis and breakdown of protein. Negative nitrogen balance is due to a greater increase in protein breakdown than that seen in synthesis. Elective surgery appears to produce a much less severe response, and most authors have reported reduction in synthesis with little or no change in catabolism (O'Keefe et al, 1974; Crane et al, 1977; Kien et al, 1978b). The reduction in whole-body protein synthesis probably reflects acute food deprivation and its effect on muscle (see Chapter 11). Clearly, elective surgery with proper pain control and maintenance of fluid balance represents a fairly minor metabolic insult. The elevation in whole-body protein synthesis and breakdown seen in severe injury and sepsis can be examined further.

It is accepted that the elevation in synthesis takes place mainly in the visceral compartment (predominantly the liver), while most of the elevation in protein breakdown is to be found in skeletal muscle. A review of the changes seen in plasma levels of hepatic export proteins after trauma has been published by Fleck et al (1985). Many of the proteins secreted by the liver have transport functions, e.g. caeruloplasmin and retinol-binding protein. Others such as α-1-antitrypsin and α-2-macroglobulin have binding properties which inhibit proteolytic enzymes and protect tissue from damage when proteases are released into the systemic circulation.

Production of cellular protein is generally elevated in liver of septic animals (Pedersen et al, 1986), and several other groups have confirmed an elevation in protein synthetic rate in liver slices taken from septic subjects (Rosenblatt et al, 1983; Loda et al, 1984; Hasselgren et al, 1986a). In tumour-bearing animals also, Warren et al (1985) have shown a significant increase in hepatocyte protein synthesis rate.

Muscle protein metabolism is dominated by a net elevation in protein breakdown (Rosenblatt et al, 1983). Jepson et al (1986) found that muscle protein breakdown increased by 60% following injection of endotoxin, and muscle protein synthesis decreased by more than 50%. Not all amino acids are released from muscle at the same rate. The branched-chain amino acids valine, leucine and isoleucine are apparently oxidized in the muscle as a source of energy (Odessey and Goldberg, 1972). In addition to this release of amino acids, muscle cells are apparently inhibited in their ability to take up amino acids in sepsis (Hasselgren et al, 1986). Total body oxidation of amino acids increases (Powell-Tuck et al, 1984). Skeletal muscle protein breakdown occurring in injured individuals is thought to confer a survival advantage, since it provides a supply of amino acids to visceral tissues for acute-phase protein synthesis. Urea synthesis increases, reflecting uptake and oxidation of amino acids by the liver. Clowes and colleagues have estimated amino acid uptake by the viscera and shown that it is enhanced in sepsis and trauma but that patients with reduced ability to clear amino acids had a significantly poorer outcome (Rosenblatt et al, 1983; Pearl et al, 1985).

A key role in the interchange of nitrogen between the periphery and the visceral compartment is played by glutamine. Following operative injury, Vinnars et al (1975) found that intracellular glutamine concentration declined by 50% in skeletal muscle. This observation has been confirmed in various centres and for different types of injury (Furst et al, 1979; Askanazi et al, 1980c; Kapadia et al, 1982; Milewski et al, 1982). In each study, a consistent fall of about 50% has been observed in intracellular glutamine concentration. It appears that the glutamine is released from muscle and is taken up by the gastrointestinal tract (Souba and Wilmore, 1983). Gut mucosal integrity is maintained in injured animals by increasing the supply of glutamine (Tsann et al, 1986). Free glutamine cannot be provided easily in currently available amino acid solutions due to instability during heat sterilization and storage. However, recent work on solutions containing alanyl–glutamine dipeptides has shown that muscle glutamine concentrations can be maintained by the use of appropriate dipeptide solutions (Furst et al, 1987). Clinical studies of the effect of these solutions on protein synthesis are necessary but the possibility that dipeptides could improve nutritional state and muscle function in stressed patients remains intriguing.

The mediators responsible for muscle proteolysis in trauma are discussed below. However, a significant correlation between plasma insulin level and nitrogen excretion led Frayn (1986) to suggest that skeletal muscle protein might be resistant to the anabolic effects of insulin after injury.

STARVATION AND THE STRESS RESPONSE

The response of the individual to starvation can be seen as a process of adaptation and conservation. In the short term, body energy requirements are met by breakdown of glycogen from liver and muscle to provide glucose. Minimum daily glucose requirements at complete rest have been calculated to be 160 g (Felig et al, 1969). The carbohydrate reserves of an average individual are thought to be at most 210 g. Glycogen stores will be exhausted within 24 hours (Cahill et al, 1966). An alternative substrate for tissues requiring glucose must be found if starvation is prolonged beyond 24 hours. Oxidation of FFAs from adipose tissue provides most of the energy in these circumstances but brain and red cells have an obligatory requirement for glucose and at least 120 g/day of new glucose must be synthesized (Reinmuth et al, 1965). The carbon required for glucose production comes mainly from amino acids and glycerol. Insulin levels fall early in starvation, and the gluconeogenic pathway is freed from the inhibitory effects of insulin (Cahill et al, 1966). Lipolysis is also stimulated by the reduction in plasma insulin, and FFAs become available for oxidation or conversion to ketones. Ketones serve to reduce brain requirements for glucose by as much as 50%. Muscle amino acids are conserved by this process (Owen et al, 1967).

At the same time as an alteration in substrate utilization is observed, REE and nitrogen excretion are reduced (Martin and Robison, 1922; Keys et al, 1950). It has been suggested that reductions in serum T3 and catecholamines may act synergistically to reduce energy expenditure in peripheral tissues (Portnay et al, 1974; Young and Landsberg, 1979). The reduction in nitrogen excretion may be mediated by ketonaemia as already mentioned. Overall the systemic response to starvation may be thought of as a co-ordinated process which acts to conserve body protein and energy stores (Table 1).

Table 1. The metabolic effects of starvation and stress.

	Starvation		Stress	
	Early	Late	Early	Late
Energy expenditure	±	−	+ +	+ +
Preferred substrate	Glucose	Fat	Fat/amino acids	Fat/amino acids
Protein synthesis	−	− −	+	−
Gluconeogenesis	−	+	+ +	+ +
Lipogenesis	+	− −	− −	+
Lipolysis	−	+ +	+ + +	+ + +
Ketogenesis	±	+ +	−	− − −
Rate of weight loss	+	+	+ +	+ + +

Obviously, the stress of injury seriously impairs the adaptive response to starvation. As already discussed, energy expenditure and net protein breakdown are elevated. The proportion of energy expenditure which is derived from oxidation of glucose is decreased, despite an elevation in glucose synthesis from amino acids, and oxidation of amino acids provides a greater proportion of body energy requirements. The drive to produce new glucose and the oxidation of amino acids may be explained, at least in part, by the failure to produce ketones in the liver (Birkhan et al, 1981). The basis of many of these effects may be mainly hormonal in nature, and they are probably a reflection of high circulating insulin levels together with the differing degrees of insulin resistance to be found in different tissues.

MEDIATORS OF THE STRESS RESPONSE

Injury causes pain, anxiety and often a variety of physical effects such as hypovolaemia and tissue damage. The psychological aspects of injury initiate a neuroendocrine response which consists of increased secretion of hypothalamic and pituitary hormones and increased activity of the autonomic nervous system. The hormonal effects of injury and sepsis have already been discussed. In recent years, however, it has been appreciated that tissue damage results in release of mediators from a variety of sources which appear to act in a co-ordinated fashion with the hormones to produce the metabolic changes associated with injury. Most interest has centred on the products of monocytes. The protein mediators produced by monocytes are collectively known as cytokines and the most thoroughly investigated of these are interleukin 1 (IL-1) and tumour necrosis factor (TNF). Many others have been described, such as the prostaglandins and leukotrienes, but this discussion will focus primarily on the interleukins and TNF. A more general review has been published by Nathan (1987).

Energy expenditure

Very little work has been produced as yet to link cytokines to alterations in energy expenditure following injury. Tocco-Bradley et al (1986, 1988) have infused murine recombinant IL-1 into rats and noted progressive elevation in temperatures associated with a decrease in REE. This finding could perhaps be explained by a reduction in activity of the animals due to central effects of the infusion. Purified murine IL-1 on the other hand increased REE. Whether the recombinant IL-1 was chemically altered in some way and had a reduced activity as a result, or whether the purified material contained some other intermediate, has yet to be resolved.

Carbohydrate metabolism

Clearly, the major controlling influences in carbohydrate metabolism in trauma are the hormones. IL-1β has recently been shown to stimulate the hypothalamic–pituitary–adrenal axis and increase circulating adrenocortico-trophin (ACTH) and cortisol (Besedovsky et al, 1986). TNF, however, produced hypoglycaemia and death when infused into rats (Ciancio et al, 1987). This response is more typical of the acute reaction to overwhelming sepsis than the hyperglycaemia which occurs after trauma.

A direct influence of IL-1 on carbohydrate metabolism has been suggested (Hill et al, 1986), and it appears that IL-1 may be more associated with the elevated glucose turnover seen in the prolonged catabolic state, while TNF may be the mediator most predominant in endotoxaemia.

Fat metabolism

Three cytokines so far have been shown to inhibit lipoprotein lipase. The most potent of these appears to be TNF (Flick and Gifford, 1984). IL-1β also has this effect (Bagby et al, 1986). IL-2 can activate lipolysis by reducing the inhibitory effect of adrenaline on hormone-sensitive lipase. The relevance of these observations to the injured patient is not yet clear, but FFA oxidation was enhanced by purified IL-1 infusion in rats (Tocco-Bradley et al, 1988) and therefore it may play a role in maintaining the drive to oxidize FFAs in stressed patients.

Protein metabolism

The role of cytokines in stimulating muscle proteolysis has received most scrutiny recently. Yang et al (1983) purified a monocyte extract and demonstrated alterations in rat protein metabolism. Muscle proteolysis was produced by another peptide, designated as proteolysis-inducing factor (Clowes et al, 1983). Recent studies with recombinant IL-1β have not been able to reproduce early findings of protein catabolism obtained with purified material, and the suspicion that several mediators were being inoculated into the animals remains strong (Flores et al, 1986; Pomposelli et al, 1987). One possibility is that the purified products were contaminated with TNF, and Flores et al (1987) have demonstrated that this cytokine does indeed have proteolysis-inducing properties. This work suggests that TNF may be the main cytokine mediator for protein breakdown in injured individuals.

A cytokine may also be responsible for stimulation of hepatic protein synthesis. IL-6, also known as interferon β-2, has recently been shown to be identical to hepatocyte-stimulating factor 1 (Gauldie et al, 1987). Nijsten et al (1987) have demonstrated that IL-6 is detectable in burns patients on admission to hospital and there is evidence that IL-6 is released into plasma in the early period following elective surgery (A. Shenkin, unpublished data).

Further studies will almost certainly identify more cytokines associated with the metabolic response to injury. How their functions will integrate with those of the hormones is still to be determined. One of the most exciting aspects of the recognition of the importance of these substances is the possibility that pharmacological manipulation of their activities will improve therapy for injured and septic patients.

MODIFICATION OF THE METABOLIC RESPONSE WITH NUTRITIONAL SUPPORT

Clearly, the stress response has profound implications for energy and protein requirements and body composition. Specific therapy to manipulate the stress response for the benefit of the patient is not yet available, and nutritional support remains the easiest way of influencing the metabolic response and preserving body tissues. From the foregoing discussion, it can be seen that the amount of energy and protein required will vary with the extent of injury. In addition, the composition of the energy and protein sources require consideration.

Calculation of daily energy requirements need not be a complicated exercise. Most surgical patients with postoperative sepsis will require about 10–20% more calories than calculated for a normal individual of similar height and weight. Accordingly, a figure of approximately 30–40 kcal kg^{-1} day^{-1} is usually satisfactory (Hill and Church, 1984). There is no advantage to be gained from provision of excess energy, since this will usually be stored as fat (Askanazi et al, 1980a). For many years energy was given exclusively as glucose, and undoubtedly glucose infusions exert a nitrogen-sparing effect in injured subjects (Moldower et al, 1980). Where all the energy expenditure was met by carbohydrate infusions, complications were noted. Carbon dioxide production increased and respiratory failure was exacerbated due to the need to increase minute ventilation to blow off the increased carbon dioxide. Excess carbohydrate was deposited in the liver as fat, and increased circulating catecholamines were noted which resulted in an elevation in energy expenditure (Elwyn et al, 1979; Nordenstrom et al, 1981a, 1983). Reduction in total number of calories provided to below $40\,kcal\,kg^{-1}\,day^{-1}$ together with the provision of a substantial proportion of these as fat has reduced the incidence of these complications. At present we would suggest that around 50% of non-protein calories be provided as lipid (Burns, 1988).

In general, nitrogen balance can be obtained by provision of about $3.0\,g\,kg^{-1}\,day^{-1}$ of amino acid, although with high levels of stress more nitrogen may be required to achieve satisfactory nitrogen retention (Birkhan et al, 1980; Cerra et al, 1983). It appears that intravenous nutrition reduces protein loss mainly by stimulating protein synthesis (Moyer et al, 1981). However, it appears that nutritional support is unable to influence the excessive degree of catabolism seen in critically ill patients (Clague et al, 1983). Alternative substrates have been suggested in an attempt to improve nitrogen retention. As already mentioned, branched-chain amino acids are an important substrate for the production of energy in skeletal muscle (Odessey and Goldberg, 1972). In addition, it has been suggested that increasing the intracellular concentration of branched-chain amino acids could stimulate muscle protein synthesis (Askanazi et al, 1980b) and indeed improved nitrogen balance has been achieved when intravenous amino acid solutions were enriched with branched-chain amino acids (Cerra et al, 1982). However, no properly controlled trials have yet been carried out which show a clinical benefit from the use of these solutions, and at present their use seems to confer theoretical rather than practical benefits and cannot be recommended.

A number of benefits have recently been noted following early introduction of enteral rather than intravenous nutritional support. Pingleton and Hadgima (1983) found a significant reduction in gastrointestinal bleeding in critically ill patients when enteral feeding was used, and anecdotal experience has suggested improved overall survival in such patients. The mechanisms responsible for this effect are as yet unclear, but it may be that patients who are able to tolerate enteral feeding are inherently less ill than patients requiring intravenous nutritional support. At present, clinical trials are needed to evaluate the role of enteral nutrition in these patients.

SUMMARY

The existence of a co-ordinated response to stress of a variety of causes has clearly been established. Basically, this consists of an elevation in energy expenditure and an increased breakdown of skeletal muscle protein. In addition, glucose level in the plasma increases as a result of increased synthesis and decreased uptake of glucose into cells. Release of fatty acid into the plasma is also increased, and an elevation in the proportion of energy derived from oxidation of fatty acids is observed. This response is qualitatively very different from that seen in simple starvation, where a progressive reduction in energy expenditure and a reduction in the synthesis of glucose allows fat to become the major energy-producing substrate and also allows sparing of body protein stores.

The mechanisms responsible for this altered pattern of metabolism are probably primarily hormonal in nature, with adrenaline, cortisol and glucagon being the major catabolic stimulants. Some evidence exists, however, for alteration in intracellular pathway metabolism. Within the past decade a new class of mediators of the stress response, the cytokines, has been recognized. These substances are protein products of circulating monocytes and the way in which they integrate into the control of the stress response has not been completely elucidated. At present there is evidence that they can stimulate production of catabolic hormones, and also they may well have direct effects in enhancing protein catabolism in muscle.

At present the main method for modification of the stress response remains the provision of energy and amino acid, either intravenously or enterally. In the present state of our knowledge, $30\text{--}40\,\mathrm{kcal\,kg^{-1}\,day^{-1}}$ would appear to be adequate for most patients, with half provided as fat. Amino acids $3\,\mathrm{g\,kg^{-1}\,day^{-1}}$ will provide adequate nitrogen. It must be said, however, that the most effective method of modifying the stress response is removal of the source of stress by surgery, antibiotics or other primary therapy.

REFERENCES

Alberti KG, Batstone GF, Foster K et al (1980) Relative role of various hormones in mediating the metabolic response to injury. *Journal of Parenteral and Enteral Nutrition* 4: 141–146.

Allsop JR, Wolfe RR & Burke JF (1978) Glucose kinetics and responsiveness to insulin in the rat injured by burn. *Surgery, Gynecology and Obstetrics* 147: 565–573.

Askanazi J, Carpentier YA, Elwyn DH et al (1980a) Influence of total parenteral nutrition on fuel utilisation in injury and sepsis. *Annals of Surgery* 191: 40–46.

Askanazi J, Carpentier YA, Michelsen CB et al (1980b) Muscle and plasma amino acids following injury: influence of intercurrent infection. *Annals of Surgery* 192: 78–85.

Askanazi J, Furst P, Michelson CB et al (1980c) Muscle and plasma amino acids after injury: Hypocaloric glucose vs amino acid infusion. *Annals of Surgery* 191: 465–472.

Bagby GJ, Corll CB, Thompson JJ & Wilson LA (1986) Lipoprotein lipase-suppressing mediator in serum of endotoxin-treated rats. *American Journal of Physiology* 251: E470–E476.

Bernard C (1877) *Leçons sur le Diabete*, pp 408–410. Paris: Librairie JB Baillière et fils.

Besedovsky H, Del Rey A, Sorkin E & Dinarello CA (1986) Immunoregulatory feedback between interleukin-1 and glucocorticoid hormones. *Science* 233: 652–654.

Bessey PQ, Waters J, Soki T & Wilmore DW (1984) Combined hormone infusion simulates the metabolic response to injury. *Annals of Surgery* 200: 264–281.

Birkahn RH, Long CL, Fitkin D, Dyger JW & Blakemore WS (1980) Effects of skeletal trauma on whole body protein turnover in man measured by L-(^{14}C)-leucine. *Surgery* 88: 294–299.

Birkahn RH, Long CL, Fitkin D, Geiger J & Blakemore WS (1981) A comparison of the effects of skeletal trauma and surgery on the ketosis of starvation in man. *Journal of Trauma* 21: 513–519.

Burns HJG (1988) Nutritional support in the perioperative period. *British Medical Bulletin* 44(2): 357–373.

Cahill GF, Herrera MG, Morgan AP et al (1966) Hormone–fuel interrelationships during fasting. *Journal of Clinical Investigation* **45:** 1751–1769.

Cannon WB & Bayliss WM (1919) Notes on muscle injury in relation to shock. *Special Reports. Medical Research Commission No. 26* **8:** 19–60.

Carpentier YA, Askanazi J, Elwyn DH et al (1979) Effects of hypercaloric glucose infusion on lipid metabolism in injury and sepsis. *Journal of Trauma* **19:** 649–654.

Cerra FB, Siegel JH, Border J & Coleman B (1979a) Correlations between metabolic and cardiopulmonary measurements in patients after trauma, general surgery and sepsis. *Journal of Trauma* **19:** 621–628.

Cerra FB, Siegel JH, Border J & Coleman B (1979b) The hepatic failure of sepsis: cellular vs substrate. *Surgery* **86:** 409–422.

Cerra FB, Upson D, Angelico R et al (1982) Branched chains support postoperative protein synthesis. *Surgery* **92:** 192–199.

Cerra FB, Mazuski J, Teasley K et al (1983) Nitrogen retention in critically ill patients is proportional to the branched chain amino acid load. *Critical Care Medicine* **11:** 775–778.

Ciancio MJ, Jones SB, Yelich MR & Filkins JP (1987) Glucoregulatory and sympathoadrenal responses to TNF in conscious rats. *Federation of Proctology* **46:** 561.

Clague MB, Keir MJ, Wright PD & Johnston IDA (1983) The effects of nutrition and trauma on whole body protein metabolism in man. *Clinical Science* **65:** 165–175.

Clowes GH, George BC, Villee CA et al (1983) Muscle proteolysis induced by a circulating peptide in patients with sepsis or trauma. *New England Journal of Medicine* **308:** 545–552.

Cooper A (1836) *Commentary on War Injuries.* London.

Crane CW, Picou D, Smith R & Waterlow JC (1977) Protein turnover in patients before and after elective orthopaedic operations. *British Journal of Surgery* **64:** 129–133.

Crile GW Jr (1899) *An Experimental Research into Surgical Shock.* Philadelphia: JB Lippincott.

Cuthbertson DP (1930) The disturbance of metabolism produced by bony and non-bony injury with notes on certain abnormal conditions of bone. *Biochemical Journal* **24:** 1244–1263.

Cuthbertson D & Tilstone W (1977) Metabolism in the post injury period. *Advances in Clinical Chemistry* **12:** 1–55.

Dale HH & Richards AN (1918) The vasodilator activity of histamine and of some other substances. *Journal of Physiology* **52:** 110–165.

Davies CL, Newman RJ, Molyneux SG & Grahame-Smith DG (1984) The relationship between plasma catecholamines and severity of injury in man. *Journal of Trauma* **24:** 99–105.

Davies JWL (1982) *Physiological Responses to Burning Injury.* New York: Academic Press.

Elwyn DH, Kinney JM, Jeevanandam M et al (1979) Influence of increasing carbohydrate intake on glucose kinetics in injured patients. *Annals of Surgery* **190:** 117–127.

Elwyn DH, Kinney JM, Gump FE, Askanazi J, Rosenbaum SH & Carpentier YA (1980) Some metabolic effects of fat infusions in depleted patients. *Metabolism* **29:** 125–132.

Exton JH, Mallette LE & Jefferson et al (1970) Role of adenosine 3,5-monophosphate in the control of gluconeogenesis. *American Journal of Clinical Nutrition* **23:** 993–1003.

Fain JN (1979) Inhibition of glucose transport in fat cells and activation of lipolysis by glucocorticoids. *Monographs in Endocrinology* **12:** 547–560.

Felig P, Parkliss E, Owen OE & Cahill GF (1969) Blood glucose and gluconeogenesis in fasting man. *Archives of Internal Medicine* **123:** 293–298.

Fleck A, Colley CM & Myers MA (1985) Liver export proteins and trauma. *British Medical Bulletin* **41:** 265–273.

Flick DA & Gifford GE (1984) Cachectin/tumor necrosis factor: Production, distribution and metabolic fate in vivo. *Journal of Immunology* **135:** 3972–3977.

Flores E, Drabik M, Bistrian BR et al (1986) The acute phase response to human recombinant mediators. *Surgical Forum* **37:** 28–30.

Flores E, Drabik M, Bistrian BR et al (1987) Synergistic effect of human recombinant mediators during the acute phase reaction. *Clinical Research* **35:** 384A.

Frayn KN (1986) Hormonal control of metabolism in trauma and sepsis. *Clinical Endocrinology* **27:** 577–599.

Frayn KN, Little RA, Stoner HB & Galasko CSB (1984) Metabolic control in non-septic patients with musculo-skeletal injuries. *Injury* **16:** 73–79.

Furst P, Bergstrom J, Holmstrom B et al (1979) Influence of amino acid supply on nitrogen and amino acid metabolism in severe trauma. *Acta Chirurgica Scandinavica* **494**(supplement): 136–138.

Furst P, Albres S & Stehle P (1987) Stress-induced intracellular glutamine depletion. The potential use of glutamine containing peptides in parenteral nutrition. In Adibi SA, Fekl W, Furst P & Oehmke M (eds) *Dipeptides as New Substrates in Nutrition Therapy*, pp 103–117. Basel: Karger.

Gagner M, Shizgal HM & Forse RA (1986) The effect of interleukin-1 and interleukin-2 on the adrenergic control of hormone-sensitive lipase in the human adipocyte. *Surgery* **100**: 298–305.

Gauldie J, Richards C, Harnish D, Lansdorp P & Baumann H (1987) Interferon β 2 B cell stimulating factor type 2 shares identity with monocyte-derived hepatocyte stimulating factor and regulates the major acute phase protein response in liver cells. *Proceedings of the National Academy of Sciences* **84**: 7251–7255.

Hansell DT, Davies JWL, Ashenkin A & Burns HJG (1986) The oxidation of body fuel stores in cancer patients. *Annals of Surgery* **204**: 637–642.

Hasselgren PO, Jagenburg R, Karlstrom L et al (1986a) Changes in protein metabolism in liver and skeletal muscle following trauma complicated by sepsis. *Journal of Trauma* **24**: 224–228.

Hasselgren PO, Talamini M, James JH & Fischer JE (1986b) Protein metabolism in different types of skeletal muscle during early and late sepsis. *Archives of Surgery* **121**: 918–923.

Heath DF & Corney PL (1973) The effects of starvation, environmental temperature and injury on the rate of disposal of glucose by the rat. *Biochemical Journal* **136**: 519–530.

Herndon JR & Riseborough EJ (1978) Alterations in serum lipid concentration following skeletal trauma. *Surgery, Gynecology and Obstetrics* **146**: 244–246.

Hill GL & Church J (1984) Energy and protein requirements in general surgical patients requiring intravenous nutrition. *British Journal of Surgery* **71**: 1–9.

Hill MR, Stith RD & McCallum RE (1986) Interleukin-1: A regulatory role in glucocorticoid-regulated hepatic metabolism. *Journal of Immunology* **137**: 858–862.

Jahoor F, Herndon DN & Wolfe RR (1986) Role of insulin and glucagon in the response of glucose and alanine kinetics in burn injured patients. *Journal of Clinical Investigation* **78**: 807–814.

Jepson MM, Pell JM, Bates PC et al (1986) The effects of endotoxaemia on protein metabolism in skeletal muscle and liver of fed and fasted rats. *Biochemical Journal* **235**: 329–336.

Kapadia CR, Muhlbacher F, Smith RJ & Wilmore DW (1982) Alterations in glutamine metabolism in response to operative stress and food deprivation. *Surgical Forum* **33**: 19.

Keys A, Brozek J, Henschel A, Mickelsen O & Taylor HL (1950) *The Biology of Human Starvation*. Minneapolis: University of Minnesota Press.

Kien CL, Young VR, Rohrbaugh DK & Burke JF (1978a) Increased rates of whole body protein synthesis and breakdown in children recovering from burns. *Annals of Surgery* **187**: 383–391.

Kien CL, Young VR, Rohrbaugh DK & Burke JF (1978b) Whole body protein synthesis and breakdown in children before and after reconstructive surgery of the skin. *Metabolism* **27**: 27–34.

Lindholm M & Rossner S (1983) Rate of elimination of the fat emulsion Intralipid from the circulation in ICU patients. *Critical Care Medicine* **10**: 740–746.

Little RA (1985) Heat production after injury. *British Medical Bulletin* **41**: 226–231.

Little RA & Stoner HB (1981) Body temperature after accidental injury. *British Journal of Surgery* **68**: 221–224.

Little RA, Stoner HB & Frayn KN (1981) Substrate oxidation shortly after accidental injury in man. *Clinical Science* **61**: 789–791.

Loda M, Clowes GHA, Dionarello CA et al (1984) Induction of hepatic protein synthesis by a peptide in blood plasma of patients with sepsis and trauma. *Surgery* **96**: 204–213.

Long CL (1983) Nutritional consideration of amino acid profiles in clinical therapy. In Blackburn GL, Grant JP & Young VR (eds) *Amino Acids: Metabolism and Medical Applications*, pp 291–307. Boston: John Wright.

Long CL (1987) Fuel preferences in the septic patient: glucose or lipid? *Journal of Parenteral and Enteral Nutrition* **11**: 333–335.

Martin CH & Robison R (1922) The minimum nitrogen expenditure of man and the biological value of various proteins for human nutrition. *Biochemical Journal* **16**: 407–447.

Meguid MM, Brennan MF, Aoki TT, Muller WA, Ball MR & Moore FD (1974) Hormone–substrate interrelationships following trauma. *Archives of Surgery* 109: 776–783.

Michelsen CB, Askanazi J, Gump FE, Elwyn DH, Kinney JM & Stinchfield FE (1979) Changes in metabolism and muscle composition associated with total hip replacement. *Journal of Trauma* 19: 29–32.

Milewski PJ, Threlfall CJ, Heath DF, Holbrook IB, Wilford K & Irving MH (1982) Intracellular free amino acids in undernourished patients with or without sepsis. *Clinical Science* 62: 83–91.

Miller HI, Issekutz B Jr, Paul P & Rodahl K (1964) Effect of lactic acid on plasma free fatty acids in pancreatectomised dogs. *American Journal of Physiology* 207: 1226–1230.

Moldower LL, O'Keefe SJD, Bothe A Jr et al (1980) In vivo demonstration of nitrogen sparing mechanism of glucose and amino acids in injured rats. *Metabolism* 29: 173–180.

Moore FD (1957) Endocrine changes after anaesthesia, surgery and anaesthetised trauma in man. *Recent Progress in Hormone Research* 13: 511–576.

Moyer F, Border JR, McMenamy R & Cerra F (1981) Multiple systems organ failure V: alterations in plasma protein profile in septic-trauma-effect of intravenous amino acids. *Journal of Trauma* 21: 645–649.

Nathan CF (1987) Secretory products of macrophages. *Journal of Clinical Investigation* 79: 319–326.

Neufeld HA, Pace JG, Kaminski et al (1980) A probable endocrine basis for the depression of ketone bodies during infectious or inflammatory state in rats. *Endocrinology* 107: 596–601.

Newsholme EA & Crabtree B (1976) Substrate cycles in metabolic regulation and in heat generation. *Biochemical Society Symposia* 41: 61–109.

Nijsten MWN, de Groot ER, ten Duis HJ, Klasen HJ, Hack CE & Aarden LA (1987) Serum levels of interleukin 6 and acute phase protein responses. *Lancet* ii: 921.

Nordenstrom J, Jeevanandam M, Elwyn D & Kinney J (1981a) Increasing glucose intake during total parenteral nutrition increases norepinephrine excretion in trauma and sepsis. *Clinical Physiology* 1: 525–534.

Nordenstrom J, Askanazi J, Elwyn DH & Kenney J (1981b) Nitrogen balance during total parenteral nutrition: glucose vs fat. *Annals of Surgery* 197: 27–33.

Nordenstrom J, Carpentier YA, Askanazi J et al (1983) Free fatty acid mobilisation and oxidation during total parenteral nutrition in trauma and infection. *Annals of Surgery* 198: 725–735.

Odessey R & Goldberg AL (1972) Oxidation of leucine by rat skeletal muscle. *American Journal of Physiology* 223: 1376–1383.

O'Keefe SJD, Sender PM & James WPT (1974) Catabolic loss of body nitrogen in response to surgery. *Lancet* ii: 1035–1038.

Owen OE, Morgan AP, Kemp HG, Sullivan JN, Herrera MG & Cahill GF (1967) Brain metabolism during fasting. *Journal of Clinical Investigation* 46: 1589–1595.

Pearl RH, Clowes GHA, Hirsch EF et al (1985) Prognosis and survival as determined by visceral amino acids and clearance in severe trauma. *Journal of Trauma* 25: 777–783.

Pedersen P, Seeman T & Hasselgren PO (1986) Protein synthesis and degradation in liver tissue following induction of septic peritonitis in rats. *Acta Chirurgica Scandinavica* 152: 29–34.

Pingleton SK & Hadgima SK (1983) Enteral alimentation and gastrointestinal bleeding in mechanically ventilated patients. *Critical Care Medicine* 11: 13–16.

Pomposelli J, Flores E, Bistrian BR et al (1987) Dose response of recombinant mediators in the acute phase response. *Clinical Research* 35: 514A.

Portnay GI, O'Brian JT, Bush J et al (1974) The effect of starvation on the concentration and binding of thyroxine and triiodothyronine in serum and on the response of TRH. *Journal of Clinical Endocrinology and Metabolism* 39: 191–194.

Powell-Tuck J, Fern E, Garlich P & Waterlow J (1984) The effect of surgical trauma and insulin on whole body protein turnover in parenterally-fed undernourished patients. *Human Nutrition. Clinical Nutrition* 38: 11–22.

Reinmuth O, Scheinberg P & Bourne B (1965) Total cerebral blood flow and metabolism. *Archives of Neurology* 12: 49–66.

Rich AJ & Wright PD (1979) Ketosis and nitrogen excretion in undernourished surgical patients. *Journal of Parenteral and Enteral Nutrition* 3: 350–354.

Robin AP, Askanazi J, Greenwood MRC, Carpentier YA, Gump FE & Kinney JM (1981)

Lipoprotein lipase activity in surgical patients: influence of trauma and infection. *Surgery* **90:** 401–408.

Roe CF & Kinney JM (1965) The caloric equivalent of fever. II. Influence of major trauma. *Annals of Surgery* **161:** 140–147.

Rosenblatt S, Clowes GHA, George BC et al (1983) Exchange of amino acids by muscle and liver in sepsis: comparative studies in vivo and in vitro. *Archives of Surgery* **118:** 167–175.

Selberg O, McMilan DC, Preston T, Shenkin A & Burns HJG (1988) Glucose-free fatty acid interactions in cancer cachexia. *Clinical Nutrition* **7**(supplement): 48.

Shaffer PA & Coleman W (1909) Protein metabolism in typhoid fever. *Archives of Internal Medicine* **4:** 538–600.

Shamoon H, Hendler R & Sherwin RS (1981) Synergistic interactions among antiinsulin hormones in the pathogenesis of stress hyperglycaemia in humans. *Journal of Clinical Endocrinology and Metabolism* **52:** 1235–1241.

Shaw JHG & Wolfe RR (1987) Free fatty acid and glycerol kinetics in septic patients and in patients with gastrointestinal cancer: the response to glucose infusion and parenteral feeding. *Annals of Surgery* **205:** 368–376.

Shaw JHF, Klein S & Wolfe RR (1985a) Assessment of alanine, urea and glucose inter-relationships in normal subjects and in patients with sepsis with stable isotope tracers. *Surgery* **97:** 557–567.

Shaw JHF, Januskiewicz J & Horsborough R (1985b) Glucose kinetics and oxidation in normal volunteers, septicaemic patients and patients with severe pancreatitis. *Circulatory Shock* **16:** 77–78.

Shuck JM, Eaton RP, Shuck LW, Wachtel TL & Schade DS (1977) Dynamics of insulin and glucagon secretion in severely burned patients. *Journal of Trauma* **17:** 706–713.

Souba WW & Wilmore DW (1983) Postoperative alteration of arteriovenous exchange of aminoacids across the gastrointestinal tract. *Surgery* **94:** 342–350.

Stoner HB (1958) Studies on the mechanism of shock. The quantitative aspects of glycogen metabolism after limb ischaemia in the rat. *British Journal of Experimental Pathology* **39:** 635–651.

Stoner HB, Frayn KN, Barton RN, Threlfall CJ & Little RA (1979) The relationships between plasma substrates and hormones and the severity of injury in 277 recently injured patients. *Clinical Science* **56:** 563–573.

Stoner HB, Little RA, Frayn KN, Elebute AE, Tresadern J & Gross E (1983) The effect of sepsis in the oxidation of carbohydrate and fat. *British Journal of Surgery* **70:** 32–35.

Tocco-Bradley R, Moldawer LL, Jones CT et al (1986) The biological activity in vivo of recombinant murine interleukin-1 in the rat. *Proceedings of the Society of Experimental Biology and Medicine* **182:** 263–271.

Tocco-Bradley R, Georgieff M, Jones CT et al (1988) Changes in energy expenditure and fat metabolism in rats infused with interleukin-1. *European Journal of Clinical Investigation* **17:** 504–510.

Traynor C & Hall GM (1981) Endocrine and metabolic changes during surgery: anaesthetic implications. *British Journal of Anaesthesia* **53:** 153–160.

Tsann LH, O'Dwyer ST, Smith RJ & Wilmore DW (1986) Preservation of small bowel mucosa using glutamine enriched parenteral nutrition. *Surgical Forum* **37:** 56–58.

Vary TC, Siegal JH, Wakatani T, Sato T & Aoyama H (1986) Effect of sepsis on activity of pyruvate dehydrogenase complex in skeletal muscle and liver. *American Journal of Physiology* **13:** 634–640.

Vinnars E, Furst P, Gump FE & Kinney JM (1975) Influence of trauma and sepsis on water and electrolytes of human muscle tissue. *Surgical Forum* **26:** 16–18.

Wangensteen OH & Wangensteen SD (1978) *The Rise of Surgery*, p 708. Minneapolis: University of Minnesota Press.

Wannemacher RW Jr, Pace JG, Beall FA et al (1979) Role of the liver in regulation of ketone body production during sepsis. *Journal of Clinical Investigation* **64:** 1565–1572.

Warren RS, Jeevanandam M & Brennan MF (1985) Protein synthesis in the tumour influenced hepatocyte. *Surgery* **98:** 275–281.

White RH, Frayn KN, Little RA et al (1987) Hormonal and metabolic responses to glucose infusion in sepsis studied by the hyperglycaemic glucose clamp technique. *Journal of Parenteral and Enteral Nutrition* **11:** 345–353.

Wilmore DW (1977) *The Metabolic Management of the Critically Ill.* New York: Plenum Medical.

Wolfe RR (1979) Burn trauma and increased glucose production. *Journal of Trauma* **19:** 898–899.

Wolfe RR, Spitzer JJ, Miller HI & Elahi D (1976) Effects of insulin infusion on glucose kinetics in normal and burned guinea pigs. *Life Sciences* **19:** 147–156.

Wolfe RR, Durkot MJ, Allsop JR & Burke JF (1979) Glucose metabolism in severely burned patients. *Metabolism* **28:** 1031–1039.

Wolfe RR, Shaw JHF & Durkot MJ (1985) Effect of sepsis on VLDL kinetics: responses in basal state and during glucose infusion. *American Journal of Physiology* **248:** 732–740.

Wolfe RR, Herndon DN, Jahoor F, Miyoshi H & Wolfe MH (1987) Effect of severe burn injury on substrate cycling by glucose and fatty acids. *New England Journal of Medicine* **317:** 403–408.

Yang RD, Moldawer LL, Sakamoto A et al (1983) Leukocyte endogenous mediator alters protein dynamics in rats. *Metabolism* **32:** 654–660.

Young JB & Landsberg L (1979) Effect of diet and cold exposure on norepinephrine turnover in pancreas and liver. *American Journal of Physiology* **236:** E524–533.

8

The aetiology and management of weight loss and malnutrition in cancer patients

M. F. VON MEYENFELDT
E. W. H. M. FREDRIX
W. A. J. J. M. HAAGH
A. C. M. J. VAN DER AALST
P. B. SOETERS

Cancer is often associated with the development of weight loss or malnutrition. This condition is generally, and often in its extreme manifestations, referred to as cancer cachexia. Whereas weight loss is an easily quantifiable entity, malnutrition is not. Accordingly, the term cancer cachexia is not a measurable entity, although most clinicians would agree that cancer cachexia may be more easily recognized than malnutrition. Thus, a discussion of the importance of malnutrition, its incidence, the factors involved in its development and the ways to treat it, should always include an effort to define this condition.

DEFINITION OF MALNUTRITION

There is constant controversy about the definition of malnutrition. Literally it means the result of feeding in insufficient quantities or of insufficient quality. However, such a definition would emphasize the role of food intake, whereas it is generally accepted that alterations in intermediary metabolism may induce important changes in body composition in patients with malignancy. Therefore, many would agree that malnutrition is a confusing word not applicable to the condition it is supposed to describe. We believe that malnutrition describes an imbalance of food (energy) intake and energy expenditure resulting in changes in body composition. Thus malnutrition may manifest itself as weight loss, but also in decreased amounts of body fat or protein stores in combination with unaltered weights. Such a definition is rather abstract and needs further quantification, but does allow assessment of the importance of malnutrition as an independent factor in the development of complications of cancer or of cancer treatment. This is in contrast to some authors who relate their definition of malnutrition to its ability to predict correctly the development of complications, as if malnutrition were the only factor important in such developments (Dionigi and Dominioni, 1986; Mullen et al, 1979). We have formulated a practicable way to quickly assess different body compartments and to combine the resulting data in one figure that represents nutritional status, or more accurately stated, catabolic state (Table 1).

Table 1. Nutritional index.

$(0.14 \times \text{Alb}) + (0.73 \times \text{TLC}) + (0.03 \times \text{PIW}) - 8.90$

values <0.14 moderate or more 'malnutrition'
values <1.31 mild or more 'malnutrition'
values ≥1.31 no signs of a catabolic state

Alb, serum albumin (g/l); TLC, total lymphocyte counts ($\times 10^9/\text{l}$); PIW, percentage of ideal body weight.

PREVALENCE OF MALNUTRITION IN CANCER PATIENTS

From the above discussion on the definition of malnutrition it may be expected that differences in the techniques used to assess nutritional status will affect many estimates of malnutrition. Thus, Müller et al (1986) found in a series of 422 patients with benign as well as malignant disease that 12% showed severe malnutrition. This estimate was based on a combination of the serum concentrations of several proteins with abnormal values. Based on a combination of clinical judgement and serum albumin levels, Detsky et al (1987a) found 3% of patients admitted for major gastrointestinal tract surgery to have severe malnutrition. In a prospective study of 100 patients, Buzby and associates (1980b) found severe malnutrition present in 9%, and moderate malnutrition in 39% when using a combination of some serum protein levels, skin test reactivity and anthropometric measures. We found, in a prospective study involving 288 patients with gastric, colon and rectal cancer, that approximately 80% showed mild malnutrition and 40% moderate malnutrition. These findings were based on a formula that considers albumin values, percent ideal body weight and total lymphocyte counts. De Wys et al (1980) pointed out that malnutrition, defined in their view by weight loss, varies greatly with the type of tumour under study. Thus, severe weight loss (> 10% of usual body weight) was present in 4–10% of patients suffering from breast cancer, non-Hodgkin's lymphoma, etc. compared to 26–38% of patients suffering from gastric or pancreatic cancer.

It is fair to state that between 3 and 38% of patients admitted for grossly similar disease show signs of severe malnutrition with up to 80% displaying mild malnutrition.

CONSEQUENCES OF THE PRESENCE OF MALNUTRITION

The presence of malnutrition has been associated by several authors with decreased performance status, increased complication rates of cancer treatment and decreased survival. Already in 1932 Warren reported that death in 22% of 500 cancer patients could be ascribed only to extreme cachexia. De Wys et al (1980) found, in a study of 3047 patients with different tumour types, a good correlation between weight loss and performance status: the majority of patients with a low performance status had lost weight, and patients suffering from severe weight loss showed a lower performance status. Weight loss has been associated in several studies with decreased responses to chemotherapy in different tumour types (Carbone et al, 1971; Bonadonna et al, 1986). This altered response rate has been thought to result from starvation-induced diversion of tumour cells from a proliferative state into a non-proliferative state (Frindell et al, 1967), thus decreasing their sensitivity to chemotherapy (Valeriote and Bruce, 1967; Bruce and Meeker, 1967), particularly when chemotherapy may induce only a moderate response rate (De Wys, 1986).

Surgical therapy complication rates of up to 70% in malnourished patients have been reported (Müller et al, 1986; Detsky et al, 1987a; Buzby et al, 1980b), with mortality reaching 90% in severely malnourished patients (Müller et al, 1986). In our institution we found the total complication rate, including minor complications such as superficial wound infection or urinary tract infection, to be unaffected by nutritional status. However, 18% of patients who showed signs of mild or greater malnutrition developed major complications, including mortality, to a more significant extent than well nourished patients (8%). Mortality in this series of 288 patients was 2% in both mildly malnourished patients and well nourished patients.

In conclusion, the presence of even mild malnutrition is associated with adverse effects on performance, response to therapy and survival.

FACTORS THAT MAY INDUCE MALNUTRITION

Disruption of the energy balance, necessary to maintain normal body composition and function may occur if energy expenditure is increased without an adequate rise of energy intake, or energy intake is lowered without adaptation of energy expenditure. Thus, maintenance of this energy balance should be conceived as a regulated system. Energy expenditure is normally quite constant since it is the result of work done to maintain basic functions and structures, and to some extent dependent on the state of health. Consequently, energy intake is the most important regulator of the system. In addition, a system may be envisaged which supplies the food intake regulator with information on energy balance and which controls hunger and satiety. Thus, the cause of disruption of the energy balance in cancer may lie either in a (relatively) increased energy expenditure, brought about by changes in intermediary metabolism and a failure to adapt to starvation, or in a (relatively) decreased food intake, brought about by a disruption of the systems that regulate food intake.

Presence and site of increased energy expenditure

Many authors have suggested that increased energy expenditure is the major contributing factor to the development of cancer-related malnutrition (Warnold et al, 1978; Bozzetti et al, 1980; Arbeit et al, 1984). Critical review of the available literature reveals that most studies were poorly controlled and more recent data obtained from well defined study groups indeed suggest that energy expenditure is generally not increased (Hansell et al, 1986). However, there are still data supporting slight but significant increments of energy expenditure in moderately depleted cancer patients, with adaptation taking place with further depletion (Lindmark et al, 1984).

We recently observed in a lung cancer patient group decreasing energy expenditure with increasing tumour stages that in itself correlated well with increasing weight loss, thus corroborating Lindmark's observation. However, in a larger group of GI-cancer patients no such adaptation could be observed. Thus, increased energy expenditure may be present in certain phases of malignant disease whether defined by tumour stage or amount of weightloss, although the magnitude of this increase seems to be very limited. Therefore, increased energy expenditure is currently not considered the most important contributor to the development of malnutrition in the cancer host (Lindmark et al, 1984; Hansell et al, 1986). In addition to overall changes in energy expenditure certain tissues or cell types may display altered energy metabolism. Thus, hepatic oxidative metabolism has been demonstrated to be depressed, presumably as an energy saving adaptation aimed at providing for the metabolic costs of increased protein synthesis activity (Lundholm et al, 1979, 1980; Karlberg et al, 1982). Furthermore, peripheral tissues as a whole did not show increased energy expenditure (Bennegard et al, 1982), although some organ-systems such as the heart, immune system, and sympathico-adrenergic system may increase their energy expenditure. Such differentiation may further contribute to the difficulty of demonstrating altered energy metabolism.

Glucose metabolism

Altered glucose metabolism in cancer patients has been recognized by several authors (Marks and Bishop, 1957; Holroyde et al, 1977; Holroyde and Reichard, 1981; Heber et al, 1982; Lundholm et al, 1982c; Kokal et al, 1983; Edén et al, 1984a). These alterations are mainly characterized by increased glucose turnover rates that have been observed both after an overnight fast and in the fed state (Edén et al, 1984a). This suggests a failure of inhibition of gluconeogenetic activity in response to feeding, which may in turn be explained by the lowered insulin response to a glucose load (Theologides et al, 1977). In addition, a decreased response to insulin administration has been reported (Lundholm et al, 1978). The increased glucose turnover may represent increased uptake in immune cells, tumour uptake or altered substrate handling in some host tissues, e.g. muscle (Burt et al, 1983). Burt and colleagues have shown increased glucose uptake and lactate release in non-cancerous tissues of cancer patients, suggesting increased gluconeogenesis through increased Cori-cycle activity. Quantitatively gluconeogenesis from lactate seems a more important energy drain than gluconeogenesis from glycerol or alanine (Lundholm et al, 1982a). It has been estimated that the increased glucose turnover rate in cancer patients may explain about half of the observed elevated energy expenditure (Edén et al, 1984b).

Lipid metabolism

Cancer has been associated with a depletion of body fat stores. Several studies employing indirect calorimetry have shown an increased whole body oxidation of lipids (Arbeit et al, 1984; Edén et al, 1985). Arbeit and colleagues (1984) described in patients suffering from metastatic disease low RQ values and increased lipid oxidation associated with lower triceps skinfold values. This would correlate well with observations suggesting an increased turnover of glycerol in cancer patients, presumably the result of increased lipolysis. The oxidation of free fatty acids, in normal individuals occurring in starvation, seems to continue in cancer patients despite the infusion of glucose (Waterhouse and Kempermann, 1971; Dempsey and Mullen, 1985). This may further explain part of the ongoing energy drain, although it has been estimated that the increased lipid turnover rate contributes little to the observed increased energy expenditure (Edén et al, 1984b).

Protein metabolism

Loss of lean body mass is a common observation in cancer (Costa, 1977). Both clinical and experimental studies have demonstrated increased protein turnover rates in cancer (Lundholm et al, 1976; Scherstén et al, 1982; Jeevanandam et al, 1984; Emery et al, 1984). Measurements of protein synthesis have demonstrated increased protein synthesis rates in hepatic tissue (Morgan and Cameron, 1973; Lundholm et al, 1979) and decreased protein synthesis in skeletal muscle (Lundholm et al, 1976). The observation in weight-losing patients that the net release of amino acids from the leg was unchanged after an overnight fast compared to weight-losing non-cancer patients or well-nourished controls (Bennegard et al, 1984) and the observation that the release of 3-methylhistidine from the leg was not increased either (Lundholm et al, 1982b) have been used to argue that decreased protein synthesis rather than increased protein degradation is responsible for the wasting of skeletal muscles. The increased hepatic protein synthesis activity seems to result mainly in the production of secretory proteins and to a lesser degree in the synthesis of structural proteins. Insulin may play a role in the induction of muscle proteolysis because the relative insulin resistance with regard to glucose uptake may induce an energy shortage in muscle tissue necessitating protein breakdown to furnish fuel, presumably by degrading especially the branched chain amino acids.

Anorexia

As for malnutrition, the definition of anorexia is difficult. In most animal studies, cancer anorexia has been defined as diminished food intake of tumour-bearing animals, when compared with the food intake of freely feeding non-tumour-bearing control animals. In human cancer, such a definition of anorexia could not apply because of the large interindividual variation of energy requirements. Weight loss (Walsh et al, 1983; Burke et al, 1980) or complaints about the loss of appetite (Trant et al, 1982; Cohn et al, 1981) have been used instead. Such definitions do not recognize the fact that weight loss may be the result of increased energy expenditure rather than decreased food intake. They also require the awareness of the patient that his or her eating behaviour has changed, which, especially in the early stages of cancer, is often not the case. We have therefore proposed a definition that considers actual food intake as a ratio of pre-illness food intake in a time period when it was presumably unaffected by disease and sufficient to maintain normal body composition and function. Such data are easily obtained through a carefully taken dietary history, and have been demonstrated to be of sufficient reliability (von Meyenfeldt and Soeters, 1985; von Meyenfeldt et al, 1988). Applying such a definition would make an estimate of the contribution of anorexia to the development of malnutrition possible, which may be valuable in predicting the effects of nutritional therapy. In a recent study of 110 patients consecutively admitted for primary treatment of gastric or colorectal cancer we found that 50% of gastric and approximately 40% of colorectal cancer patients ate less than 80% of their pre-illness total energy intake. Thus defined, the groups of anorectic patients were smaller than if defined by the presence of weight loss, abnormal nutritional status, or abnormal appetite.

As no consensus on the definition has been reached, the role of anorexia in the development of malnutrition may only be assessed indirectly (Hansell et al, 1986; Lindmark et al, 1984).

Several theories have been put forward with regard to the mechanisms underlying the development of cancer anorexia. These theories require the existence of a control system that regulates energy balance. The observations that body composition both in animals and in humans remains relatively constant over longer periods of time and under different conditions, and that an individual becomes hungry and starts eating or notices satiety, leading to cessation of eating, suggest the existence of both long- and short-term feed-back control of our hypothetical food intake control system (von Meyenfeldt et al, 1986). It seems as if this concept would indeed be able to incorporate many of the processes proposed over the years to play a role in the control of food intake (Morley and Levine, 1983). How the system fails and induces anorexia remains unknown (Morrison, 1976; von Meyenfeldt et al, 1986).

How does cancer induce metabolic alterations?

It is not known whether all tumours induce malnutrition to a similar degree or in a similar way. Thus, it is not certain that cancer-related malnutrition is a single entity. The observation, however, that even a tumour burden of only 0.1% of host weight is able to induce metabolic alterations contributing to malnutrition signifies the concept that it cannot be the energy drain or tumour metabolism itself that is causing malnutrition. Therefore, Theologides (1977) put forward a theory claiming that tumours produce small peptides and other products that may alter normal metabolic processes. These products would induce the observed metabolic derangements. More recently the identification of macrophage products capable of inducing metabolic alterations in both infectious and neoplastic diseases, and often referred to as TNF or cachectin, has created enormous activity in exploring the true role of these products (Beutler and Cerami, 1987). Although no detectable increments of TNF levels were found in cancer patients (Scuderi et al, 1986), other findings provide circumstantial evidence for TNF or cachectin activity in cancer, e.g. increased net efflux of amino acids from peripheral tissue after the administration of TNF in a pattern very similar to that observed in cancer (Warren et al, 1987), or increased release of TNF by monocytes obtained from patients with cancer (Aderka et al, 1985).

TREATMENT OF MALNUTRITION

Aims for treatment

If an abnormal nutritional status is harmful it seems reasonable to assume that nutritional support would counteract its detrimental influence. Nutritional support may be given parenterally or enterally, either by the oral route or through a tube inserted on different sites into the upper GI tract. In general, the aims of such support may be defined as:

1. reduction of treatment associated morbidity and mortality;
2. improved response to chemo- or radiotherapy;
3. improved overall survival;
4. avoidance or limitation of adverse effects of nutritional support.

In our opinion it is not relevant to aim for improvement of nutritional status as the definition of nutritional status is not clear. Consequently the relationship between nutritional status and the outcome of the treatment of cancer is uncertain. Although some association between the presence of malnutrition and poor outcome is accepted, no method of describing nutritional status achieves a 100% correct identification of the patient who will have a poor outcome. Achieving predictive accuracy with nutritional assessment alone is not possible because many factors, such as age, tumour stage, tumour type, type of treatment, etc. will influence the outcome of treatment. As malnutrition is a factor that may be influenced, nutritional support is an attractive treatment modality. Thus, its value should not be measured by its ability to improve nutritional status, but rather by its ability to reduce the incidence and severity of undesirable, adverse effects of treatment and so improve outcome.

Value of nutritional support

Assessment of the value of nutritional support is only possible if the methods used are adequate. One may formulate the basic requirements of such assessment as follows:

1. The study should include all patients fitting the descriptive criteria of the study population, but
2. The study should clearly define exclusion criteria.
3. The study should stratify for nutritional status using a parameter, or set of parameters, that describes an impairment of the nutritional status, and preferably has been proven to characterize a population at risk, and
4. The study should randomize only within the risk group.
5. The study should evaluate strictly defined goals, and not improvement of nutritional status.
6. The study should include proper pre-trial statistical considerations, that will calculate the required numbers of trial patients needed to prove the hypothesis as it was conceived at the start of the trial.

In trying to answer the questions formulated to describe the aims of nutritional support it is helpful to divide the trials into the following clinical categories: perioperative support, support as an adjunct to chemotherapy, or to radiotherapy, and see how well they fulfil the criteria stated above.

Nutritional support as an adjunct to radiotherapy

In this area relatively few studies (Valerio et al, 1978; Solassol et al, 1979; Solassol and Joyeux, 1979) fulfil the criteria described above and no benefit of nutritional support could be demonstrated. There is one intriguing observation in the paper of Solassol et al (1979) that shows increased survival of patients receiving TPN apparently undergoing multimodality treatment in a randomized study. However, the study design and study population are poorly described and this conclusion may be wrong. The same paper reports significantly fewer interruptions of the planned radiotherapy course in the TPN-supported group, however, without affecting total dose. Thus, it is fair to state that the quality of the studies hardly allows any conclusion to be drawn, making it very difficult to assess the success of nutritional support as adjuvant therapy. It seems as if no reduction of treatment-induced morbidity or mortality and no improved response to therapy or survival may be gained with the administration of nutritional support, although no harmful effects were observed.

Nutritional support as an adjunct to chemotherapy

Eight papers report the effects on response to therapy, therapy toxicity or survival, of nutritional support as an adjunct to chemotherapy, as they were collected in prospective randomized trials in adult patients. These studies are summarized in Table 2 and include patients with lung cancer, cancer of colon and rectum, lymphoma, sarcoma and testicular malignancies. In no paper is there a clear description given of whether all patients fulfilling the inclusion criteria are indeed entering the study, thereby precluding the introduction of a selection bias. Only Clamon et al (1985) report clearly the

Table 2. Summary of papers reporting on the effects of nutritional support as an adjunct to chemotherapy in prospective trials in adult patients.

Authors (year)	Tumour type	All patients selected?	Exclusion criteria?	Stratified for nutritional status	Randomization	Defined goals	Pretrial statistical consideration	n	Results
Clamon et al (1985)	small cell lung	yes?	yes	yes	yes	yes	no	119	No significant benefit regarding – survival – response to therapy – amelioration of toxicity – ability to deliver chemotherapy } no identifiable subgroups that may benefit from adjuvant nutrition
Valdivieso et al (1981)	small cell lung	yes?	no	yes	yes	±	no	49	No significant benefit regarding – hematological toxicity – GI toxicity – infectious morbidity Tendency towards higher CR-response in nutritional support group Preservation of body weight, skin test reactivity
Jordan et al (1981)	adenocarcinoma lung	yes?	no	no	semi	±	no	65	Decreased survival in nutritional support group No protection from leukopenia or neutropenia No protection against GI or myelosuppression toxic effects
Serrou et al (1981)	small cell lung	no	no	no	yes	yes	no	11	No effect regarding CR response rate nausea vomiting myelosuppression
Nixon et al (1981)	colon	yes?	no	yes	yes	yes	no	50	Decreased survival in IVH group No effect on nutritional status parameters No effect on hematological parameters No effect on chemotherapy tolerance
Popp et al (1983)	lymphoma	yes?	no	no	yes	±	no	42	No effect on survival No effect on chemotherapy dose
Shamberger et al (1984)	sarcoma	yes	no	no	yes	yes	no	32	No difference in length of myelosuppression No survival advantage No therapeutic advantage Improved nitrogen balance
Samuels et al (1981)	testis	yes	yes	yes	yes	yes	no	30	No improvement of hematological parameters Slight increase of infections in nutritional support group No difference in response rates

GI, gastrointestinal; CR, chemotherapy; IVH, intravenous hyperalimentation.

exclusion criteria used. Most trials do not stratify for the condition that is to be treated, as if all patients undergoing some form of chemotherapy are at risk and susceptible to a reduction of that risk by administering nutritional support. It may be argued, however, that the administration of chemotherapy induces harmful metabolic aberrations and therefore preventive nutritional support is warranted. This assumption has yet to be proven. Although all trials are randomized, Jordan et al (1981) included a group added to the study population in a non-randomized fashion. Furthermore, all authors describe more or less clearly defined goals, but in no study was an attempt made to quantify the potential benefits, thereby allowing a pre-trial statistical evaluation calculating the required number of patients to prove the assumed benefits. As a consequence most trials are too small to provide any answer. Reviewing the results, despite the conceptual flaws summarized above, reveals no positive effect of nutritional support. Although Shamberger et al (1984) observed significantly improved nitrogen balances and Valdivieso et al (1981) reported a preservation of body weight and skin test reactivity in the nutritional support groups, neither study could demonstrate any beneficial effect with respect to response to therapy, therapy toxicity or survival. All other authors either do not mention an effect or report no effect of nutritional support on nutritional status parameters. Moreover, Jordan et al (1981) and Nixon et al (1981) observed decreased survival rates in the nutritional support groups in their studies which are somewhat complicated by the fact that patients in the nutritional support groups had a higher incidence of metastatic disease than the control patients had. It seems fair to conclude that routine nutritional support as an adjunct to chemotherapy of several malignancy types cannot be advocated. Even in a well designed trial in small cell lung cancer patients Clamon et al (1985) were not able to observe any beneficial effect.

Perioperative nutritional support

Six trials studying the effects of perioperative nutrition have been published (Table 3). Regarding patient selection, only the trials of Holter and Fischer (1977), Thompson et al (1981) and Müller et al (1982) fulfilled the criterion of no selection. In addition, Müller et al (1982) used obstruction as an exclusion criterion. All other authors either did not state inclusion criteria, or stated that they handpicked patients to enter their trial. Holter and Fischer (1977) and Thompson et al (1981) described the use of a risk criterion to select patients who were, on the basis of an impaired nutritional status, at risk for postoperative complications. Both groups used weight loss, but did not establish in their own patients that this criterion indeed defined those at risk. Holter and Fischer (1977) and Thompson et al (1981) were the only authors to describe an apparently well nourished group that served to demonstrate the standard treatment risks. Most authors included a no-treatment arm in their studies.

Heatley et al (1979) studied the addition of parenteral nutrition to an enteral nutrition regimen and Lim et al (1981) reported on the use of parenteral nutrition as opposed to gastrostomy feeding. Both groups appar-

Table 3. Summary of trials* studying the effects of perioperative nutrition.

Authors (year)	All patients selected?	Risk criterion	Standard treatment risk control	No-treatment arm	No treatment – quickly operated	Clearly defined goals	Pre-trial statistical consideration	n	Morbidity/ mortality of treatment decreased
Holter & Fischer (1977)	GI cancer	weight loss	yes	yes	yes	?	insufficient	84	n.s.
Moghissi et al (1977)	oesophageal cancer only dysphagia patients	no	no	yes	no	no	insufficient	15	no
Heatley et al (1979)	?	no	no	no	no	no	insufficient	75	n.s.
Thompson et al (1981)	all	weight loss	yes	yes	?	yes	insufficient	41	n.s.
Lim et al (1981)	selection	no	no	no	no	±	insufficient	24	n.s.
Müller et al (1982)	all patients	no	no	yes	no	yes	sufficient	125	$P < 0.05$†

* Survival was not studied in any of these trials. No adverse effects of nutritional support were seen.
† For both major complications and mortality.

ently assumed a positive effect of preoperative nutrition being present. Only Holter and Fischer (1977) reported that patients in the no-treatment arm were quickly operated upon. Thompson et al (1981) were not specific on this, and Müller et al (1982) reported that control patients were kept in the hospital on a regular hospital diet for a period of time that turned out to be similar to that of the parenterally fed patients. Thompson et al (1981) and Müller et al (1982) set clearly defined treatment goals: decreased morbidity and mortality of surgical treatment, but only the latter group applied a proper pre-trial statistical consideration to this goal. In conclusion, the trials of Holter and Fischer (1977) and Thompson et al (1981) were in concept the best trials, but both were inconclusive because of insufficient statistical considerations. Müller's trial (1982) was complete in this regard, but it remains disturbing that a risk group was not defined, and that control patients were left in the hospital for the same time period as parenterally fed patients, uncontrolled for their dietary intake, and thus probably starving.

Again, the design of the studies described above hardly allows any conclusion. The Müller et al trial (1982) concluded that preoperative nutritional support resulted in significantly fewer major complications and lower mortality, thereby confirming the tendency observed by Holter and Fischer (1977). All other trials did not show a significant support for adjuvant nutritional therapy. A recently published review on this subject, with an additional meta-analysis of the trial results, concluded that results published up to the present do not justify the routine use of preoperative nutritional support, although the tendency towards lower morbidity and mortality rates seems to indicate that certain subgroups, not yet defined, may benefit from such a regimen (Detsky et al, 1987b). Long-term effects on survival have not been reported, but may be present because observations in our institution suggest a significant correlation between plasma total protein and survival in patients undergoing colon or rectum resections for adenocarcinoma (Wiggers, 1987).

Effects of nutritional support on tumour growth

It is of obvious concern that, with the administration of nutritional support to patients suffering from a malignancy, stimulation of tumour growth may take place. A multitude of animal studies (Steiger et al, 1975; Cameron and Pavlat, 1976; Daly et al, 1978a; 1978b; 1980; Buzby et al, 1980a; Cameron, 1981; Kishi et al, 1982; Popp et al, 1983; Hasegawa et al, 1984; Torosian et al, 1984; King et al, 1985) have addressed this subject by assessing tumour volume, tumour weight (relative to carcass weight), mitotic activity, RNA, DNA or protein synthesis and changes in cell cycle activity.

Stimulation of tumour growth was observed in most studies, but to an extent not more than the rate of weight gain or nitrogen retention in the tumour host (Daly et al, 1978a and 1978b; Daly et al, 1980; Buzby et al, 1980a) or to a greater advantage of the tumour (Steiger et al, 1975; Cameron et al, 1976 and 1981; Popp et al, 1983; Torosian et al, 1984). However, no significant stimulation of tumour growth was observed by Kishi et al (1982), Hasegawa et al (1984) and King et al (1985). Nutrition-induced effects on the tumour–host relationship may further be derived from the observations that protein deprivation results in reduced liver RNA and protein content with tumour RNA and protein content remaining unaffected (Munro and Clark, 1959; Ota et al, 1977). Shortage of one or more amino acids has been described to reduce tumour growth (Bounous et al, 1981). In addition, a stimulatory effect of arginine-enriched amino acid solutions on macrophage phagocytic activity has been described. This observation was thought to be responsible for the parallel observation of reduced tumour growth and development of metastases (Tachibana et al, 1985). In general it seems as if tumour tissue is able to accumulate nitrogen efficiently and to maintain a normal growth rate as long as a balanced diet is administered. Applying these animal observations to cancer patients is not correct, because the ratio of tumour weight to host carcass weight and the time period of nutritional therapy relative to their lifespan are longer in animals than in humans. Tumour doubling time is shorter in animals compared to humans and most experimental tumours are not arising spontaneously but are artificially induced. No paper has reported a significant tumour growth stimulation in patients (Terepka and Waterhouse, 1956; Mullen et al, 1980; Nixon et al, 1981; Ota et al, 1984; Shamberger et al, 1984). More recently tumour growth under the influence of a nutritional regimen was studied employing a cell-kinetic analysis of tumour biopsies (Dionigi et al, 1987). The number of patients studied was very small, but the application of such techniques may provide an answer to the question of nutrition-induced (excessive) tumour growth. Current opinion is that no tumour growth stimulation has been observed in cancer patients receiving nutritional support.

SUMMARY

Abnormal values of parameters generally associated with description of protein or energy stores are often observed in cancer patients. The aetiology of these abnormal values is not clear, but seems to include insufficient energy intake absolutely (anorexia), or relative to energy needs (increased energy expenditure). In addition, the ability of some tissues to acquire nitrogen and energy seems to be changed when cancer is present. The resulting status described by abnormal values of protein or energy store parameters is often incorrectly referred to as malnutrition. Incorrect because many factors other than nutrition are related to the development of this condition. However, the presence of the so-called malnutrition is associated with increased morbidity, decreased survival and decreased tolerance to cancer therapy. Whether nutritional therapy is able to reverse these adverse effects by malnutrition remains unproven: most trials performed in an attempt to prove such restoration of the individual's ability to withstand cancer and its treatment, display such conceptual flaws that a convincing answer cannot be given. On the other hand, a deleterious effect of nutritional support has not been observed. More, and clinically relevant, research needs to be performed in this field.

REFERENCES

Aderka D, Fisher S, Levo Y et al (1985) Cachectin tumour necrosis factor production by cancer patients. *Lancet* **ii:** 1190.

Arbeit JM, Lees DE, Corsey R & Brennan MF (1984) Resting energy expenditure in controls and cancer patients with localized and diffuse disease. *Annals of Surgery* **199:** 292–298.

Bennegard K, Edén E, Ekman L, Scherstén T & Lundholm K (1982) Metabolic balance across the leg in weight-losing cancer patients compared to depleted patients without cancer. *Cancer Research* **42:** 4293–4299.

Bennegard K, Lindmark L, Edén E, Svaninger G & Lundholm K (1984) Flux of amino acids across the leg in weight-losing cancer patients. *Cancer Research* **44:** 386–393.

Beutler B & Cerami A (1987) Cachectin: More than a tumor necrosis factor. *New England Journal of Medicine* **316:** 379–385.

Bonadonna G, Valagussa P & Santoro A (1986) Alternating non-cross-resistant combination chemotherapy or MOPP in stage IV Hodgkin's disease: a report of 8-year results. *Annals of Internal Medicine* **104:** 739–746.

Bounous G, Sadarangani C, Pang KC & Kongsharn PAL (1981) Effect of dietary amino acids on tumor growth and cell-mediated immune responses. *Clinical and Investigative Medicine* **4:** 109–115.

Bozzetti F, Pagnoni AM & Del Vecchio M (1980) Excessive caloric expenditure as a cause of malnutrition in patients with cancer. *Surgery, Gynecology and Obstetrics* **150:** 229–234.

Bruce WR & Meeker BE (1967) Comparison of the sensitivity of hematopoietic colony-forming cells in different proliferative states to 5-fluorouracil. *Journal of the National Cancer Institute* **38:** 401–405.

Burke M, Bryson EI & Kark AE (1980) Dietary intakes, resting metabolic rates, and body composition in benign and malignant gastrointestinal disease. *British Medical Journal* **280:** 211–215.

Burt ME, Aoki TT, Gorschboth CM & Brennan MF (1983) Peripheral tissue metabolism in cancer-bearing man. *Annals of Surgery* **198:** 685–691.

Buzby GP, Mullen JL, Stein TP et al (1980a) Host-tumor interaction and nutrient supply. *Cancer* **45:** 2940–2948.

Buzby GP, Mullen JL, Matthews DC, Hobbs CL & Rosato EF (1980b) Prognostic nutritional index in gastrointestinal surgery. *American Journal of Surgery* **10:** 53–63.

Cameron JL (1981) Effect of total parenteral nutrition on tumor-host responses in rats. *Cancer Treatment Reports* **65 (supplement):** 93–99.

Cameron JL & Pavlat WA (1976) Stimulation of growth of a transplantable hepatoma in rats by parenteral nutrition. *Journal of the National Cancer Institute* **56:** 597–601.

Carbone PP, Kaplan HS, Musshoff K, Smithers SW & Tubiana M (1971) Report of the committee on Hodgkin's disease staging classification. *Cancer Research* **31:** 1860–1861.

Clamon JH, Feld R, Evans WK et al (1985) Effect of adjuvant central in i.v. hyperalimentation on the survival and response to treatment of patients with small cell lung cancer: a randomized trial. *Cancer Treatment Reports* **69:** 167–177.

Cohn SH, Gartenhaus W, Vartsky D et al (1981) Body composition and dietary intake in neoplastic disease. *American Journal of Clinical Nutrition* **34:** 1997–2004.

Costa G (1977) Cachexia, the metabolic component of neoplastic diseases. *Cancer Research* **37:** 2327–2335.

Daly JM, Reynolds HM, Rowlands BJ et al (1978a) Nutritional manipulation of tumor-bearing animals: effects on body weight, serum protein levels and tumor growth. *Surgical Forum* **29:** 143–144.

Daly JM, Copeland EM & Dudrick SJ (1978b) Effect of intravenous nutrition on tumor growth and host immunocompetence in malnourished animals. *Surgery* **84:** 655–658.

Daly JM, Copeland EM, Dudrick SJ & Delaney JM (1980) Nutritional repletion of malnourished tumor-bearing and non-tumor-bearing rats: effects on body weight, liver, muscle and tumor. *Journal of Surgical Research* **28:** 507–518.

Dempsey DT & Mullen JL (1985) Macronutrient requirements in the malnourished cancer patient. *Cancer* **55:** 290–294.

Detsky AS, Baker JP, O'Rourke K et al (1987a) Predicting nutrition-associated complications for patients undergoing gastrointestinal surgery. *Journal of Parenteral and Enteral Nutrition* **11:** 440–446.

Detsky AS, Baker JP, O'Rourke K & Goel V (1987b) Perioperative parenteral nutrition: a meta-analysis. *Annals of Internal Medicine* **107:** 195–203.

DeWys WD (1986) Weight loss and nutritional abnormalities in cancer patients: incidence, severity and significance. *Clinics in Oncology* **5:** 251–261.

DeWys WD, Begg C, Lavin PT et al (1980) Prognostic effect of weight loss prior to chemotherapy in cancer patients. *American Journal of Medicine* **69:** 491–497.

Dionigi R & Dominioni L (1986) Predictive indices for the identification of high risk patients. *European Surgical Research* **18:** 201–206.

Dionigi P, Jemos V, Cebrelli T, Danova M et al (1987) Nutritional support and tumor cell proliferation in patients with gastric cancer: a cytofluorometric study. *Clinical Nutrition (special supplement)* **6:** 113.

Edén E, Edström S, Bennegard K, Scherstén T & Lundholm K (1984a) Glucose flux in relation to energy expenditure in malnourished patients with and without cancer during periods of fasting and feeding. *Cancer Research* **44:** 1718–1724.

Edén E, Ekman L, Bennegard K, Lindmark L & Lundholm K (1984b) Whole body tyrosine flux in relation to energy expenditure in weight-losing cancer patients. *Metabolism* **33:** 1022–1027.

Edén E, Edström S, Bennegard K, Lindmark L & Lundholm K (1985) Glycerol dynamics in weight-losing cancer patients. *Surgery* **97:** 176–184.

Emery PW, Edwards RHT, Rennie MJ, Souhaami RL & Halliday D (1984) Muscle-protein synthesis measured in vivo in cachectic cancer patients. *British Medical Journal* **289:** 584–586.

Frindell E, Malaise EP, Alpen E & Tubiana M (1967) Kinetics of cell proliferation of an experimental tumor. *Cancer Research* **27:** 1122–1131.

Hansell DT, Davies JWL & Burns HJG (1986) The relationship between resting energy expenditure and weight loss in benign and malignant disease. *Annals of Surgery* **203:** 240–245.

Hasegawa J, Okada A, Nakao K & Kawashima Y (1984) Does total parenteral nutrition (TPN) really promote tumor growth? A morphometric study. *Cancer* **54:** 1739–1746.

Heatley RV, Williams RHP & Lewis MH (1979) Pre-operative intravenous feeding—a controlled trial. *Postgraduate Medical Journal* **55:** 541–545.

Heber D, Chlebowski RT, Ishibashi DE, Herrold JN & Block JB (1982) Abnormalities in glucose and protein metabolism in non-cachectic lung cancer patients. *Cancer Research* **42:** 4815–4819.

Holroyde CP & Reichard GA (1981) Carbohydrate metabolism in cancer cachexia. *Cancer Treatment Reports* **65:** 55–59.

Holroyde CP, Myers RN, Smink Rd et al (1977) Metabolic response to total parenteral nutrition in cancer patients. *Cancer Research* **37:** 3109–3114.

Holter AR & Fischer JE (1977) The effects of perioperative hyperalimentation on complications in patients with carcinoma and weight loss. *Journal of Surgical Research* **23:** 31–34.

Jeevanandam M, Horowitz GD, Lowry SF & Brennan MF (1984) Cancer cachexia and protein metabolism. *Lancet* **i:** 1423–1426.

Jordan WM, Valdivieso M, Frankmann C et al (1981) Treatment of advanced adenocarcinoma of the lung with florafur, doxorubicin, cyclophosphamide and cisplatin FACP and intensive i.v. hyperalimentation. *Cancer Treatment Reports* **65:** 197–205.

Karlberg I, Ekman L, Edstrom S, Scherstén T & Lundholm K (1982) Re-utilization of amino acid carbons in relation to albumin turnover in non-growing mice with sarcoma. *Cancer Research* **42:** 2284–2288.

King WWK, Boelhouwer RU, Kingsworth AN et al (1985) Total parenteral nutrition with and without fat as substrate for growth of rats and transplanted hepatocarcinoma. *Journal of Parenteral and Enteral Nutrition* **9:** 422–427.

Kishi T, Iwasawa Y, Hiroshi I & Chibata I (1982) Nutritional responses of tumor-bearing rats to oral or intravenous feeding. *Journal of Parenteral and Enteral Nutrition* **6:** 295–300.

Kokal WA, McCulloch A, Wright PD & Johnston IDA (1983) Glucose turnover and recycling in colorectal carcinoma. *Annals of Surgery* **198:** 601–604.

Lim STK, Choa RG, Lam KH, Wong J & Ong GB (1981) Total parenteral nutrition versus gastrostomy in the preoperative preparation of patients with carcinoma of the oesophagus. *British Journal of Surgery* **68:** 69–72.

Lindmark L, Bennegard K, Edén E (1984) Resting energy expenditure in malnourished patients with and without cancer. *Gastroenterology* **87**: 402–408.

Lundholm K, Bylund AC, Holm J & Scherstén T (1976) Skeletal muscle metabolism in patients with malignant tumour. *European Journal of Cancer* **12**: 465–473.

Lundholm K, Holm G & Scherstén T (1978) Insulin resistance in patients with cancer. *Cancer Research* **38**: 4665–4670.

Lundholm K, Ekman L, Edström S et al (1979) Protein synthesis in liver tissue under the influence of a methylcholanthrene-induced sarcoma in mice. *Cancer Research* **39**: 4657–4661.

Lundholm K, Karlberg I, Scherstén T (1980) Albumin and hepatic protein synthesis in patients with early cancer. *Cancer* **46**: 71–76.

Lundholm K, Bennegard K, Edén E, Edström S & Scherstén T (1982a) Glucose metabolism in cancer disease. In Wesdorp RIC & Soeters PB (eds) *Clinical Nutrition 81*, pp 153–160. Edinburgh: Churchill Livingstone.

Lundholm K, Bennegard K, Edén E et al (1982b) Efflux of 3-methylhistidine from the leg in cancer patients who experienced weight loss. *Cancer Research* **42**: 4807–4811.

Lundholm K, Eström S, Karlberg I, Ekman L & Scherstén T (1982c) Glucose turnover, gluconeogenesis from glycerol and estimation of net glucose cycling in cancer patients. *Cancer* **50**: 1142–1150.

Marks PA & Bishop JS (1957) The glucose metabolism of patients with malignant disease and of normal subjects as studied by means of an intravenous glucose tolerance test. *Journal of Clinical Investigation* **36**: 254–264.

Meyenfeldt von MF & Soeters PB (1985) Anorexia in cancer. In Bozzetti F & Dionigi R (eds) *Nutrition in Cancer and Trauma Sepsis*, pp 54–67. Basel: Karger.

Meyenfeldt von MF & Soeters PB (1986) Mechanisms of anorexia in cancer and potential ways for intervention. In Calman KC & Fearon KCH (eds) *Clinics in Oncology*, pp 293–307. Philadelphia: W. B. Saunders Company.

Meyenfeldt von MF, Visser GJ, Buil-Maassen R, Wesdorp RIC & Soeters PB (1988) Food intake and nutritional status in patients with newly detected gastric or colorectal cancer. *Clinical Nutrition* **7**: 85–91.

Moghissi K, Hornshaw J, Teasdale PR & Dawes EA (1977) Parenteral nutrition in carcinoma of the oesophagus treated by surgery: nitrogen balance and clinical studies. *British Journal of Surgery* **64**: 125–128.

Morgan WW & Cameron IL (1973) Effect of fast growing transplantable hepatoma on cell proliferation in host tissue of the mouse. *Cancer Research* **33**: 441–448.

Morley JE & Levine AS (1983) The central control of appetite. *Lancet* **i**: 398–401.

Morrison SD (1976) Control of food intake in cancer cachexia: a challenge and a tool. *Physiology & Behavior* **17**: 705–714.

Mullen JL, Gertner MH, Buzby GP, Goodhart GL & Rosato EF (1979) Implications of malnutrition in the surgical patient. *Archives of Surgery* **114**: 121–125.

Mullen JL, Buzby GP, Gertner MH et al (1980) Protein synthesis dynamics in human gastrointestinal malignancies. *Surgery* **87**: 331–338.

Müller JM, Dients C, Brenner U & Pichlmaier H (1982) Preoperative parenteral feeding in patients with gastrointestinal carcinoma. *Lancet* **i**: 68–71.

Müller JM, Keller HW, Brenner U, Walter M & Holzmüller W (1986) Indications and effects of preoperative parenteral nutrition. *World Journal of Surgery* **10**: 53–63.

Munro HN & Clark CM (1959) The influence of dietary protein on the metabolism of ribonucleic acid in rat hepatoma. *British Journal of Cancer* **13**: 324–335.

Nixon DW, Moffitt S, Lawson DH et al (1981) Total parenteral nutrition as an adjunct to chemotherapy of metastatic colorectal cancer. *Cancer Treatment Reports* **65**: 121–128.

Ota DM, Copeland EM, Strobel HW et al (1977) The effect of protein nutrition on host and tumor metabolism. *Journal of Surgical Research* **22**: 181–188.

Ota D, Nishoka K, Foulkes M & Grossie B (1984) Nutritional parameters affecting erythrocyte polyamine levels in cancer patients. *Journal of Clinical Oncology* **2**: 1157–1164.

Popp MB, Fisher RI, Wesley R, Aamodt R & Brennan MF (1981) A prospective randomized study of adjuvant parenteral nutrition in the treatment of advanced diffuse lymphoma: influence on survival. *Surgery* **90**: 195–203.

Popp MB, Wagner SC & Brito OJ (1983) Host and tumor responses to increasing levels of intravenous nutritional support. *Surgery* **94**: 300–308.

Samuels ML, Selig DE, Ogden I et al (1981) I.V. hyperalimentation and chemotherapy for Stage II testicular cancer: a randomized study. *Cancer Treatment Reports* **63**: 615–627.

Scherstén T, Bennegard K, Ekman L et al (1982) Protein metabolism in cancer. In Wesdorp RIC & Soeters PB (eds) *Clinical Nutrition 81*, pp 143–153. Edinburgh: Churchill Livingstone.

Scuderi P, Lam KS, Ryan KJ et al (1986) Raised serum levels of tumor necrosis factor in parasitic infections. *Lancet* **ii:** 1364–1365.

Serrou B, Cupissol D, Plagne R et al (1981) Parenteral intravenous nutrition as an adjunct to chemotherapy in small cell anaplastic lung carcinoma. *Cancer Treatment Reports* **65:** 151–155.

Shamberger RC, Brennan MF, Goodgame JT et al (1984) A prospective, randomized study of adjuvant parenteral nutrition in the treatment of sarcomas: results of metabolic and survival studies. *Surgery* **96:** 1–12.

Solassol CI & Joyeux H (1979) Artificial gut with complete nutritive mixtures as a major adjuvant therapy in cancer patients. *Acta Chirurgica Scandinavica* **Supplementum 494:** 186–187.

Solassol CI, Joyeux H & Dubois J-B (1979) Total parenteral nutrition (TPN) with complete nutritive mixtures: an artificial gut in cancer patients. *Nutrition and Cancer* **1:** 13–17.

Steiger E, Oram-Smith J, Miller E, Kuo L & Vons HM (1975) Effects of nutrition on tumor growth and tolerance to chemotherapy. *Journal of Surgical Research* **18:** 455–461.

Tachibana K, Mukai K, Hiraoka I, Moriguchi S, Takama S & Kishino Y (1985) Evaluation of the effect of arginine enriched amino acid solution on tumor growth. *Journal of Parenteral and Enteral Nutrition* **9:** 428–434.

Terepka AR & Waterhouse C (1956) Metabolic observations during the forced feeding of patients with cancer. *American Journal of Medicine* **20:** 225.

Theologides A (1977) Cancer cachexia. In Winick M (ed) *Current Concepts in Nutrition* **6**, pp 75–94. New York: Wiley.

Theologides A, McHugh RB & Lindall AW (1977) Post-hypophysectomy insulin response in patients with advanced breast cancer. *Medical and Pediatric Oncology* **3:** 93–99.

Thompson BR, Julian TB & Stremple JF (1981) Perioperative total parenteral nutrition in patients with gastrointestinal cancer. *Journal of Surgical Research* **30:** 497–500.

Torosian MH, Tsou KC, Daly JM et al (1984) Alteration of tumor cell kinetics by pulse total parenteral nutrition: potential therapeutic implications. *Cancer* **53:** 1409–1415.

Trant AS, Serin J & Douglass HO (1982) Is taste related to anorexia in cancer patients? *American Journal of Clinical Nutrition* **36:** 45–58.

Valdivieso M, Bodey GP, Benjamin RS (1981) Role of intravenous hyperalimentation as an adjunct to intensive chemotherapy for small cell bronchogenic carcinoma. *Cancer Treatment Reports* **65:** 145–150.

Valerio D, Overett L, Malcolm A et al (1978) Nutritional support of cancer patients receiving abdominal and pelvic radiotherapy: a randomized prospective clinical experiment of intravenous feeding. *Surgical Forum* **29:** 145–148.

Valeriote FA & Bruce WR (1967) Comparison of the sensitivity of hematopoietic colony-forming cells in different proliferative states to vinblastine. *Journal of the National Cancer Institute* **38:** 393–399.

Walsh TD, Bowman KB & Jackson GP (1983) Dietary intake of advanced cancer patients. *Human Nutrition: Applied Nutrition* **37A:** 41–45.

Warnold I, Lundholm K & Scherstén T (1978) Energy balance and body composition in cancer patients. *Cancer Research* **38:** 1801–1807.

Warren RS, Starnes F, Gabrilove JL, Oettgen HF & Brennan MF (1987) The acute metabolic effects of tumor necrosis factor administration in humans. *Archives of Surgery* **122:** 1396–1400.

Warren S (1932) The immediate causes of death in cancer. *American Journal of the Medical Sciences* **184:** 610–615.

Waterhouse D & Kempermann JH (1971) Carbohydrate metabolism in subjects with cancer. *Cancer Research* **31:** 1273–1278.

Wiggers T (1987) The no-touch isolation technique in colon cancer. Report on a multicentre study with analyses of prognostic factors. Thesis, University of Limburg, The Netherlands.

9

Nutritional management of paediatric patients

FORRESTER COCKBURN
JOHN EVANS

Failure to provide adequate nutrition for the normal infant and child can result in permanent defects in growth and development. These defects affect not only physical growth and development, but also the intellectual, emotional and social development of the child. Failure to provide adequate nutrition for the sick or abnormal child, particularly during periods of prolonged hospital care away from family support can result in physical, intellectual and emotional handicaps.

METABOLIC REQUIREMENTS OF CHILDREN

Growth of the body and its individual organs requires a balanced supply of all nutrients together with efficient removal of all metabolic waste products to allow effective cellular division and tissue growth to occur. The more immature the child the lower are tissue 'reserves' of nutrients and the shorter the period before tissue catabolism will commence. A 1 kg preterm infant will enter a catabolic state within 2 to 3 hours unless a balanced supply of nutrients is started. It is estimated that in acute starvation, fed water alone, the 1 kg preterm infant will survive 3 to 4 days, the 3.5 kg term infant 30 days and the 30 kg adult male 90 days. Chronic undernutrition in the adult once corrected can result in a return to normality, but in the infant and child will result in permanent deficits. More immature infants are ill adapted to tissue catabolism because of the anatomical and functional immaturity of their body organs particularly skin, lung, liver, kidney, endocrine and nervous systems. States of starvation which result in tissue catabolism and an increase in metabolic waste production must be avoided. The key to successful nutrition in children is a balanced supply of all nutrients to maintain an anabolic state and reduce to a minimum the need to excrete urea, carbon dioxide, heat and other products which result from tissue catabolism.

It would be wrong to assume that for any individual nutrient there would be a sufficient body store of that nutrient to allow the child to compensate for a limited dietary intake. All nutrients must be given, otherwise there will be induced a degree of tissue catabolism to provide the rate-limiting nutrient, be it an individual amino acid, a mineral or a vitamin. Supplying excessive amounts of individual nutrients, e.g. an amino acid, will equally inhibit peptide and protein synthesis, cellular division and tissue growth and maturation.

Which foods provide a balanced supply of nutrients? For the normal mature infant human milk is the evolutionary ideal food, but for the preterm infant and the infant with inherited or acquired abnormalities of tissue function specialized foods and feeding methods may prove essential for the child's undamaged survival and growth to maturity. Table 1 gives an indication of the nutritional requirements for the healthy growing infant and child. Conditions which create metabolic stress such as surgery, burns, trauma and sepsis can greatly increase these requirements. The requirements given in Table 1 are for total parenteral nutrition, but are based on the enteral requirements and may be used as a guide for enteral feeding.

Table 1. Allowances per kg bodyweight per day for total parenteral nutrition in infants and children (sufficient for growth in all but severe stress conditions). (After Cockburn, 1984).

Age (years)	0–1	1–6	6–12	12–18
Water (ml)	120–150	90–120	60–90	30–60
Energy (MJ)	0.38–0.50	0.31–0.38	0.25–0.31	0.13–0.25
Energy (kcal)	90–120	75–90	60–75	30–60
Glucose (g)	12–20	6.0–12.0	3.0–6.0	2.0–4.0
Fat (g)	2.5–4.0	2.0–3.0	2.0–3.0	2.0–2.5
Amino acids (g)	2.0–3.0	1.5–2.5	1.3–2.0	1.0–1.3
Sodium (nmol)	1.0–2.5	1.0–2.0	1.0–2.0	1.0–1.5
Potassium (mmol)	2.0–2.5	1.0–2.0	0.9–2.0	0.7–1.2
Calcium (mmol)	0.5–1.0	0.3–0.7	0.2–0.7	0.11–0.20
Magnesium (mmol)	0.15–0.40	0.08–0.20	0.06–0.20	0.04–0.08
Phosphorus (mmol)	0.4–0.8	0.20–0.50	0.18–0.50	0.15–0.25
Iron (μmol)	2.0–3.0	1.5–2.5	1.5–2.5	1.0–1.5
Copper (μmol)	0.2–0.4	0.1–0.3	0.1–0.3	0.07–0.12
Zinc (μmol)	0.5–0.7	0.4–0.5	0.4–0.5	0.2–0.4
Manganese (μmol)	0.8–1.0	0.7–0.9	0.7–0.9	0.6–0.8
Chlorine (mmol)	1.8–4.3	1.5–2.5	1.5–2.5	1.3–2.3
Iodine (μmol)	0.03–0.05	0.02–0.04	0.02–0.04	0.015–0.03
Vitamins (water-soluble)				
Thiamine (mg)	0.05	—	—	0.02–0.04
Riboflavine (mg)	0.10	—	—	0.03–0.05
Nicotinamide (mg)	1.00	—	—	0.20–0.50
Pyridoxine (mg)	0.10	—	—	0.03–0.05
Folic acid (μg)	20.00	—	—	3.00–6.00
Cyanocobalamin (μg)	0.20	—	—	0.03–0.10
Pantothenic acid (mg)	1.00	—	—	0.20–0.50
Biotin (μg)	30.00	—	—	5.00–10.00
Ascorbic acid (mg)	3.00	—	—	0.50–1.00
Vitamins (fat-soluble)				
Retinol (μg)	100.00	—	—	10.00–25.00
Cholecalciferol (μg)	2.50	—	—	0.04–1.00
Phytylmenaquinone (μg)	50.00	—	—	2.00–10.00
α-Tocopherol (mg)	3.00	—	—	1.50–2.00

MODIFIED FEEDS FOR INFANTS WITH CONGENITAL ABNORMALITIES OF DIGESTION AND ABSORPTION (See Table 2)

Management of the very low birth weight preterm infant might involve complete parenteral nutrition or the use of specialized preterm formulas and fresh or pasteurized human milk given by nasogastric or nasojejunal infusions or a combination of these methods (Turner and Cockburn, 1988). Children with inherited metabolic defects such as phenylketonuria, galactosaemia or

Table 2. Composition of specialized infant feeding formulae (values are g/100 ml of standard concentration).

	Protein	Fat	Carbohydrate	Comments
Formula S (Cow and Gate)	2.2 Soya protein Methionine	3.3 Vegetable oils	7.3 Glucose syrup solids	218 mosmol/kg
Wysoy (Wyeth)	2.1 Soya protein Methionine	3.6 Oleic/corn/ coconut oils	6.9 Sucrose Corn syrup solids	242 mosmol/kg
Isomil (Abbott)	1.8 Soya protein Methionine Carnitine/taurine	3.7 Corn/coconut oils	6.9 Corn syrup solids Sucrose	250 mosmol/kg
Prosobee (Mead Johnson)	2.0 Soya protein Methionine	3.6 Corn/coconut oils	6.6 Glucose syrup	160 mosmol/kg
Pregestimil (Mead Johnson)	1.9 Casein hydrolysate Tyrosine/cystine Tryptophan	2.7 Corn oil MCT oil Lecithin	6.4 Glucose syrup solids Modified tapioca starch	338 mosmol/kg
Neocate (15% w/v) (Scientific Hospital Supplies)	2.0 L-Amino acids	3.5 Pork/beef/ coconut oil	8.4 Maltodextrin	320 mosmol/kg
Galactomin 17 'New formula' (Cow and Gate)	1.9 Casein	3.4 Vegetable oils	7.5 Glucose syrup	211 mosmol/kg Trace element and vitamin supplemented
Galactomin 19 'New formula' (Cow and Gate)	2.0 Casein and L-cystine	4.2 Vegetable oils	6.8 Fructose	445 mosmol/kg Trace element and vitamin supplemented
Portagen* (Mead Johnson)	2.5 Casein	3.4 MCT/corn oil	8.2 Sucrose Corn syrup solids	264 mosmol/kg High protein

* Not recommended for infants less than 6 months old.
MCT, medium-chain triglycerides.

maple syrup urine disease can avoid the major handicaps of their deficient tissue enzymes by taking diets modified to reduce or exclude the relevant substrates—phenylalanine, lactose and the branched chain amino acids, leucine, isoleucine and valine.

Disorders of carbohydrate digestion and absorption

Apart from sucrase-isomaltase deficiency, these are unusual or rare problems, but the response to the correct diagnosis and appropriate diet is often dramatic and very rewarding. None of the standard infant feeding formulas recommended for infants in the United Kingdom contains sucrose, and many proprietary infant weaning foods are also sucrose free. Prior to the major changes that took place in infant feeding practices during the early 1970s sucrose was frequently given to bottle-fed infants during the first few months of life and those with sucrase-isomaltase deficiency sometimes presented with severe watery diarrhoea and failure to thrive. This is now an unusual presentation and infants with this problem tend now to present with milder symptoms when mixed feeding containing sucrose is introduced to their diet. However, some individuals with sucrase-isomaltase deficiency appear to be very sensitive to the glucose polymers (e.g. malto dextrins) present in some standard bottle feeds such as Ostermilk Complete Formula (Farley), Progress (Wyeth) and Milumil (Milupa), but also in several specialized infant feeding formulas. They are also freely used as a calorie supplement in the form of Maxijul (SHS) and Caloreen (Roussel) (Dossetor and Connell, 1981). However, sucrose restriction alone is usually sufficient and later in childhood need only be as strict as is required to produce a satisfactory bowel motion and absence of abdominal pain. As with any dietary regimen in childhood behavioural problems and deliberate diet breaking may occur and be difficult to manage and so the observation that the yeast *Saccharomyces cerevisiae* improves sucrose digestion in this disorder may prove to be helpful (Harms et al, 1987).

The rare infant with true congenital lactase deficiency will respond to a lactose-free formula. Pregestimil (Mead Johnson), Wysoy (Wyeth), Formula S (Cow and Gate) and Isomil (Abbott) would all be suitable, but they are modified with respect to their protein as well as carbohydrate composition. Galactomin 17 (Cow and Gate) was the formula often used in the past, but it is being reformulated to reduce its protein concentration and make it complete without the addition of major minerals, trace elements and vitamins.

Infants with glucose and galactose malabsorption thrive with fructose as the sole dietary carbohydrate. There is, however, no satisfactory ready-made fructose formula suitable for young infants. Galactomin 19 (Cow and Gate) is no longer readily available and was unsatisfactory because of its high protein content and deficiency in trace elements and vitamins. A formula based on comminuted chicken, arachis oil, minerals and vitamins with a variable carbohydrate content (see Table 3) can be used with fructose as the source of the carbohydrate. Whilst the feed is nutritionally satisfactory it is complex and time consuming to prepare.

A possible congenital fructose absorption defect has been described

Table 3. Comminuted chicken meat mixture. (After Larcher et al, 1977).

Comminuted chicken (Cow and Gate)	30 g
Glucose polymer (Maxijul—SHS)	10 g
50% Arachis oil emulsion (Calogen—SHS)	3 ml
Metabolic mineral mixture (SHS)	0.8 g (maximum of 8 g/day)
Water to make up to	100 ml

Note:
(i)   Carbohydrate can be glucose, fructose or mixture.
(ii) Fat can be increased to 6 ml/100 ml of feed.
(iii) Calcium gluconate added to provide extra calcium.
(iv) Ketovite tablets (3) and Ketovite liquid (5 ml) required daily.

Standard feed osmolality 221 mosmol/kg.
'Mixture' fed at 200 ml/kg actual body weight starting with dilute mixture and increasing
  concentrations gradually.

(Barnes et al, 1983) and would respond to a sucrose-free infant formula and the exclusion of fructose foods such as fruit, peas and honey.

Disorders of fat digestion and absorption

The use of formulas with part or all of the fat as medium chain triglyceride (MCT) has been advocated in infants with pancreatic exocrine failure, intestinal lymphangiectasia, abetalipoproteinaemia and deficiency of bile salts. There are, however, several hazards with the use of MCT formulas or MCT supplements to standard feeds. Abdominal pain, borborygmi and diarrhoea may occur particularly during the initial period of introduction. Essential fatty acid (EFA) deficiency may develop and be symptomatic if sufficient essential long chain fat is not provided (Dodge et al, 1975). It has also been suggested that MCT may exacerbate the tendency for some patients with abetalipoproteinaemia to develop micronodular cirrhosis (Partin et al, 1974). The absorption of MCT is impaired with pancreatic lipase deficiency and improved with its replacement (Durie et al, 1980). The use of MCT diets would appear to be clearly indicated for treating congenital intestinal lymphangiectasia (Tift and Lloyd, 1975) and probably reduce the intestinal protein and lymphocyte loss in addition to improving fat absorption.

Severe protracted diarrhoea in infancy (SPDI)

Some infants with this condition have a congenital and familial disorder. Those with a family history tend to have the worst prognosis (Candy et al, 1981). The aetiology of SPDI is multifactorial and includes defects of the enterocyte cytoskeleton and brush border enzymes and transport mechanisms, food protein-induced enteropathies, immunodeficiency, autoimmune mechanisms, pancreatic exocrine failure and gastrointestinal infection. Whatever the aetiology the severe malnutrition secondary to the initiating disorder leads to a vicious cycle of events (Rossi and Lebenthal, 1984) which involves impaired local humoral and cell-mediated immunity, reduced pancreatic secretion, ineffective villus repair, small bowel bacterial overgrowth, reduced duodenal bile salt concentration and deficient brush border hydrolysis. The resultant protein-energy malnutrition (see Figure 1) requires, at least initially, a period of parenteral nutrition, but as soon as possible some enteral feeding should be established and can then be gradually increased. Lactose and multiple food protein intolerance is common in these infants and so their enteral feeds must be hypoallergenic and lactose free. A protein hydrolysate such as Pregestimil is often tolerated although the casein-derived peptides contained in this preparation may still lead to intolerance in some infants (Kuitunen et al, 1975). Pregestimil and other protein hydrolysate formulas are also expensive and are often initially unpalatable to all but the smallest infants.

The comminuted chicken-based formula pioneered at the Hospital for Sick Children, Great Ormond Street, London (Larcher et al, 1977) is a modular feed which allows variation in both the concentration and type of fat, carbohydrate and minerals to suit the requirements for individual patients (see Table 3). The principal drawbacks with this formula are the time required for its preparation and its viscosity and lumpiness which make bottle and tube feeding troublesome. Despite some skill and training being

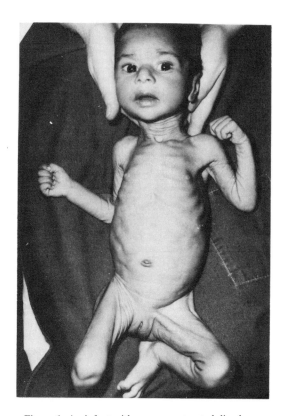

Figure 1. An infant with severe protracted diarrhoea.

required in its formulation we have successfully used it on an out-patient basis, with the parents mixing the formula on the directions of a paediatric dietitian.

Infants with small bowel disorders are very sensitive to high osmolality feeds (>500 mosmol/kg) and this is a major problem with elemental diets such as Vivonex (Norwich Eaton Limited). However, by gradually increasing the concentration and using a continuous gastric infusion, results comparable with the use of Pregestimil have been achieved (Lloyd-Still et al, 1985). Neocate (SHS) is an elemental formula with an amino acid and fatty acid distribution similar to the protein and fat of human breast milk. It has a relatively low osmolality (320 mosmol/kg). We have sometimes found it successful when given as a constant intragastric infusion when protein hydrolysates and the comminuted chicken formula have not been tolerated.

Indications for nutritional support

To wait for a clinical or biochemical indicator of tissue catabolism to appear is in most circumstances an admission of failure; a failure to anticipate the need for additional or alternative feeding for the child. The younger, smaller and less mature the child the more important is it to anticipate and to meet these needs. Measurements of body length up to the age of 2 years and height thereafter, related to a knowledge of parental stature, will give one measure of growth adequacy. These measures are related to body weight and to head circumference. With prolonged malnutrition or undernutrition there may be body weight loss (negative weight velocity) or reduced weight gain (reduced weight velocity for age).

Acute weight loss over a few days is usually related to loss of body water and dehydration. During sub-acute and chronic weight loss there is a loss of body fat which can be measured by skinfold thickness measurements and loss of muscle protein can be estimated from reductions in mid-arm circumference measurements.

Measurements of concentrations of individual minerals and vitamins in plasma, white blood cells and urine may show major deficiencies of these nutrients and altered plasma amino acid patterns together with the ratio of urinary 3-methylhistidine: creatinine or negative nitrogen balance can give some indication of protein malnutrition. It is much easier and better, however, to calculate and to ensure an adequate and complete nutrient intake for every child and to observe carefully the clinical progress of the child. During prolonged parenteral nutrition there is need to have more regular biochemical assessments (Cockburn, 1986).

The indications for the introduction of parenteral nutrition are based on a balance of risks. When the risk to the growth and wellbeing of an infant or child outweighs the risks of parenteral nutrition then parenteral nutrition should be given. This implies the need for good clinical judgement. The previously healthy boy who develops appendicitis, is mildly ketotic but not dehydrated, will not require complete parenteral nutrition, but may benefit from a preoperative infusion of 10% dextrose. The 1 kg preterm infant requiring gastrointestinal surgery should be established on parenteral nutrition preoperatively to prevent the development of a catabolic crisis. If sufficient nutrient intake to prevent tissue breakdown can be achieved by the enteral route then parenteral nutrition should not be used. When total parenteral nutrition is essential the gut mucosa is inadequately nourished. The introduction or reintroduction of enteral feeding should be achieved at the earliest possible opportunity in order to allow the luminal aspect of the gut to function (Aynsley-Green, 1988).

GROWTH AND ITS ASSESSMENT IN CHILDREN WITH GASTROINTESTINAL DISORDERS

Assessment

Growth failure is an important and common presenting feature of gastro-intestinal disease in childhood. It is also a good index of response, or lack of it, to treatment. The most useful anthropometric measurements are weight, height (supine length for children less than 2 years old), skin fold thickness and mid-arm circumference. It is essential that the measurements can be made with accuracy and with a small inter-observer error, as the most useful parameter is the velocity of growth. The equipment produced by Holtain Limited of Crosswell, Crymmych, Dyfed, Wales is satisfactory for obtaining supine length (Infantometer), standing height (Stadiometer) and skin fold thickness (Holtain Caliper). For weighting, beam balances are superior to spring balances and a satisfactory damping system is necessary as children will rarely keep perfectly still during the weighing procedure.

Charts showing standards for British children for height and weight (absolute and velocity) and also for skin fold thickness are available from Castlemead Publications, Swains Mill, 4a Crane Mead, Ware, Hertford-shire, England. The charts have been produced from work of Tanner and Whitehouse (Tanner et al, 1966; Tanner and Whitehouse, 1975). Percentiles for the onset of stages of puberty are also shown on the height and weight charts. For boys the assessment is for penile stage, pubic hair and testicular volume and in girls stages of breast development, pubic hair and menarche. Clinical stages of puberty taken in conjunction with a radiological measurement of skeletal maturity (Tanner et al, 1983) form an essential assessment in later childhood, particularly for patients with chronic inflammatory bowel disease and cystic fibrosis.

Aetiology of growth failure

There are probably three major reasons why growth failure is seen in paediatric gastrointestinal disease. They are malnutrition, chronic inflam-mation and the effects of treatment.

Malnutrition is the net result of the reduced intake of calories, protein and essential nutrients associated with anorexia and vomiting, combining with the gastrointestinal losses from impaired digestion, malabsorption and protein-losing enteropathy. A number of hormonal changes have been found in children with prolonged malnutrition. Hintz and colleagues observed low plasma concentrations of somatomedin-C/insulin-like growth factor I (IGF-1), whereas growth hormone was increased and a somatomedin inhibitor was present in 30% of their malnourished patients (Hintz et al, 1978). Somatomedin values increased after treatment. Whether these hormonal changes are a primary cause of the growth failure is not yet clear.

Chronic inflammation in the gastrointestinal tract in childhood Crohn's disease and in the respiratory tract in cystic fibrosis was previously thought to be the most important aetiological factor leading to growth failure in these diseases. Chronic inflammation, as in childhood rheumatoid arthritis, can undoubtedly contribute to short stature (Byron et al, 1983). However, there is now substantial evidence that in chronic inflammatory bowel disease and cystic fibrosis malnutrition is the prime cause of suboptimal growth. (Rosenthal et al, 1983; Parsons et al, 1983).

Impaired growth in coeliac disease was clearly recognized by Samuel Gee in the first full clinical description of the condition (Gee, 1888), 'while the disease is active, children cease to grow; even when it tends slowly to recover, they are left frail and stunted'. Young and Pringle (1971) found 55% of 110 children with coeliac disease were less than the 3rd centile for height. Whilst in many patients there is obvious malnutrition from anorexia and malabsorption, occasionally growth failure is seen without gastrointestinal symptoms (Groll et al, 1980).

There is usually excellent catch-up growth in childhood coeliac disease following the introduction of a strict gluten-free diet (Young and Pringle, 1971). However, with some gastrointestinal disorders the treatment itself may be a significant cause of poor growth. Until recently many children with cystic fibrosis were advised to take a low fat diet (see Chapter 1). This deprived them of an important concentrated source of calories and exacerbated their tendency to nutritional dwarfism (Pencharz, 1983). Clinically evident essential fatty acid deficiency is rarely seen in enterally fed children, but when it does occur growth impairment is a prominent feature. Dodge et al (1975) described both clinical and biochemical essential fatty acid deficiency in a child with cystic fibrosis who had been prescribed an artificial diet which was inadvertently deficient in linoleic acid.

At diagnosis many children with Crohn's disease are short (Raine, 1984). Treatment with corticosteroids is likely to exacerbate the growth problems in children with inflammatory bowel disease (Berger et al, 1975).

Nutritional therapy in paediatric Crohn's disease

Dietary treatment in paediatric Crohn's disease is now established as a major mode of therapy particularly because of the beneficial effects on growth and delayed puberty.

There are three principal aims. First, it is essential to ensure an adequate intake of calories and protein which in the face of malabsorption and enteric protein loss may need to be 20 to 40% above the normal requirements (Motil et al, 1982). The second aim is to prevent or correct a deficiency of major and trace elements particularly iron, magnesium, potassium, zinc and vitamins especially vitamins D, A and B. The third aim is to induce a 'remission' in the activity of the disease. This last aspect is the most controversial. Most studies have utilized elemental diets but early reports were mostly anecdotal. In a randomized control study of 17 children with Crohn's disease an elemental diet was found to be as effective as corticosteroids with the added advantage of improved growth (Sanderson et al, 1987). The diet chosen in this study contained a mixture of amino acids and oligopeptides whilst most previous studies, both in children and adults, had utilized a pure amino acid based elemental formula. Koretz and Mayer (1980) have ably questioned the specific value of an elemental diet and it may well be that whole protein/polymeric diet may be equally valuable and would certainly be cheaper, more palatable and have fewer side-effects.

SUPPLEMENTAL NUTRITION BY TUBE FEEDING IN CHILDREN WITH CYSTIC FIBROSIS

The steadily improving survival for children with cystic fibrosis has stimulated a rethinking of several aspects of their management. One such area is the severe nutritional dwarfism common in late childhood cystic fibrosis. This was accepted by some as of little consequence when death before adolescence was the rule, but certainly not now with at least 60% survival to the age of 16 years (Phelan and Hey, 1984). A markedly reduced adult stature and delayed or incomplete development of secondary sexual characteristics may be associated with psychiatric disorders (Kraemer et al, 1978). There have been several excellent reviews of nutritional supplementation in cystic fibrosis (Anon, 1986; Soutter et al, 1986) and there is little doubt that in the short term, growth can be improved by increasing the calorie and protein intake. In our own clinic we have made careful assessments of dietary intake and frequently find that children are consuming well below the Recommended Daily Allowance (RDA) for their age. We do not restrict fat and rarely find that this gives rise to gastrointestinal symptoms provided the patient has an adequate intake of pancreatic enzymes preferably using the newer microsphere preparations. Acute infection, purulent secretions from the upper and lower respiratory tracts, the sheer bulk of oral medication, behavioural problems and frank depression are some of the factors responsible for poor food intake. Calorie loss from malabsorption can rarely be completely prevented even with generous supplementation with pancreatic enzymes and H_2 receptor antagonists. Exacerbating the problems of poor intake and malabsorption is the high resting energy expenditure, which has been found even when there is no evidence of acute respiratory infection (Vaisman et al, 1987).

The assistance of a paediatric dietitian experienced in dealing with cystic fibrosis is invaluable, not only to assess nutrient intake, but to advise on a varied palatable high energy diet using, if necessary, concentrated calorie and/or protein supplements. Whilst oral intake can usually be improved in the short term, sustaining it, particularly during periods of infection, is difficult to achieve. It is then that we resort to tube feeds. We have used nasogastric tubes passed each evening at home by parent or patient rather than gastrostomy or jejunostomy feeding favoured in North America. The children and parents become very proficient at both placing the tube correctly and safely administering the feeds (Figure 2). The high caloric density and minimal side-effects of Ensure Plus (Abbott) have encouraged us to continue its use as a standard tube feed rather than using an elemental, peptide or MCT preparation. The feeds are usually delivered as a continuous pump-driven infusion over 2 to 4 hours late in the evening when the children are doing homework, reading or watching TV. Pancreatic enzymes are taken at the beginning and during the feed. A flexible regimen with one or two evenings off per week for 'social engagements' and breaks for short holidays improves compliance. A portable battery-driven pump allows some degree of freedom of movement. We have not encountered problems with pulmonary aspiration, abdominal pain, diarrhoea or distal ileal obstruction. One child who was receiving oral prednisolone for allergic bronchopulmonary aspergillosis developed diabetes mellitus soon after supplemental nasogastric feeds were commenced, but when the steroid treatment was discontinued his glucose intolerance was no longer a clinical problem. There is often dramatic improvement in weight velocity and, in

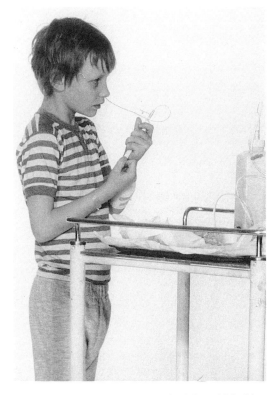

Figure 2. Self-intubation for nasogastric tube feeds in a child with cystic fibrosis.

some children, height velocity after this form of nutritional supplementation, but the final effect on adult stature is not known and the finding by
Yassa et al (1978) that bone age advanced more rapidly than height age
during periods of nutritional supplementation requires further study.
Evidence of a useful improvement in pulmonary function or exercise
tolerance has not yet been clearly demonstrated in a controlled trial.

Gastro-oesophageal reflux appears to occur more commonly in children
with cystic fibrosis than in normal children (Thomas et al, 1985). We have
therefore been discouraged from using nasogastric tube feeding at night
when the patient is at home for fear of pulmonary aspiration. Jejunostomy
and possibly gastrostomy may reduce the likelihood of this problem, but we
have been reluctant to subject our patients to an invasive procedure,
particularly one involving a general anaesthetic which often adversely
affects their pulmonary disease. Gastrostomy tubes can, however, be placed
percutaneously under a local anaesthetic and using endoscopic guidance
(Gauderer et al, 1980) with apparently minimal complications.

TECHNICAL ASPECTS OF ENTERAL NUTRITION IN CHILDREN

Enteral nutrients may be given orally or by tubes placed via the nasogastric
or nasojejunal routes and by gastrostomy and jejunostomy. Anorexia from
disease and the unpalatability of many specialized infant formulas are
frequent limitations to oral nutrition. Even quite young infants will sometimes feed better from a cup and spoon than by teat and bottle, but some
form of tube feeding is often required, at least initially. This is especially
likely if dyspnoea and weakness are present. Enterostomy feeding is not
often utilized in the UK unless there are special anatomical or surgical
problems as, for example, with oesophageal atresia.

Equipment and administration

Tubes made from polyurethane or silicone rubber are non-reactive and do
not stiffen during use. Polyurethane tubes are firmer and less comfortable,
but easier to pass and less likely to become occluded during suction. The
softer fine-bore silicone rubber tubes can be passed more easily with the aid
of a stylet, but this increases the risk of intubating the trachea or perforating
the wall of the intestine. In young infants a size 5 FG tube is usually
satisfactory and in older children a size 8 FG or 10 FG. Larger bore tubes will
allow a faster delivery of feed and are usually easier for self-intubation.

Feeds may be delivered intermittently or continuously, utilizing gravity or
a pump. Peristaltic or syringe pumps designed for intravenous infusions may
be used, but care is required to prevent the accidental connection to an
intravenous line. This is less likely since the introduction of connections
which are incompatible with intravenous cannulae. A useful portable
enteric pump is manufactured by Viomedex. There are two versions. One
will deliver between 10 and 80 ml/hour (within 10 ml increments) and the

other up to 225 ml/hour with a minimum of 50 ml/hour and then 25 ml/hour increments.

Continuous infusions are not only usually tolerated better than bolus feeds, but, in young infants, also result in improved absorption of fat and nitrogen (Parker et al, 1981). A gradual increase in the concentration of the feed over 5 to 10 days will often reduce or avoid osmotic diarrhoea, vomiting and abdominal pain.

Care should be taken when using feeds that have a tendency to separate, such as pasteurized human breast milk, as significant energy loss may result from fat or protein remaining within the tubing of continuous infusion sets (Brooke and Barley, 1978).

TECHNICAL ASPECTS OF PARENTERAL NUTRITION IN CHILDREN

Access to the vascular system is relatively easy with needle, cannula or catheter, but always introduces risks of infection, trauma, haemorrhage, thrombosis and tissue damage. Always consider the balance of risk to the child. Once a decision to give parenteral nutrition is taken the decision as to the site of access must be taken. This will depend on the size and maturity of the child and the likely duration of therapy.

Site of access

1. Umbilical artery

Catheterization of the umbilical artery in the first days after birth is readily achieved using a 3.5 FG end-holed umbilical arterial catheter fitted with a Luer lock. The authors' preference is to situate the catheter tip within the descending aorta at L3/4 level and the catheter can remain in situ for a week or more. There have been occasional reports of peripheral vascular occlusion with limb ischaemia and infarction from this technique and, rarely, an aortic saddle embolus has formed. Injection of drugs or withdrawal of blood samples through the catheter may predispose to these complications as does stopping the infusion for any length of time. It is preferable to maintain the continuous infusion of feeding solutions alone and obtain blood samples and inject drugs via a separate vascular access. As umbilical arterial catheterization has been suggested as one of the many factors involved in encouraging necrotizing enterocolitis in low birth weight infants the route should only be used if really necessary and for as brief a period of time as possible.

2. Peripheral veins

Teflon cannulas of 24 or 26 gauge can be inserted into peripheral veins on the scalp, dorsum of hand or foot, ventral aspect of wrist, antecubital fossa or the long saphenous vein at the ankle. Fixation of the cannula must be firm allowing visibility of the skin puncture site in order that signs of leakage or extravasation of fluids into the tissues can be observed. Splinting of the limb with a padded splint will help prevent dislodgement of the cannula by a vigorous infant. Peripheral veins may last from 24 to 72 hours and the appearance of redness around the entry site or increased pressure readings from the delivery pump are indications for cannula removal.

3. Peripheral vein access with silastic catheter placement in central vein

After skin preparation with Betadine and alcohol an appropriate vein on the scalp, external jugular or antecubital fossa is punctured with a 19-gauge needle. When a free flow of blood is obtained a radio-opaque silastic catheter gauge 23 is inserted through the needle and advanced along the vein into the right atrium. Graduated markings on the catheter allow accurate placement and the final position can be checked radiologically. The needle is then withdrawn over the catheter and the catheter connected to the intra-venous infusion system using the detachable Luer lock compression hub (Vygon* ECC neonatal silicone catheter). The whole procedure must be carried out with strict asepsis and scrupulous after care of the site of insertion is essential to prevent infection. These catheters can remain in situ for long periods of time and their average useful life is between 3 to 4 weeks (Griffith et al, 1984).

4. Central vein

Where periods of prolonged parenteral nutrition are anticipated or in the event of failure to gain access to a peripheral vein, central venous catheteriza-tion is necessary. Several techniques are available. Percutaneous puncture of subclavian or internal jugular vein using a Seldinger technique will allow central venous access, but for prolonged infusions there is increased risk of infection because of the lack of a subcutaneous tunnel and the greater difficulties involved in obtaining catheter fixation. A modified Seldinger technique may be used with subcutaneous tunnelling of the catheter (Gauderer et al, 1982). After careful skin preparation two small incisions are made, one just below the clavicle, the second medial to the nipple and with the help of a trocar (Vygon Life-Cath-Broviac Type) the Broviac catheter is introduced until the fixation cuff is within the subcutaneous tunnel. The subclavian vein is entered using the needle supplied through the upper incision and a guide wire is inserted and the needle withdrawn. The dilator and sheath are pushed over the guide wire into the vessel and the guide wire and dilator are then removed while the Broviac catheter is passed through the sheath and into the vein. The sheath is then pulled apart and gently removed allowing the insertion of the remainder of the catheter. The fixation cuff is then positioned just within the exit wound.

A third method is the direct surgical exposure of central veins using a 'cut-down' technique. The external jugular vein can be exposed surgically

* Vygon (UK) Limited, Bridge Road, Cirencester, Gloucester, GLY 1PT.

and used as the entry point for a Broviac or Hickman catheter which is advanced to the right atrium (El-Gohary, 1985). A subcutaneous tunnel can then be created and led onto the anterior chest wall. Some recommend bringing the tunnel through to the dorsum at the level of the 8th thoracic vertebra (Hoelzer et al, 1986).

The internal jugular vein and the long saphenous vein in the upper thigh are other sites used for a direct surgical introduction of a paediatric Broviac catheter. Any catheter fed into a central vein should be treated with great respect. Fixation at the exit site must be firm and is usually achieved by suture. The area is covered with a sterile transparent adhesive dressing (Opsite, Smith and Nephew).

Pumps and filters

Great accuracy is required when giving fluids to small infants. For the small quantities required by immature infants syringe pumps such as the Treonic* with a range of infusion rates between 0.1 and 99 ml/hour are used. The IVAC† 560565 variable pressure pumps, which allow monitoring of the rate, total fluid volume infused and pressure at the site of delivery will infuse at rates between 1 ml and 999 ml/hour.

It is our custom to use an i.v. filter/air eliminator with a 0.2 micron removal rating for protein and carbohydrate solutions used. These filters remove particulate debris, microbial contaminants and air bubbles and are replaced daily with the giving sets. Intralipid and blood cannot be delivered through these filters.

Home parenteral nutrition

When prolonged parenteral nutrition is necessary in the infant or child consideration should be given to providing this treatment at home. This will reduce the stress caused by prolonged separation from parents and siblings in hospital and will often considerably reduce the stress on parents. Before embarking on home parenteral nutrition the infant or child should be well stabilized on the parenteral regimen and the parents have to be intellectually and emotionally able to cope with the discipline required for day-to-day management of the techniques. This usually requires a period of training of several days with regard to pump function, the giving sets and sterile techniques required for catheter care and changing the infusates. Parents should be taught how to manage emergency problems such as catheter fracture or blockage and signs of sepsis should be explained. A parenteral nutrition team is involved in the preparation for home nutrition and parental support. Health visitors, district nurses, general practitioners, dietitians and social workers are involved at different times in the management and must be kept informed about the ongoing and future management plans. A home teaching service may be necessary for a child on long-term home parenteral

---

* Vickers Medical, Priestly Road, Basingstoke, Hants, England.
† IVAC Corporation, San Diego, California.

nutrition. Of great value in home management is the specialized liaison nurse who can visit regularly and advise these families. This nurse would normally be based in a children's hospital and visit the home on several occasions before the child is discharged in order to ensure that the general hygiene and refrigeration and communication systems are adequate. The hospital pharmacy would normally supply the intravenous solutions with the electrolyte concentrations being changed according to the instructions of the supervising physician or surgeon. The nutrient containers are collected twice weekly from the pharmacy and stored in the domestic refrigerator.

There has to be considerable flexibility with regard to the timing of the infusion and it is usual for most, if not all, of the nutrition to be delivered during the sleeping hours leaving the patient free for normal daytime activities. Regular monitoring of the child's growth and general physical health together with biochemical assessments are made. A routine monthly biochemical profile including zinc, copper and magnesium estimation together with a three monthly analysis for chromium, selenium and manganese provide a routine check on trace mineral status. Monthly assessment of haemoglobin and red cell indices together with a total white count and differential is helpful. For an insight into the effect of home total parenteral nutrition we would recommend reading the article by Mr Liam Liston entitled *Paediatric HTPN: A Father's View* (1987). Patients on a home parenteral nutrition programme may show considerable catch-up in weight and height (Ralston et al, 1984) and our own experience together with that of others (Cannon et al, 1980) is that there is considerable improvement in the behaviour and cheerfulness of the children together with improved weight gain and development. The initial effort necessary to set up the programme within an individual home and to train the parents is more than balanced by the marked improvement in the wellbeing of the child after returning home. There is also an important added advantage in that the parents' morale improves enormously once they take more responsibility for the care of their own child in their own home.

REFERENCES

Anon (1986) Supplementary nutrition in cystic fibrosis. *Lancet* **i:** 249–251.

Aynsley-Green A (1988) The adaptation of the human neonate to extrauterine nutrition: a prerequisite for postnatal growth. In Cockburn F (ed.) *Fetal and Neonatal Growth*, pp 153–193. Chichester: John Wiley & Sons.

Barnes G, McKellar W & Lawrance S (1983) Detection of fructose malabsorption by breath hydrogen test in a child with diarrhoea. *Journal of Pediatrics* **103:** 575–577.

Berger M, Gribetz D & Korelitz B (1975) Growth retardation in children with ulcerative colitis: the effect of medical and surgical treatment. *Pediatrics* **55:** 459–467.

Brooke OG & Barley J (1978) Loss of energy during continuous infusions of breast milk. *Archives of Disease in Childhood* **53:** 344–345.

Byron MA, Jackson J & Ansell BM (1983) Effect of different corticosteroid regimens on hypothalamic–pituitary–adrenal axis and growth in juvenile chronic arthritis. *Journal of the Royal Society of Medicine* **76:** 452–457.

Candy D, Larcher VF, Cameron DJS et al (1981) Lethal familial protracted diarrhoea. *Archives of Disease in Childhood* **56:** 15–23.

Cannon RA, Byrne WJ, Ament ME, Gates B, O'Connor M & Fonkalsrud EW (1980) Home parenteral nutrition in infants. *Journal of Pediatrics* **96:** 1098–1104.

Cockburn F (1986) Practical aspects of paediatric nutrition. In Woolfson AMJ (ed.) *Biochemistry of Hospital Nutrition*, pp 232–248. London: Churchill Livingstone.

Dodge JA, Salter DG & Yassa JG (1975) Essential fatty acid deficiency due to artificial diet in cystic fibrosis. *British Medical Journal* **2:** 192–193.

Durie PF, Newth CJ, Forstner GG & Gall DG (1980) Malabsorption of medium-chain triglycerides in infants with cystic fibrosis: correction with pancreatic enzyme supplements. *Journal of Pediatrics* **96:** 862–864.

Dossetor JFB & Connell MD (1981) Sucrase-isomaltase deficiency: difficulties in diagnosis. *Archives of Disease in Childhood* **56:** 653–654.

El-Gohary MA (1985) The external jugular vein—a simple access to the central venous system. *British Journal of Parenteral Therapy* **6:** 154–156.

Gauderer MWL, Ponsky JL & Izant RJ (1980) Gastrostomy without laparotomy: a percutaneous endoscopic technique. *Journal of Pediatric Surgery* **15:** 872–875.

Gauderer MW, Stellato TA & Izant RJ (1982) Broviac silastic catheter insertion in children: a simplified direct subclavian approach. *Journal of Pediatric Surgery* **17:** 580–584.

Gee SJ (1888) On the coeliac affection. *St Bartholomew's Hospital Reports* **24:** 17–20.

Griffith CDM, Quayle AR, Clark RG & Gurnell P (1984) Home parenteral nutrition in Sheffield 1978–1983. *Journal of the Royal College of Surgeons of Edinburgh* **29:** 335–338.

Groll A, Candy DCA, Preece MA, Tanner JM & Harries JT (1980) Short stature as the primary manifestation of coeliac disease. *Lancet* **ii:** 1097–1099.

Harms H-K, Bertele-Harms R-M & Bruer-Kleis D (1987) Enzyme substitution therapy with the yeast sacchromyces cerevisiae in congenital sucrase isomaltase deficiency. *New England Journal of Medicine* **316:** 1306–1308.

Hintz R, Suskind R & Amatayakul K (1978) Plasma somatomedin and growth hormone values in children with protein calorie malnutrition. *Journal of Pediatrics* **92:** 153–156.

Hoelzer DJ, Brian MB & Mussemeche CA (1986) Selective placement of the Broviac catheter in the infant. *Journal of Pediatric Surgery* **21:** 159–160.

Koretz L & Meyer JH (1980) Elemental diets—facts and fantasies. *Gastroenterology* **78:** 393–410.

Kraemer R, Rudeberg A, Hadorn B & Rossi E (1978) Relative underweight in cystic fibrosis and its prognostic value. *Acta Paediatrica Scandinavica* **67:** 33–37.

Kuitunen P, Viskapori JK, Savilahti E & Pelkonen P (1975) Malabsorption syndrome with cow's milk intolerance: clinical findings and course in 54 cases. *Archives of Disease in Childhood* **50:** 351–356.

Larcher VF, Shepherd DR, Francis DEM & Harries JT (1977) Protracted diarrhoea in infancy. Analysis of 82 cases with particular reference to diagnosis and management. *Archives of Disease in Childhood* **52:** 597–605.

Liston L (1987) Paediatric HTPN: a father's view. *Intensive Therapy and Clinical Monitoring* **8:** 186–196.

Lloyd-Still JD, Smith AE, Sullivan DK & Cooper RA (1985) Comparison of protein hydrolysates and elemental diets in the intractable diarrhoea syndrome of infancy. In Lifshitz F (ed.) *Nutrition for Special Needs in Infancy*, pp 193–199. New York: Marcel Dekker.

Motil K, Grand RJ, Maletskos CG et al (1982) The effect of disease, drugs and diet on whole body protein metabolism in adolescents with Crohn's disease and growth failure. *Journal of Pediatrics* **101:** 345–351.

Parker P, Stroop S & Greene H (1981) A controlled comparison of continuous versus intermittent feeding in the treatment of infants with intestinal disease. *Journal of Pediatrics* **99:** 360–364.

Parsons HG, Beaudry P, Dumas A & Pencharz PB (1983) Energy needs and growth in children with cystic fibrosis. *Journal of Pediatric Gastroenterology and Nutrition* **2:** 44–49.

Partin JS, Partin JC, Schubert WK & McAdams AJ (1974) Liver ultrastructure in abetalipoproteinaemia. Evolution of micronodular cirrhosis. *Gastroenterology* **67:** 107–118.

Pencharz PB (1983) Editorial. Energy intakes and low fat diets in children with cystic fibrosis. *Journal of Pediatric Gastroenterology and Nutrition* **2:** 400–401.

Phelan P & Hey E (1984) Cystic fibrosis mortality in England and Wales and in Victoria, Australia 1976–80. *Archives of Disease in Childhood* **59:** 71–73.

Raine PAM (1984) BAPS Collective Review. Chronic inflammatory bowel disease. *Journal of Pediatric Surgery* **19:** 18–23.

Ralston CW, O'Connor MJ, Ament M, Berquist W & Parmalee AH (1984) Somatic growth and developmental functioning in children receiving prolonged home total parenteral nutrition. *Journal of Pediatrics* **105:** 842–846.

Rosenthal SR, Snyder JD, Hendricks KM & Walker WA (1983) Growth failure and inflammatory bowel disease: approach to treatment of a complicated adolescent problem. *Pediatrics* **72:** 481–490.

Rossi TM & Lebenthal E (1984) Pathogenic mechanisms of protracted diarrhoea. In Barness LA (ed.) *Advances in Pediatrics Vol. 31,* pp 593–633. Chicago: Year Book Medical Publishers.

Sanderson IR, Udeen S, Davies PSW, Savage MO & Walker-Smith JA (1987) Remission induced by an elemental diet in small bowel Crohn's disease. *Archives of Disease in Childhood* **61:** 123–127.

Soutter VL, Kristidis P, Grucia MA & Gaskin KJ (1986) Chronic undernutrition/growth retardation in cystic fibrosis. *Clinics in Gastroenterology* **15:** 137–155.

Tanner JM & Whitehouse RH (1975) Revised standards for triceps and subcapsular skinfolds in British children. *Archives of Disease in Childhood* **50:** 142–145.

Tanner JM, Whitehouse RH & Takaish M (1966) Standards from birth to maturity for height, weight, height velocity and weight velocity: British children 1965 Parts I and II. *Archives of Disease in Childhood* **41:** 454–471 and 613–635.

Tanner JM, Whitehouse RH, Cameron N et al (1983) *Assessment of Skeletal Maturity and Prediction of Adult Height,* 2nd edition. London: Academic Press.

Thomas D, Rothberg RM & Lester LA (1985) Cystic fibrosis and gastrooesophageal reflux in infancy. *American Journal of Diseases of Children* **139:** 66–67.

Tift WL & Lloyd JK (1975) Intestinal lymphangiectasia. Long term results with an MCT diet. *Archives of Disease in Childhood* **50:** 269–276.

Turner TL & Cockburn F (1988) *Craig's Care of the Newly Born Infant.* London: Churchill Livingstone.

Vaisman N, Pencharz PB, Corey M, Canny GJ & Hahn E (1987) Energy expenditure of patients with cystic fibrosis. *Journal of Pediatrics* **111:** 496–500.

Yassa JG, Prosser R & Dodge JA (1978) Effects of an artificial diet on growth of patients with cystic fibrosis. *Archives of Disease in Childhood* **53:** 777–783.

Young WF & Pringle EM (1971) 110 children with coeliac disease. *Archives of Disease in Childhood* **46:** 421–436.

10

Problems and organization of a home parenteral nutrition service

P. BURGESS
M. H. IRVING

Home parenteral nutrition has now progressed from being an experimental technique for the treatment of patients with intestinal failure, to an efficient service available at several specialist centres in the UK. This advance is the result of an increased understanding obtained from a quarter of a century of clinical experience in hospitals all over the world.

Total parental nutrition (TPN) is now the standard treatment for patients with acute intestinal failure who temporarily are unable to receive enteral nutrition, because of loss of gastrointestinal continuity following surgical operations or because of extensive bowel disease. Acute intestinal failure of this kind is caused by conditions such as acute pancreatitis, small bowel fistula, sub-total gut resections and paralytic ileus. Parenteral nutritional support is necessary only whilst the primary disease state is treated and until the underlying condition has resolved or until intestinal adaptation has occurred, following which normal enteral nutrition can be re-established. Most such patients receive TPN as an in-patient until normal enteral function is restored.

However, a smaller group of such patients will require long-term or even permanent support, which in order to allow a more normal life-style, has to be provided on a home basis. These patients suffer from chronic intestinal failure following total or near total small bowel resection, extensive small bowel involvement by Crohn's disease or motility disorders due, for example, to scleroderma. Patients with high output jejunal fistula may also require prolonged parenteral support to counter the excessive losses of fluid and electrolytes seen in this group of patients.

The relevant historical background to clinically useful parenteral nutrition dates back to the reports of Dudrick et al (1968), who demonstrated that normal metabolism and growth could be maintained by parenteral nutrition. Shortly afterwards, the first patient to be treated by home parenteral nutrition (HPN) was discharged using an ateriovenous shunt for access to the circulation (Shils et al, 1970). The first report of HPN via a central route was by Scribner in 1974, who described 165 patients treated through a silicone rubber catheter inserted into the subclavian vein with its tip in the superior vena cava. This catheter, developed by Broviac and colleagues (1973), could be left in situ for prolonged periods, and was anchored in the subcutaneous tissues by an integral Dacron cuff which surrounded the proximal end of the catheter.

The demonstrable success of this technique led to the wider use of HPN and many centres have now reported their experience with home programmes. It is clear from these reports that careful patient selection is the most important requirement for successful HPN. Additionally, the concentration of these programmes within recognized nutritional centres appears to be a major factor in guaranteeing success. Such centres allow the accumulation of clinical and nursing expertise and enable pharmaceutical, biochemical and dietetic support to be provided, services which also are important for an efficient HPN programme.

INDICATIONS FOR HOME NUTRITIONAL SUPPORT

If progressive weight loss leading to death is to be prevented, patients with chronic intestinal failure require long-term nutritional support which may be temporary or permanent. The majority of patients with chronic intestinal failure will ultimately regain normal intestinal function and hence will be able to return to normal enteral nutrition. However for those patients with continuing disease or with an inadequate remnant of small bowel, permanent parenteral nutrition is the only option for survival.

In Britain, the principal indications for HPN are total or sub-total small bowel resection for Crohn's disease, volvulus of the small intestine or mesenteric infarction (Table 1), all of which present obvious indications for nutritional support. There are however other less frequent causes of intestinal failure in which the decision to institute treatment may raise ethical considerations. Thus for example, radiation enteritis following treatment of pelvic malignancy may result in intestinal failure. When the underlying malignancy has successfully been treated, the decision to institute HPN is relatively straightforward. However the same problem in the presence of incurable malignancy poses a difficult ethical dilemma.

Examination of figures from the United States of patients receiving HPN shows that there has been a change in the indications for treatment since 1978. At that time the commonest indications were inflammatory bowel disease and mesenteric infarction which accounted for 68% of patients whilst malignancy accounted for only 17% of patients' treatment. However, by 1986, the number of patients on HPN with malignant disease increased to nearly equal those with inflammatory bowel disease (Howard et al, 1986). In comparison, the United Kingdom HPN register, which recently reported on 200 patients from 28 centres, has shown that the indications for HPN have not changed significantly over the last six years (Table 1) with Crohn's disease remaining the most frequent.

PATIENT SELECTION AND TRAINING

Several factors have now been identified which have to be considered in

Table 1. Comparative indications for home parenteral nutrition.

	Rault & Scribner (1977)	Ladefoged & Jarnum (1978)	Byrne et al (1979)	Fleming et al (1980)	UK HPN Register Irving (1982)	UK HPN Register Mughal & Irving (1986)	Howard et al (1986) (National Registry 1983)
Number of patients	51	19	105	21	35	193	465
Conditions treated	%	%	%	%	%	%	%
Crohn's disease	25.5	65	41	66	56	46	20
Ulcerative colitis		10		5	3	4	
Short bowel syndrome (trauma, vascular, volvulus)	39	20	15	19	17	7	10
Radiation enteritis	10		8.5		6	6	
Pseudo-obstruction	9		8.5	5	3	5	5
Systemic sclerosis	9				9	3	
Intestinal fistula (non-Crohn's)	2		4		3		
Malignant disease			9.5			6	44
Others	12	5	13.5	5	14	23	17

addition to the underlying disease when considering a patient's suitability for HPN. The aim of HPN should be to maintain the patient at home on parenteral nutrition, largely independent of the clinicians and nursing staff involved in the HPN programme. Obviously, review and monitoring of the patient's nutritional and metabolic status will be necessary but this should not intrude frequently into the patient's life.

The most important factor in successfully achieving this aim is the training of the patient by the nutritional support team. Success in training is related to the age of the patient, his motivation, manual dexterity and general health. Surprisingly, intelligence is not a particularly important factor. Training of the patient requires dedicated single-mindedness on the part of the nutritional unit nursing staff. The results can to some extent be measured by the subsequent rates of catheter-related infection.

Patients with significant degrees of cardiac, respiratory and renal failure, mental disorders and terminal illness are generally excluded from consideration for HPN. The effects of age appear to be independent of the patient's social or educational background. Patients over 60 years of age tend to achieve less independence than younger patients. The majority of patients commencing HPN are within the second to fourth decades of life, representing the peak incidence of inflammatory bowel disease, and they are obviously the most adaptable when it comes to learning new techniques.

It is necessary for the patient to have a degree of manual dexterity and good eyesight in order to manage the daily tasks involved in HPN. Problems may be mitigated to some degree by the presence of strong family support, which may even extend to the day-to-day care being undertaken by a spouse or relative.

Some assessment of the potential success of HPN for a given patient can be provided by reference to the performance status of previously studied groups of patients (Table 2). It is our belief that HPN generally should be avoided in patients who are unlikely to be able to maintain themselves on the treatment. Similarly, caution should be exercised in initiating HPN in those patients who on past evidence will progress from being in categories I or II to III and IV as a result of underlying disease or concomitant pathology. However it must be admitted that it is often difficult to predict for a given patient how they will manage with the problems of HPN and what will be the outcome. This often only can be determined after a period of in-patient observation to assess the patient's overall capabilities before embarking on training for HPN.

Table 2. Assessment of performance status of HPN patients (from the UK HPN Register 1986).

Group	Performance status	Number of patients
I	At work full time or looking after family unaided	87
II	At work part time or looking after family with help	43
III	Unable to work, but able to cope with HPN unaided and go out occasionally	50
IV	Housebound. Needs major assistance	15

At Hope Hospital, patients referred from other centres as possible candidates for HPN are admitted for assessment to a purpose-built four bed nutritional unit. Further management of their underlying disease process may be required before the HPN programme can be instituted. This may necessitate surgical intervention to resect diseased bowel, drain intraabdominal abscesses or control multiple fistulae. When stabilized, the patient's nutritional requirements are assessed together with the appropriateness of parenteral as opposed to enteral nutrition. If, following vigorous attempts at enteral feeding, the patient remains in intestinal failure and dependent upon intravenous feeding, a decision is made to institute HPN. Training is given in the aseptic management of the feeding line by the nutritional unit nursing staff, a process which may take up to two weeks to complete.

Most patients have Broviac or Hickman type catheters inserted into either the subclavian or internal jugular vein and subcutaneously tunnelled to emerge through the skin overlying the sternum. Patients are taught how to set up infusions and manage their catheter, and to recognize complications and their management. They are assisted in these tasks by an illustrated manual prepared by the unit staff. A home visit is arranged to assess the availability of adequate space, hygienic work surfaces, and washing facilities. Automatic infusion pumps, trolleys and essential disposables are provided along with refrigeration facilities.

The contents of 3-litre bags containing the prescribed nutritional requirements are infused over a 12 to 18 hour period to give maximum independence. During the day the patient is free from the infusion system, the catheter being 'locked' with heparinized saline to prevent clotting.

In those patients who are malnourished and weak following surgery or prolonged illness, training has to be delayed until the patient can cope. Frequently such patients have also to learn how to manage a stoma, which is an added burden and a potent source of catheter sepsis.

COMPLICATIONS

The main complication encountered during HPN is related to the feeding catheter. There does not appear to be a limit to the lifespan of well managed silicone-based catheters as they are robust and not prone to fracture. Blockage by clot or lipid can be prevented by accurate flushing of the catheter with heparinized saline after infusions. Should a catheter become blocked by clot, it can be cleaned by the instillation of urokinase into the lumen (Glyn et al, 1980).

Thrombosis within subclavian veins associated with the use of central lines probably results from inaccurate positioning of the tip of the catheter. It should ideally lie in the superior vena cava or right atrium. Hence accurate placement with X-ray image intensifier control is mandatory. Reduction in the dextrose content of the feeding regimens is also a factor which has resulted in a lower incidence of thrombosis. Atrial clots secondary to long-term indwelling catheters may be under-reported and it is recommended that regular echocardiography be performed in patients receiving HPN (Chamsi-Pasha and Irving, 1987). Routine venography has shown that 50% of patients on long-term parenteral nutrition have evidence of venous thrombosis (Ladefoged et al, 1981), but it is only clinically apparent in less than 5% of patients (Ryan et al, 1974).

Catheter sepsis is almost always the result of breach of the aseptic technique taught to the patient. This allows colonization of the catheter by skin commensal organisms such as *Staphylococcus aureus* and *epidermis*, although any organism will take advantage of poor aseptic technique. Management of an infected catheter depends upon the presentation of the condition. The majority of line infections, when proven by microbiological culture, can be dealt with by specific antibiotic treatment and 'locking' of the catheter with antibiotics combined with urokinase. When successful this allows salvage of the catheter but if the infection persists, it has to be replaced. The emphasis however must be upon prevention of line infections. A meticulous aseptic protocol combined with the use of occlusive dressings over skin entry sites has been shown to be completely successful in preventing catheter sepsis. The UK HPN register records only 0.35 episodes of catheter infection per year. The lowest rate is recorded by those units with the most experience of HPN.

Parenteral nutrition is associated with a degree of hepatic dysfunction as seen by abnormalities in the so-called 'liver function tests'. Many of these changes have been shown to be related to the dextrose content of TPN regimens. With the introduction of an increased proportion of the calories being provided by fat emulsion the degree of hepatic disturbance has fallen. There is a correlation between hepatic dysfunction and the duration of infusion of parenteral regimens within a 24 hour period, reduction of which appears to reduce the rise in serum liver enzymes. Persistent changes in liver function which do not respond to changes in the feeding regimen are almost always a result of sepsis.

Parenteral nutrition regimens routinely include trace elements, fat and water soluble vitamins. Deficiencies are therefore uncommon during HPN. However, high output fistulas are often associated with increasing losses of trace elements particularly zinc and regular monitoring of trace metal levels is essential for patients on HPN.

SOCIAL EFFECTS OF HOME PARENTERAL NUTRITION

Patients who ultimately receive HPN have often spent many months as in-patients debilitated by their disease, poor nutritional status and the after-effects of surgery. As a result, many have become institutionalized and have lost their employment. This is reflected in the dependence upon hospital staff which these patients may exhibit. This is particularly evident when family support is lacking or has failed secondary to the patients long-term ill-health.

Restoration of physical independence through HPN can, therefore, have a tremendous impact on life-style. Many patients return to their original full-time employment or careers although others will have lost their skills due to frequent hospital admissions. Many take up household duties, relying on the spouse to provide an income to the family.

Sleep patterns may be disturbed by nocturnal HPN feeding regimens. The act of eating with the family may be disrupted and this may cause psychological disturbances. Where patients are able to eat without excessive loss of fluid and electrolytes, they should be encouraged to do so, not only to stimulate adaptation but also to stimulate normal daily activity.

Assessment of life quality has been attempted by structured interviews of patients on HPN as described by Ladefoged (1981). These studies were based on the following criteria:

1. No major physical complaints
2. No major psychological symptoms
3. No substantial restriction in social and leisure time activities
4. Ability to accept HPN
5. Overall satisfaction with the conditions of life

Applying these categories, a third of all patients were felt to have a poor quality of life, which appeared to be independent of age, sex, primary disease, the presence of a stoma or the duration of HPN. This underlines the importance of careful patient selection for consideration for HPN.

The experience with patients from the United Kingdom HPN register suggests that careful selection has resulted in the majority of patients treated remaining independent, and able to work full time or care for their families (Table 2). When assessment of quality of life is related to the indication for HPN, it is apparent that patients with Crohn's disease or postoperative short bowel symptoms have the best outcome (Table 3). Simply stated, patients with a healthy body but a diseased bowel have a better outcome than patients whose diseased bowel is but a manifestation of a generalized disorder.

Of the first 200 HPN patients registered in the UK from 1977 to 1986, over 50% have ceased treatment because of resumption of normal oral nutrition due to intestinal adaptation or remission of their underlying disease.

Table 3. Quality of life grades and relation to indications for HPN (from Mughal and Irving, 1986).

Disease	Quality of life grades			
	1	2	3	4
Crohn's disease	52	18	19	1
Mesenteric vascular disease	9	5	10	3
Volvulus and postoperative short bowel	7	3	3	0
Malignant disease	2	3	2	4
Pancreatitis and malabsorption	0	2	3	2
Pseudo-obstruction	2	5	2	0
Radiation enteritis	5	2	4	1
Ulcerative colitis	2	1	3	1
Scleroderma	1	2	0	3
Other	7	2	4	0
Total	87	43	50	15

Mortality rates for patients on HPN vary, but range from 1 in 8 to 1 in 40 patient years. The wide range reflects the criteria for patient selection for HPN, and the increasing numbers of patients with malignant disease in some series. The main cause of morbidity is catheter sepsis. Of the 34 deaths recorded from the UK HPN register to 1986, 10 were catheter related resulting from overwhelming sepsis, the remainder being principally the result of progression of underlying disease.

ORGANIZATION AND PROVISION OF NUTRIENT DELIVERY

Within the United Kingdom, provision of parenteral nutrition to patients in both hospital and home is usually under the control of the hospital pharmacy departments of the National Health Service. Many pharmacies can now provide parenteral nutrition regimens in self contained 3-litre bags which can be modified as prescribed for individual patient needs. These are issued under prescription to the patient along with dressing packs, antiseptic solutions, syringes and needles and other disposables required. Delivery of supplies to the patient's home is organized by the hospital. However, an increasing proportion of patients are supplied by a commercial service provided by one of the major pharmaceutical companies. This approach may set the pattern for the future as hospital pharmacies find the burden of increasing numbers of patients on HPN difficult to cope with. The whole question of funding of the HPN service has not yet been resolved within the UK. Only in a few regions is it regarded as a regional specialty receiving direct funding.

Centralization of HPN management to single regional centres has the advantage of standardizing regimens and equipment used and allows accurate cost evaluation of HPN facilities provided. It also allows negotiation with pharmaceutical and equipment suppliers to obtain significant cost reductions for bulk ordering of requirements.

COSTS

In the United Kingdom, the cost of maintaining a patient on home parenteral nutrition now reaches £25000 per annum for the supply of nutrients, essential equipment, dressings, etc. In the United States, figures of $40000–$90000 are quoted (Baptista et al, 1984). These approximate costs do not take into account the extra financial requirements to cover services from professional staff, which are difficult to quantify. The cost of providing home parenteral nutrition is 25–50% less than that incurred by parenteral nutrition within a hospital environment.

Hope Hospital currently has 35 patients on HPN. The North Western Regional Health Authority at present allocates funding to maintain 10 patients based on the Nutrition Unit at Hope Hospital. The remainder receive their financial support from other regions or through the Family Practitioner Committee. The cost to the State of HPN can be expected to increase, with the demand for HPN estimated to be two patients per million population, representing an extra 100 cases per year. However only half of these patients will need to stay on treatment for more than a year.

The patient on HPN in the UK does not incur any financial burden from this treatment. This is borne entirely by the Health Service in contrast to the United States where 26% of patients are contributing to the cost of their treatment, accounting for 1% to 64% of the patient's annual income (Robb et al, 1983).

The annual bill to the National Health Service for HPN is above £6 million per annum. However, if home parenteral nutrition returns a patient to an active working existence within a community, then the treatment becomes more cost effective. The alternative costs, namely those of treating patients in hospital, are substantially higher. When HPN not only releases a hospital bed but enables a patient to be returned to the community to lead a useful alternative existence, then the costs are certainly justified.

SUMMARY

Home parenteral nutrition services have revolutionized the treatment, and improved the survivial, of patients with prolonged or permanent intestinal failure. Without such a programme, these patients either would be condemned to continuous in-patient parenteral nutrition or to death.

The indications for HPN in the UK remain predominantly intestinal failure resulting from inflammatory bowel disease, and major small bowel resection. Nearly 50% of patients receiving HPN will ultimately have normal intestinal function restored and thus be able to return to enteral feeding. This knowledge is reflected in the selection criteria for instituting HPN. The use of HPN in patients with malignant disease poses significant ethical questions.

The success of HPN is dependent upon the organization of nutritional units to allow centralization of HPN programmes and to provide the necessary support to patients. It is clear that not all patients will benefit from HPN, and it is only by careful assessment of patients, based on the experience of specialized nutritional units, that a rational HPN service can be provided.

REFERENCES

Baptista RJ, Lahey MA, Bistrian BR et al (1984) Periodic reassessment for improved, cost-effective care in home total parenteral nutrition: a case report. *Journal of Parenteral and Enteral Nutrition* **8:** 708–710.

Broviac JW, Cole JJ & Scribner BH (1973) A silicone rubber atrial catheter for prolonged parenteral alimentation. *Surgery, Gynecology and Obstetrics* **136:** 602–606.

Broviac JW & Scribner BH (1974) Prolonged parenteral nutrition in the home. *Surgery, Gynecology and Obstetrics* **139:** 24–28.

Byrne WJ, Ament ME, Burke M & Fonkalsrud E (1979) Home parenteral nutrition. *Surgery, Gynecology and Obstetrics* **149:** 593–599.

Chamsi-Pasha H & Irving MH (1987) Right atrial thrombus: a complication of total parenteral nutrition in an adult. *British Medical Journal* **295**: 308.

Dudrick SJ, Wilmore DW, Vars HM & Rhoads JE (1968) Long term total parenteral nutrition with growth, development and positive nitrogen balance. *Surgery* **64**: 134–142.

Fleming CR, Witzke DK & Beart RW (1980) Catheter-related complications in patients receiving home parenteral nutrition. *Annals of Surgery* **192**: 593–599.

Glyn MFX, Langer B & Jeejeebhoy KN (1980) Therapy for thrombotic occlusion of long-term intravenous alimentation catheters. *Journal of Parenteral and Enteral Nutrition* **4**: 387–390.

Howard L, Heaphey LL & Timchalk M (1986) A review of the current national status of home parenteral nutrition and enteral nutrition from the provider and consumer perspective. *Journal of Parenteral and Enteral Nutrition* **10**: 416–424.

Irving MH (1982) The United Kingdom home parenteral nutrition register. *Gut* **23**: A438.

Ladefoged K (1981) The quality of life in patients on permanent home parenteral nutrition. *Journal of Parenteral and Enteral Nutrition* **5**: 132–137.

Ladefoged K & Jarnum S (1978) Long term parenteral nutrition. *British Medical Journal* **2**: 262–266.

Ladefoged K, Efsen F, Christofferson JK & Jarnum S (1981) Long term parenteral nutrition. II Catheter-related complications. *Scandinavian Journal of Gastroenterology* **16**: 913–919.

Mughal M & Irving MH (1986) Home parenteral nutrition in the United Kingdom and Ireland. *Lancet* **ii**: 383–387.

Rault RMJ & Scribner BH (1977) Parenteral nutrition in the home. In Jerzy BH (ed) *Progress in Gastroenterology*, Volume III, pp 545–562. New York: Glass, Grune and Stratton.

Robb R, Brakebill J, Ivey M et al (1983) Subjective assessment of patient outcomes on home parenteral nutrition. *American Journal of Hospital Pharmacy* **40**: 1646–1650.

Ryan JA, Abel RM, Abbott WM et al (1974) Catheter complications in total parenteral nutrition. *New England Journal of Medicine* **290**: 757–761.

Shils ME, Wright WL, Turnbull A et al (1970) Long term parenteral nutrition through an external arteriovenous shunt. *New England Journal of Medicine* **283**: 341–344.

11

Regulation of muscle protein turnover: possible implications for modifying the responses to trauma and nutrient intake

PETER J. GARLICK
HENRY J. G. BURNS
ROBERT M. PALMER

As the preceding chapters have shown, injured or infected patients suffer considerable loss of body protein reserves and undergo alterations in their energy requirements. Despite the apparent similarity of their state to starvation, they often fail to respond adequately to provision of nutrients alone. A variety of ways of modifying the stress response are therefore being sought that might improve the traumatized patient's ability to utilize infused or ingested nutrients.

A major component of the stress response is the loss of muscle, which compromises rehabilitation and might even contribute to mortality. In this chapter we have examined a number of factors that might alter the accretion or loss of protein by skeletal muscle as possible ways of improving muscle gain during nutritional support. We start with a summary of the normal physiological regulation of muscle protein balance and turnover, mostly derived from work on animal models, and use this as a basis for a discussion of modifiers of these control processes that have potential therapeutic value.

PHYSIOLOGICAL CONTROL OF MUSCLE PROTEIN BALANCE

In this summary of the major determinants of muscle protein gain or loss we consider first the supply of nutrients, the level of activity or work and the physiological or pathological state. This is followed by an outline of the main humoral factors that alter muscle protein metabolism, i.e. hormones and amino acids. Finally the prostaglandins are discussed, as these appear to be involved in mediating a number of the above factors. A summary of the effects observed in animal models is shown in Table 1.

Nutrient supply

Food deprivation results in an immediate and progressive decrease in the

Table 1. Summary of effects of various factors on muscle protein synthesis and breakdown measured in animal models.

	Synthesis	Breakdown
Physiological states		
Food deprivation (acute)	↓	?
Starvation	↓	↑
Disuse atrophy	↓	↑
Work hypertrophy	↑	↑
Infection	↓ ?	↑
Hormones		
Insulin	↑	↓
Corticosteroids	↓	↑
Glucagon	↓	
Growth hormone	↑	
Thyroid hormones	↓	↓
Androgens	↑ ?	?
Catecholamines (β-agonists)	→	↓
Amino acids		
Branched chains	↑	↓
Prostaglandins		
PGF$_{2\alpha}$	↑	→
PGE$_2$	→	↑

Arrows indicate direction of change, when there is a reasonable consensus in the literature, question marks indicate lack of agreement and spaces are used when there is inadequate information. For more details see appropriate sections of text.

rate of muscle protein synthesis (Waterlow et al, 1978). In growing rats a 40% fall has been demonstrated only 12 hours after the removal of food (Garlick et al, 1983). This effect varies in magnitude in different muscles, fast twitch muscles such as soleus being rather resistant and slow twitch muscles like gastrocnemius and plantaris being more sensitive (Preedy and Garlick, 1983). Sensitivity also depends on the age of the animals: in one-year-old female rats no effect of an overnight fast on muscle protein synthesis was observed (Baillie et al, 1988). How much this is a general property of adults is not yet clear, as an overnight fast has been reported to cause a 50% fall in thigh muscle protein synthesis in young adult humans (Cheng et al, 1987; Halliday et al, 1988).

As fasting progresses there are further decreases in the rate of muscle protein synthesis. In young rats it may fall as low as 28% of the fed value by 4 days. This decrease was shown to be accompanied by a decrease in the amount of RNA (ribosomes) in the muscle, as well as a fall in the rate of protein synthesis per ribosome (Millward et al, 1976). During the first 2 days no loss of protein from the muscles was detected, and balance was maintained by a decline in the rate of degradation (Millward et al, 1976). There was then a rapid loss of protein brought about by a large increase in the rate of protein degradation (Millward et al, 1976). The period of starvation before this secondary rise in breakdown has been shown to depend on the age and the body fat content of the animal (Goodman et al, 1980).

The changes brought about by fasting can be reversed by provision of nutrients; when 12-hour or 4-day starved animals are refed there is a rapid recovery in muscle protein synthesis within the first hour (Garlick et al, 1983; Millward et al, 1983). Furthermore, it has been reported that in fasted surgical patients muscle protein synthesis was higher when enteral nutritional support was given during the preceding week (Ward et al, 1983).

Activity

In addition to nutritional influences, the activity of muscle has an important influence on the maintenance of its mass. Experimental manipulation of the nerve supply, activity, workload and degree of stretch can lead to changes in the rate of growth or atrophy of individual muscles (Brevet et al, 1976; Goldspink, 1977; Booth and Watson, 1985), and disuse is well known to result in a decrease in muscle mass (Goldberg et al, 1974; Jaspers and Tischler, 1984).

The mechanisms of disuse atrophy have been studied in a variety of models, e.g. the loss of neuronally induced contractility by denervation (Buse et al, 1965; Turner and Garlick, 1974; Goldspink, 1976, 1978a; Goldspink et al, 1983). Different muscles appear to respond to denervation in different ways; in some experiments a true atrophy occurred, while in others growth slowed or was even transiently stimulated. Thus unilateral phrenicectomy of the diaphragm resulted in an elevated rate of growth and protein synthesis for a short period followed by an increase in degradation and muscle atrophy (Turner and Garlick, 1974). In other studies of denervated leg muscles (Goldspink, 1977, 1978a), those that were held in a shortened position showed elevated rates of protein degradation and atrophied, whilst those in a stretched position also showed increased rates of degradation but hypertrophied. In this instance the increase in muscle protein resulted from a larger increase in the rate of synthesis.

Limb immobilization by the use of plaster casts has also been used to maintain muscles in either a shortened or stretched position (Goldspink, 1977, 1978b). Even in fully innervated muscles, immobilization in a shortened position led to atrophy as a result of decreases in rates of protein synthesis and increases in breakdown.

Disuse is well recognized to cause muscle wasting in man. In a study of the effect of leg immobilization after tibial fracture, Gibson et al (1987) showed that protein synthesis in the immobilized muscle was lower than that on the opposite side. Estimates of the rate of muscle protein breakdown suggested that it was little affected by immobilization.

Work-induced hypertrophy of specific muscles has also been examined in a number of models. For example, an increase in the weight load on chicken wing muscles led to an increase in muscle growth (Laurent et al, 1978a, 1978b; Holly et al, 1980). A widely used model is the tenotomy of a specific muscle (e.g. the gastrocnemius) which results in the atrophy of that muscle and a hypertrophy of the synergists, soleus and plantaris (Goldberg, 1967; Mackova and Hnik, 1973; Goldspink et al, 1983; McMillan et al, 1987). Generally these studies have shown hypertrophy to be achieved by an increase in the rate of muscle protein synthesis, which may be accompanied by a proportionately smaller rise in the rate of protein degradation.

Pathological states

The rapid development of muscle wasting following trauma or sepsis has been recognized for many years (Cuthbertson, 1930; Duke et al, 1970). The main reason for the muscle protein loss in infection or with experimental endotoxaemia is a rise in the rate of protein breakdown, which has been demonstrated both in vivo and in vitro (Baracos et al, 1983; Clowes et al, 1983; Jepson et al, 1986). The changes in protein synthesis are less clear, however, and there are reports that rates are increased (Pomposelli et al, 1985), unchanged (Baracos et al, 1983) or decreased (Fern et al, 1985; Jepson et al, 1986). In the latter two studies the decrease in synthesis was aggravated by anorexia, but was still marked in animals that were pair fed or fasted.

With scald injury in rats, similar effects have been observed on protein breakdown, which was elevated in muscle of the injured limb, but not in uninjured muscle (Shangraw and Turinsky, 1984). Protein synthesis in the injured limb was elevated, but to a smaller degree than breakdown, resulting in rapid protein loss. An increase in synthesis was also noted on the uninjured side, but only in soleus and not in plantaris muscle. The increase in synthesis of the injured muscle might be related to the repair process, while that on the uninjured side could have resulted from increased workload.

Hormones

Insulin

The long-term effects of insulin deficiency on muscle protein metabolism have been studied in animals made diabetic with either alloxan or strepto-zocin. A pronounced inhibition of synthesis when measured in vitro or in vivo has been demonstrated (Pain and Garlick, 1974; Flaim et al, 1978; Pain et al, 1983). The effect on protein breakdown is variable, depending on the time after induction of diabetes. Initially, there is a rapid loss of muscle protein, which is accompanied by an increase in the rate of proteolysis (Flaim et al, 1978; Pain et al, 1983). If the animals survive, however, they start to grow again, albeit slowly, and at this time there is a decrease in muscle proteolysis (Millward et al, 1976; Pain et al, 1983).

Acute effects of insulin have also been demonstrated in muscle from non-diabetic animals. When insulin was added to the medium of incubated or perfused muscle preparations from fasted animals there was an increase in protein synthesis and a decrease in breakdown (Fulks et al, 1975; Frayn and Maycock, 1979; Li et al, 1979; Preedy and Garlick, 1983). In preparations from fed animals the same effects were not observed (Li et al, 1979), leading to the suggestion that the increase in plasma insulin concentration might be responsible for the increase in muscle protein synthesis on feeding. Indeed, when postabsorptive or 4-day starved rats were refed after injection of anti-insulin serum to eliminate the food-induced rise in plasma insulin, there was no increase in muscle synthesis, suggesting that the normal rise in synthesis on refeeding required insulin (Millward et al, 1983; Preedy and Garlick, 1986). Furthermore, infusion of insulin into postabsorptive rats in vivo increased the rate of muscle protein synthesis, but had no effect on fed animals (Garlick et al, 1983). In postabsorptive rats the response was rapid (about 10 min), but to be effective the plasma concentration of the hormone needed to be higher than normal fed values. This relative insensitivity to insulin suggested that it was not the only factor involved in the stimulation of muscle protein synthesis by feeding.

In postabsorptive man the effect of infusing insulin is also anabolic, but the mechanism appears to be different, involving only a decrease in muscle protein breakdown. Measurement of the balance of amino acid and label across the forearm while infusing [^{3}H]phenylalanine has been used to assess muscle protein turnover (Gelfand and Barrett, 1987). In postabsorptive subjects there was a net loss of phenylalanine from the forearm, but on infusion of insulin this was reversed, as a result of a decrease in muscle protein breakdown, with no change in synthesis. The apparent difference in mechanism between the studies in rats and man might relate to the fact that the rats were young and growing whilst the human subjects were adult.

Corticosteroids

The biochemistry of the catabolic action of these hormones has been studied mainly in animal tissues. Addition of corticosteroid hormones to the incubation medium has been shown to inhibit protein synthesis in incubated rat and rabbit muscle (McGrath and Goldspink, 1982; Reeds and Palmer, 1984). Measurements in rats in vivo have also shown a decrease in muscle protein synthesis after injection of corticosterone (Garlick et al, 1987). Both in vitro and in vivo, about 3–4 hours of exposure to the hormone were required for the effect to become apparent. Longer term treatment results in a continued fall in synthesis as a result of a progressive loss of ribosomes, in addition to a low rate of protein synthesis per ribosome (Odedra et al, 1983). Increases in muscle protein degradation have also been noted, but these are less important in relation to the loss of muscle protein than the decrease in synthesis (Odedra and Millward, 1982; Tomas et al, 1984).

Glucagon

Although glucagon is catabolic to muscle, its site of action has been considered to be in the liver, through a stimulation of gluconeogenesis. However, high concentrations of the hormone have been shown to inhibit muscle protein synthesis in isolated muscle preparations in vitro (Beatty et al, 1963; Preedy and Garlick, 1988a). Furthermore, infusion of glucagon into growing rats depresses muscle protein synthesis measured in vivo. This effect occurs at plasma concentrations within the pathophysiological range, takes between 1 hour and 6 hours to develop, is opposed by small increases in insulin concentration, and occurs by a mechanism that does not appear to involve amino acid depletion through stimulated liver gluconeogenesis (Preedy and Garlick, 1985, 1988a). High concentrations of glucagon in starvation, diabetes or trauma might therefore be important in the muscle protein loss occurring in these conditions.

Growth hormone

Hypophysectomy in rats results in diminished growth, associated with decreases in protein synthesis, ribosome content and protein synthesis per ribosome in skeletal muscle (Flaim et al, 1978; Brown et al, 1981). Furthermore, exposure of incubated diaphragm muscles from hypophysectomized rats to growth hormone (GH) results in an acute stimulation of protein synthesis (Kostyo and Nutting, 1974), an effect that has been attributed to the 'insulin-like' action of the hormone (Cameron et al, 1988). Longer-term treatment with GH results in growth promotion, which has been shown to involve an increase in muscle protein synthesis (Pell and Bates, 1987).

Thyroid hormones

Thyroidectomy of animals has been shown to cause a decrease in muscle protein synthesis, measured both in vivo and in vitro, as a result of loss of ribosomes rather than a decrease in the rate of synthesis per ribosome (Flaim et al, 1978; Brown et al, 1981). Replacement of triiodothyronine restored rates of protein synthesis to normal. Thyroidectomy also lowered, and T3 treatment increased, rates of protein degradation. The changes in protein synthesis and breakdown therefore occur in parallel, with higher plasma levels of T3 resulting in higher levels of protein turnover (Brown and Millward, 1983).

Gonadal steroids

The effects of gonadal steroids on muscle protein metabolism in animal studies have been shown to be complex and to vary depending on many factors, including the sex and age of the animal and the particular muscle under study.

Most work has concentrated on the anabolic action of androgens, since with many mammalian species the male is larger than the female. Administration of testosterone to male experimental animals has not been shown to have any consistent effect on muscle growth or protein turnover (Grigsby et al, 1976; Dohm et al, 1979), but in young female rats a stimulation of muscle growth has been observed (Martinez et al, 1984). This was brought about by an increase in protein synthesis accompanied by a smaller increase in protein breakdown. Synthetic androgens have also been shown to have anabolic effects in female rats, but apparently by different mechanisms. Stanozolol caused an increase in muscle protein synthesis with no change in breakdown (Bates et al, 1987), whilst trenbolone had no effect on synthesis but decreased breakdown (Vernon and Buttery, 1978). It has been suggested that the anabolic actions of androgens might be mediated either by stimulating the production of GH (Jansson et al, 1983) or by interfering with the catabolic action of corticosteroids (Mayer and Rosen, 1977).

Catecholamines

Although adrenaline is commonly considered to be 'catabolic', in rat skeletal muscle in vitro it has been shown to inhibit the release of free amino acids, and hence to prevent protein loss (Garber et al, 1976). This effect was observed at physiological concentrations, could be reproduced by the β-agonist iso-prenaline (isoproterenol *USP*) and was blocked by the β-antagonist pro-pranolol. In the perfused rat hind-quarter, isoprenaline was shown to act by suppressing protein breakdown, without affecting synthesis (Jefferson et al, 1977). A similar effect of noradrenaline on amino acid release from incubated muscle has also been demonstrated, but this was believed to be through stimulation of the β- rather than the α-adrenergic receptor, because the concentration required was very high (Garber et al, 1976). Furthermore, the α-agonist phenylephrine, and the α-antagonist, phentolamine, were without effect. However, in another study with perfused rat muscle phentolamine has been shown to inhibit protein synthesis (Preedy and Garlick, 1988b).

Amino acids

Although muscle protein balance is clearly dependent on amino acid supply, either from the diet or when given parenterally, their detailed mode of action has been less clear. Studies in isolated muscles have shown that additions of high concentrations of amino acid mixtures to the medium stimulate protein synthesis and inhibit degradation (Fulks et al, 1975; Li and Jefferson, 1978). This effect appears to require only the branched-chain amino acids (BCAAs), in particular leucine (Buse and Reid, 1975; Fulks et al, 1975; Li and Jefferson, 1978). Subsequent studies have shown that the inhibition of breakdown is brought about by the keto acid derived from leucine (α-keto isocaproate), but that the stimulation of synthesis depends on the amino acid itself (Tischler et al, 1982).

The physiological role of these effects has been more difficult to define, and studies of the response of nitrogen balance or muscle protein turnover to administration of BCAAs in vivo have been conflicting, both in man and animals (Adibi, 1980; Walser, 1984). Recent data have suggested that amino acids act synergistically with insulin in mediating the stimulation of muscle protein synthesis by food intake, as infusion of amino acids into post-absorptive rats increased the sensitivity of muscle protein synthesis to insulin (Figure 1a) (Preedy and Garlick, 1986; Garlick and Grant, 1988). Experiments with infusion of various amino acid mixtures in combination with glucose (to raise plasma insulin levels) have shown that the effect of amino acids can be attributed mainly to the branched chains (see Figure 1b). This would help explain why reports of the response to BCAAs are not

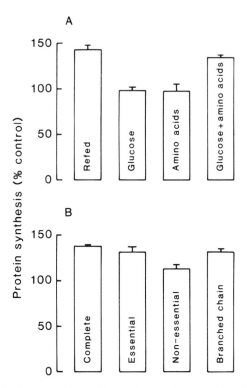

Figure 1. Combined effects of amino acids and insulin (generated by glucose infusion) on muscle protein synthesis in postabsorptive rats. (**a**) Effect of 1 hour of refeeding or intravenous infusion of glucose, a mixture of amino acids (Synthamin 17) or a mixture of glucose plus amino acids. The bars represent fractional rates of muscle protein synthesis expressed as percentages of saline-infused controls. Data from Garlick et al (1983) and Preedy and Garlick (1986). (**b**) Effect of infusing glucose plus a complete amino acid solution (Synthamin 17), essential amino acids, non-essential amino acids or only the branched-chain amino acids. Results are expressed as percentages of rates in controls given glucose alone. Data from Garlick and Grant (1988).

consistent, since it would depend not only on leucine but also on the degree of saturation of the insulin effect.

Glutamine is also an amino acid that has attracted attention. It has been known for many years that it must be added to the medium for optimal growth of cultured cells (Eagle et al, 1956). Recent evidence suggests a relationship between the muscle glutamine content and muscle protein synthesis rate in vivo in various normal and pathological states (Rennie et al, 1986). Furthermore, the experimental manipulation of the glutamine content of muscle in the perfused rat hind-limb altered the rate of protein synthesis (Rennie et al, 1986).

THE ROLE OF PROSTAGLANDINS IN THE CONTROL OF MUSCLE PROTEIN BALANCE

Prostaglandins are metabolites, via the cyclo-oxygenase pathway, of the ω6 fatty acid, arachidonic acid. Along with the other eicosanoids, thromboxanes, prostacyclins and leukotrienes, they have been implicated in the control of a very wide range of metabolic processes, both in normal tissues and in pathological states. In many cases, pairs of eicosanoids exert opposing influences on a metabolic process. For example, in the circulatory system thromboxane A_2 mediates platelet aggregation and is a potent vasoconstrictor; prostacyclin prevents platelet aggregation and is vasodilatory (Moncada and Vane, 1980). In particular, the prostaglandins have been implicated as mediators in the control of muscle protein metabolism by four of the factors discussed above, namely activity or workload, insulin, the glucocorticoids and infection.

Activity

Two observations have linked levels of PGE_2 and $PGF_{2\alpha}$ to the hypertrophy or atrophy of muscle that occurs as a result of increased use or disuse. Firstly, denervation of the gastrocnemius muscle of one limb of rats caused muscle atrophy and increased the PGE and PGF content of the muscles; electrical stimulation of the muscle retarded muscle atrophy and reduced the PGE content (Jaweed et al, 1981). Secondly, the increase in protein synthesis induced by the intermittent stretching of isolated intact muscles was blocked by indomethacin, an inhibitor of prostaglandin synthesis, and was mimicked by addition of arachidonic acid or $PGF_{2\alpha}$ (Smith et al, 1983).

Insulin

The involvement of prostaglandins in the action of insulin was suggested by the demonstration that insulin-induced increases in protein synthesis in isolated muscle were also blocked by indomethacin (Reeds and Palmer, 1983). This possible mediating role for prostaglandins in the action of insulin was confirmed by experiments in vivo (Reeds et al, 1985) showing that the stimulation of protein synthesis in postabsorptive rats by insulin infusion was also blocked by indomethacin.

Glucocorticoids

A reduction in the activity of phospholipase A_2, reducing the availability of arachidonic acid for prostanoid synthesis, is known to underlie the anti-inflammatory action of the glucocorticoids. A reduction in $PGF_{2\alpha}$ has also been implicated in the glucocorticoid-induced reduction in the rate of protein synthesis (Reeds and Palmer, 1984). However, these changes, although closely correlated, are possibly not causally related. The reasons for this are that non-steroidal anti-inflammatory drugs (NSAIDs), which are equally effective in reducing prostaglandin release, do not inhibit protein synthesis. Furthermore, the $\omega 3$ fatty acids, which also induce a significant reduction in $PGF_{2\alpha}$ production by competition for the cyclo-oxygenase enzymes, also fail to inhibit basal rates of protein synthesis (Palmer and Wahle, 1986).

Pathological states

It is now recognized that fever induced by infection or by the administration of microbial toxins may be initiated by the release of interleukin 1 from leukocytes (Dinarello and Wolff, 1982). Elevated rates of proteolysis in such conditions are accompanied by a dramatic rise in PGE_2 release from muscle, while addition of PGE_2 to isolated muscles has been shown to stimulate protein degradation (Rodemann and Goldberg, 1982). Furthermore, addition of indomethacin blocked the increase in both proteolysis and prostaglandin release (Baracos et al, 1983). Similarly, sepsis following *Streptococcus pneumoniae* infection in rats caused muscle wasting and this was reduced by indomethacin (Ruff and Secrist, 1984).

Effects of inhibiting prostaglandin synthesis on muscle metabolism

Studies on the effect of NSAIDs on the growth of normal muscle or on work- or overload-induced hypertrophy are few and contradictory. Using a model involving suspension-induced atrophy of the hind-limb muscle of rats, Templeton et al (1986) showed that the subsequent ability of the soleus muscle to hypertrophy was blocked by indomethacin. The drug also modified the membrane phospholipid composition of the muscle, reducing the phosphatidylethanolamine content. Hypertrophy of the plantaris muscle was investigated by McMillan et al (1987). In these experiments

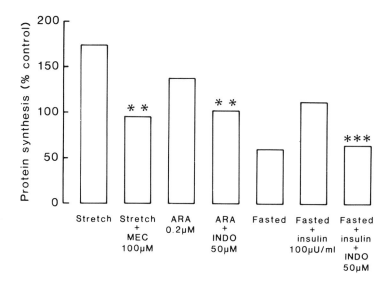

Figure 2. Effects of non-steroidal anti-inflammatory drugs on the stimulation of protein synthesis. Bars represent fractional rates of protein synthesis expressed as a percentage of the controls and show reversal of the effects of: (a) intermittent stretch by meclofenamate (MEC) (Palmer et al, 1983); (b) arachidonic acid (ARA) addition by indomethacin (INDO) (Smith et al, 1983); (c) insulin by indomethacin (Reeds and Palmer, 1983). Significance of the effect of the NSAID $** p < 0.01$; $*** p < 0.001$.

hypertrophy of the plantaris of one limb was achieved by tenotomy of the gastrocnemius. Dietary administration of fenbufen greatly reduced prosta-glandin excretion but had no effect on the ability of the plantaris to hyper-trophy. However, the drug did induce changes in the muscles, specifically in the RNA content of the plantaris of both limbs (Figure 2). The conclusion was drawn that although the ability of the muscle to accrete protein was unaffected by the drug, the mechanism by which growth occurred had altered.

PHARMACOLOGICAL MANIPULATION OF RESPONSES TO INJURY AND NUTRIENT INTAKE

The inability of severely stressed patients to respond to provision of nutrients has prompted several groups to attempt to alter the stress response pharmacologically in an effort to minimize the nutritional consequences of the illness. An extremely diverse range of techniques have been employed to modify the injury response and these are now briefly reviewed.

Non-steroidal anti-inflammatory drugs (NSAIDs)

Clinical use of NSAIDs in the control of protein loss was proposed previously by Baracos et al (1983). Since the NSAIDs would tend to reduce both $PGF_{2\alpha}$ and PGE_2 production, their action might be presumed to result in an undesirable decrease in protein synthesis, as well as a beneficial decrease in degradation. This might not be the case, however. Protein synthesis and degradation appear to be stimulated by factors which induce a small increase in $PGF_{2\alpha}$ and PGE_2 release respectively. However, the effect on protein synthesis seems to be reversed when PGF_2 production is further elevated (Reeds and Palmer, 1986), whereas a pathologically high release of PGE_2 tends to produce a further increase rather than a reduction in protein degradation. Thus there is reason to surmise that NSAIDs might be beneficial in limiting muscle wasting by reducing protein degradation in pathological conditions. Indeed, very recently, apparently beneficial effects of indomethacin following surgery have been reported: regular postoperative doses of the drug not only reduced fever but also resulted in an 18% reduction in nitrogen loss (Asoh et al, 1987). All patients in this study recovered uneventfully, and while those treated with NSAIDs showed a significant reduction in pyrexia, no clinical benefit of the drug was identified.

Whilst the reported effects of NSAIDs on protein turnover give reason to hope that these drugs may be of benefit in the reduction of muscle wasting, there are also reasons for caution. Apart from their known side-effects, such as gastric ulceration, there is also evidence that indomethacin may be ineffective in blocking rates of protein synthesis or degradation if the elevation in the rate has already occurred before administration of the drug. Thus the stimulatory effect of insulin on protein synthesis was inhibited by indomethacin only if indomethacin was present at the start of the incubation, suggesting that the prostaglandins may be involved only at an early stage in the response to the hormone (Palmer et al, 1986). Of greater relevance are the analogous observations that indomethacin administered to rats before endotoxin inhibited the onset of fever, the increase in PGE_2 and the increased rate of proteolysis. When indomethacin was administered 2 hours after endotoxin or to muscles removed from previously endotoxin-treated rats, PGE_2 production was inhibited but the elevated rate of protein breakdown was unaffected (Fagan and Goldberg, 1985). Both these observations suggest that administration of NSAIDs to patients after the onset of pathological changes in protein breakdown may be ineffective. Thus, patients may be exposed to potentially harmful side-effects of these drugs without hope of clinical benefit.

The animal studies have also shown that NSAIDs can interfere with the normal physiological responses to work and insulin. For example, the stimulation of muscle protein synthesis by food intake depends on a normal response to insulin (see above), which can be blocked by indomethacin (Reeds et al, 1985). This has led to studies in fasting rats, showing that the response of muscle to refeeding is also blocked by the drug (McNurlan et al, 1987). However, this effect on the acute response to food intake in rats does not appear to interfere with protein retention during feeding in man. In healthy human volunteers a single dose of indomethacin did not affect nitrogen balance or whole-body protein synthesis and breakdown rates in either the fed or fasted states (McNurlan et al, 1987). Furthermore, in elderly patients taking NSAIDs chronically for arthritis, withdrawal of treatment for 1 week did not affect nitrogen balance or whole-body protein turnover rates (Gann et al, 1988). Although this suggests that NSAIDs might not interfere with the ability of patients to retain protein during nutritional support, it should be borne in mind that prostaglandins are involved in both catabolic and anabolic processes, and not all of the effects of NSAIDs might therefore be beneficial. At present, routine clinical use of these drugs in an attempt to improve nutritional state cannot be recommended.

Insulin infusion

Since insulin is anabolic in muscle, the question arises whether it will also improve nitrogen balance. This was examined by Woolfson et al (1979) in burned patients, and they concluded that additional insulin was only of value in those subjects who were very highly traumatized with nitrogen excretions in excess of 30 g/day. With inflammatory bowel disease, patients receiving total parenteral nutrition (TPN) (Powell-Tuck et al, 1984) showed no effect of additional insulin on nitrogen balance or on whole-body rates of protein synthesis and breakdown measured with [^{15}N]glycine. Indeed, as indicated in Chapter 4, infusion of insulin in stressed patients is positively harmful. An increased synthesis of triglycerides will result in adipose tissue deposition (Jeejeebhoy et al, 1976), and increased glucose oxidation will cause an elevation in oxygen consumption and carbon dioxide production, both of which may be harmful to the stressed patient (Askanazi et al, 1981). The ability of insulin to prevent release of amino acids from skeletal muscle may in itself be clinically harmful, since muscle amino acids are required for synthesis of hepatic proteins following injury (Moldawer et al, 1980).

Insulin, therefore, has no clinical role to play in the reversal of the stress response, and while it will continue to be given in physiological doses in diabetic patients, its use as a pharmacological manipulating agent is to be avoided.

Branched-chain amino acids

The last few years has seen considerable interest in the use of branched-chain amino acid (BCAA) enriched solutions for TPN, following reports described above that they can stimulate protein synthesis and inhibit degradation in isolated muscle incubated in vitro. The clinical use of BCAAs has been reviewed extensively (Adibi, 1980; Smith and Elia, 1983; Walser, 1984; Brennan et al, 1986) and will not be dealt with in detail here. A workshop sponsored by the American Society for Parenteral and Enteral Nutrition (Brennan et al, 1986) has reached the following conclusions regarding the use of BCAAs in trauma or sepsis. They point out that studies in septic primates have suggested that the use of BCAA-enriched solutions might lessen the caloric requirements for maintaining nitrogen balance. Furthermore, some clinical studies have also shown a positive benefit from using BCAA-enriched solutions on parameters of nitrogen metabolism, but these have generally been seen only in the most severely ill patients. However, as little major effect on outcome has yet been demonstrated, the conclusion of the workshop was that no widespread application of BCAA formulations could be endorsed.

It might seem surprising that despite the unquestioned effects of BCAAs on protein balance in muscle from growing animals in vitro, they have no clear benefits in patients. Firstly, it is possible that this apparent discrepancy results from the use in laboratory studies of growing animals which might not be comparable with adult patients: in one study with perfused rat muscle, an effect of BCAAs was noted with young rats but not with older animals (Li and Jefferson, 1978). Secondly, as discussed above, present evidence suggests that the BCAAs are involved in mediating the normal physiological response of muscle to feeding. Increasing BCAA concentrations above the normal fed levels may not show any additional positive effect if protein synthesis is already maximally stimulated. As one of the actions of BCAAs appears to be to enhance the sensitivity of muscle protein synthesis to insulin, the effects of BCAAs might only be observable when the response to insulin is submaximal. By analogy, exogenous insulin only stimulates muscle protein synthesis in rats when plasma concentrations of the hormone are low (e.g. in fasting), and has no additional, stimulatory effect in fed animals (Garlick et al, 1983). In patients, insulin-resistant states might provide the circumstances where additional insulin or BCAAs might be effective. For example, it was noted earlier that insulin only appears to affect nitrogen balance in patients who are very severely traumatized, and it is also in very severely ill patients that BCAAs have their most pronounced effect. Could the interaction between BCAAs and insulin seen in animal studies be the key to explaining these two observations? More detailed knowledge of the mechanisms involved would be needed to answer this question, but in the future such knowledge might help us to derive clinical benefit from the use of BCAAs.

Other potential modifying agents

A number of other agents have been used to modify the metabolic effects of injury, although these are not known to have specific effects on muscle protein metabolism.

Naftidrofuryl, which appears to improve the entry of carbohydrates into the tricarboxylic acid cycle, may improve nitrogen balance in surgical patients (Burns et al, 1981), although this has not been confirmed in subsequent studies.

Brackett et al (1985) have used a combination of H_1- and H_2-histamine receptor antagonists in experimental animals subjected to endotoxaemia. They noted that most of the metabolic abnormalities commonly seen in these animals were minimized by the use of this therapy. Clinically, Shaw and Wolfe (1988) have measured glucose kinetics in surgical patients receiving the H_2-blocker ranitidine. They found no alteration in glucose metabolism in these patients, but they did note a reduction in net protein catabolism in patients who were either fasting or receiving parenteral nutrition. They considered that this significant reduction in protein catabolism was independent of humoral effects, and have postulated that stimulation of the H_2-receptor in surgical patients in some way leads to increased protein catabolism.

These authors, in addition, examined the effects of infusion of the endorphin blocking agent naloxone. This substance was similar to ranitidine in that it had no effect on glucose turnover but produced a significant decrease in net protein catabolism. It is possible, therefore, to postulate that a number of factors such as endorphins or histamine are involved in some, as yet unknown, mechanism controlling the release of amino acids from muscle protein. Further investigation in this area may well prove fruitful in attempts to improve the nutritional status of injured patients.

Manipulation of the adrenergic system

The importance of adrenaline as a mediator of the stress response has been underlined by Bessey et al (1984) and the effect of catecholamines on protein turnover has already been described. Clinically, two possibilities exist for altering the effects of catecholamines after injury. Production of the hormones in surgical patients may be abolished by spinal anaesthesia or, alternatively, β-adrenergic blockade may be used to lessen the effects of adrenaline on muscle cells.

Spinal anaesthesia

The possibility that the metabolic response to injury could be mediated by neurological pathways was first suggested at the beginning of this century by George Crile (Crile, 1910). He hypothesized that peripheral nerve block might reduce the disruptive effect on the organism of an injury and hence improve outcome. Evidence that this theory might have some validity came in 1934, when it was demonstrated that spinal anaesthesia in experimental animals reduced mortality following blunt hind-limb trauma (O'Shaughnessy and Slome, 1934). Since then, several studies have provided evidence that both the peripheral and central nervous systems can modify the hormonal response to trauma.

Many studies have confirmed the observation that spinal or epidural anaesthesia can reduce the cortisol response to surgery (Gordon et al, 1973; Cosgrove and Jenkins, 1974; Brandt et al, 1976). Similarly, output of catecholamines from the adrenal medulla has also been modified by spinal anaesthesia (Engquist et al, 1980; Pflug and Halter, 1981). The consequence of this reduction in adrenal output is that spinal anaesthesia reduces or completely blocks the usual hyperglycaemic response to injury (Brandt et al, 1976; Moller et al, 1984). The reduced adrenaline response following surgery under spinal anaesthesia results in a reduction in glycogenolysis and glucose release from the liver. In addition, Brandt et al (1977) have suggested that neural blockade can reduce plasma insulin levels during surgery. This, however, is probably an effect of the reduction in plasma glucose rather than a cause of it. A reduction in glycogenolysis may also be brought about by blockade of the afferent sympathetic pathways to the liver. Lautt (1983) has suggested that this is an important mechanism for release of glucose from glycogen stored in the liver. These observations suggest that patients undergoing surgery under spinal or epidural anaesthesia are more likely to remain normoglycaemic, and insulin requirements, especially in diabetics or those receiving intravenous nutrition preoperatively, may be less than anticipated.

Reduced levels of plasma free fatty acids have been observed during surgery undertaken with regional anaesthesia (Cooper et al, 1979). Hallberg and Oro (1965), however, only observed this effect when the level of analgesia was in the high thoracic region (T1–T3). Plasma levels of free fatty acids are thought to be directly proportional to the degree of lipid turnover, and therefore this observation indicates a probable reduction in fatty acid mobilization and utilization in patients undergoing spinal anaesthesia. It is possible, therefore, that by reducing lipid turnover, spinal anaesthesia can maintain body fat stores after elective surgery.

Little data are available on the effects of spinal or epidural anaesthesia on protein turnover in surgical patients. However, Brandt et al (1978) reported a highly significant improvement in 5-day cumulative postoperative nitrogen balance in patients undergoing pelvic surgery when analgesia was provided by continuous infusion of bupivacaine into the epidural space.

Shaw et al (1987) have recently reported an 11% reduction in net protein catabolism and a 20% reduction in glucose turnover in a group of patients who had undergone surgical procedures under epidural anaesthesia. The effect of regional anaesthesia on energy expenditure is unclear. Wilmore (1976) was unable to demonstrate any alteration in resting energy expenditure in a burned patient given a spinal anaesthetic. At least two studies have reported a reduction in postoperative oxygen consumption following surgical procedures in patients receiving epidural analgesia (Renck, 1969; Fournell et al, 1980). Hakansson et al (1985) did not identify any alteration in oxygen consumption following cholecystectomy in regional analgesia patients. The normal increase in energy expenditure which might be expected in these patients is small, and given the 5% error in the measurement of energy expenditure which might be expected to be seen in their technique, it is not surprising that they found no difference between general anaesthesia and epidural analgesia patients.

These alterations in the hormonal and substrate response to injury following epidural or spinal analgesia are consistent with the view that the response to injury can be modified and ameliorated by regional anaesthesia. However, it appears that the degree of analgesia obtained is critical in producing improvements in the metabolic patterns seen after injury. Thus, while studies published on lower abdominal surgical procedures show good efficacy of regional analgesia, studies carried out on more major upper abdominal procedures have shown only marginal improvements in the metabolic changes (Kehlet, 1984). It is thought that the difficulty in obtaining a sufficiently complete neural block in the upper abdomen accounts for this difference. Tsuji et al (1980) showed a much greater inhibition of the metabolic response when a coeliac plexus block was added to epidural analgesia. Kehlet and Schulze (1986) have suggested that for epidural analgesia to be effective during abdominal surgery, the proximal level of analgesia must extend upwards to at least T4, which is the upper limit for entry of afferent sympathetic fibres from the splanchnic nerves into the spinal chord.

It is clear that neural pathways play an important role in the co-ordination of the metabolic response to injury, but while substrate and hormone levels within the plasma can be modified as a result of neural blockade, as yet no study has shown any significant clinical benefit in terms of morbidity or mortality resulting from manipulation of the metabolic response in this fashion.

Adrenergic blockade

The evidence that spinal anaesthesia can reduce the extent of the metabolic response to injury is strong. It is likely that one factor causing this reduced response is the inhibition of release of catecholamines from the adrenal gland. A number of authors have extended this concept and have attempted to inhibit adrenal function by the use of α- or β-adrenergic blockade. Allison et al (1969) used phentolamine to block the α-adrenergic effects of noradrenaline in injured patients. They were unable to find any effect of adrenergic blockade on insulin response to a glucose infusion. However, Fahmy and Battit (1975) found that phentolamine administration inhibited the hyperglycaemia associated with surgery. Nakao and Miyata (1977) were unable to confirm this. β-Adrenergic blockade, however, seems to be more successful in modifying the effects of injury. Administration of propranolol in high doses produced a reduction in plasma glucose, plasma lactate and free fatty acids (Tsuji et al, 1980). Propranolol at a lower dose only reduced plasma free fatty acid levels. Studies on the elevated energy expenditure of injury have shown that β-adrenergic blockade can reduce hypermetabolism significantly, while α-adrenergic blockade has no effect on oxygen consumption in burned patients (Wilmore et al, 1974a). Shaw and Wolfe (1988) have reported that infusion of the β-adrenergic agonist salbutamol resulted in a significant increase in glucose turnover and the rate of free fatty acid appearance in the plasma. It had no effect on protein metabolism.

It appears, therefore, that adrenaline is a more potent inducer of the metabolic abnormalities associated with trauma than noradrenaline. This appears to be inconsistent with the evidence from rat models suggesting that adrenaline is anabolic, and its role in trauma may be more related to its effects on carbohydrate and fat metabolism. However, the effect of adrenergic blockade on protein turnover and nitrogen balance in traumatized patients remains uninvestigated. The laboratory studies already mentioned suggest that reduced protein synthesis might be an α-adrenergic effect (Preedy and Garlick, 1988b).

β-Adrenergic agonists

Clenbuterol is one of a series of β-agonists that have been shown in animal studies to increase muscle mass and decrease body fat (Emery et al, 1984; Reeds et al, 1986; Williams et al, 1987). It is also capable of reversing the muscle protein loss that occurs after denervation (Maltin et al, 1986). Although clenbuterol produces the classical β-adrenergic effects on the cardiovascular and respiratory systems, and is used clinically as an anti-asthmatic and antidepressant, its growth-promoting action does not appear to be β-mediated, since it is not inhibited by β-blockade (Reeds et al, 1988). Its potential for improving livestock production has therefore been considered (Williams, 1987). To our knowledge, several groups are intending to study the effect of clenbuterol treatment on nitrogen loss from catabolic patients, but as yet there appear to be no published data on the clinical benefits of this potentially very useful drug.

Hypothermia

Clinical observation led Johnston et al (1986) to conclude that expected catabolic responses were not as highly developed in patients who underwent major cardiac surgical procedures. These patients usually receive high-dose narcotic anaesthesia with neuromuscular blockade, and in addition undergo a period of cardiopulmonary bypass with hypothermia. These workers investigated in a group of laboratory animals the nitrogen balance responses to standard surgical stress associated with hypothermic anaesthesia. They concluded that hypothermia led to a significant reduction in nitrogen excretion, and a reduction in the release of nitrogen by forearm muscle. The patients received high-dose fentanyl anaesthesia. Fentanyl has been shown to reduce renal function in patients undergoing cardiac surgery (Stanley et al, 1980) and therefore the results of this study could not be conclusively related to hypothermia. Our own group (Taggart et al, 1988) has examined the effects of two levels of intraoperative hypothermia—28°C and 20°C—on the catabolic response to cardiac surgery. Basically, the greater the degree of hypothermia, the less whole-body protein turnover is affected. Whole-body protein synthesis falls by a greater extent in the warmer group, and whole-body protein catabolism is affected similarly at both temperatures. Net protein balance, therefore, was significantly better in patients under-going surgery at the lower temperature.

The mechanism by which hypothermia modifies the protein response to surgery is, as yet, uncertain. Cytokines, such as IL-1, IL-6 and cachectin, may well be less efficiently released from activated macrophages at a lower temperature. Alternatively, the secretion of adrenaline, cortisol and glucagon may be modified, and this possibility is under active investigation. Whatever the explanation, it is of interest that a short period of hypothermia which occurs at the time of injury, but does not extend into the postoperative period, seems to provide significant amelioration of the metabolic effects of injury on protein metabolism.

Steroid hormones

Johnston and Chenneour (1963) used a single dose of anabolic steroid to treat patients undergoing elective surgery. This produced a significant improvement in postoperative nitrogen imbalance, an observation which has been confirmed by subsequent studies (Tweedle et al, 1973; Blamey et al, 1984). Yule et al (1981) gave anabolic steroids to surgical patients receiving intravenous nutrition. They were unable to demonstrate any effect of these anabolic steroids on body composition, and similarly Lewis et al (1981) were unable to demonstrate improved nitrogen balance in patients receiving a combination of anabolic steroids and intravenous feeding. The alterations seen in muscle amino acid composition following injury were modified by anabolic steroids (Michelsen et al, 1982), and the possibility that they encouraged enhanced uptake by muscle of amino acids from plasma was suggested by Young et al (1983). We have been unable to demonstrate any effect of stanozolol on postoperative carbohydrate or fat oxidation rate, although we did find some evidence to suggest that postoperative nitrogen excretion in patients undergoing surgery for gastric cancer was improved. No clinical benefit of the anabolic steroid was observed in this study (Hansell et al, 1987). The inconsistent effects of anabolic steroids on nitrogen metabolism in patients are in line with the variable effects seen in animal muscles discussed above.

The decrease in muscle protein synthesis observed following cortico-sterone therapy has already been mentioned. Blocking of the adrenal pro-duction of cortisol following injury with the anaesthetic induction agent etomidate is a theoretical possibility but the increased mortality observed in young trauma patients with continuous infusions of this drug makes such a course potentially hazardous.

Inhibition of glucagon synthesis

Shaw and Wolfe (1988) have inhibited glucagon release from the pancreas in severely ill surgical patients. This manoeuvre produced a 14% reduction in the net rate of protein breakdown. Normoglycaemia was maintained by infusion of exogenous insulin.

Growth hormone

Wilmore et al (1974b) first suggested the use of growth hormone as an anabolic agent in burned patients. They demonstrated an improved nitrogen balance with the use of hormone prepared from human pituitary material. The subsequent development of recombinant DNA techniques has greatly increased the availability of this hormone, and Ward et al (1987) have demonstrated improved protein synthesis following the administration of growth hormone to surgical patients. Again, the clinical relevance of this observation is unclear, and no routine use of growth hormone can, as yet, be advised.

CONCLUSIONS

Clearly there have been a number of attempts to ameliorate the harmful effects of the metabolic response to injury and sepsis. Nutritional support is certainly the most widely practised in clinical terms, but as other authors in this volume have argued, very few studies showing clear-cut benefit in clinical terms from nutritional support have been identified. In Chapter 2 it is pointed out that most complications of surgery are related to poor technique, advanced tumours or pre-existing medical problems, such as coronary artery disease or chronic bronchitis. As yet, the benefits to be derived from the use of pharmacological methods to alter muscle protein synthesis have not been significant enough to alter outcome from surgery. In these circumstances it has proven to be extremely difficult to convince clinicians that adrenergic blockade, non-steroidal anti-inflammatory drugs or indeed preoperative parenteral nutrition should be used routinely in the malnourished patient. We would agree with the vast majority of clinicians that attempts to manipulate the metabolic response in this way are not routinely indicated. It remains a priority, therefore, for research workers in the field to continue to apply lessons learned from studies on animals to the clinical situation. In our brief outline of what is known from animal studies of the regulation of muscle protein turnover, a number of pharmacological and other potentially beneficial treatments were indicated, only a few of which have been investigated thoroughly in a clinical context. Hence additional, carefully controlled, clinical studies will still be needed to prove or disprove the benefits claimed for any of the specific methods of treatment discussed in this chapter.

SUMMARY

The physiological control of muscle protein balance has been reviewed. In addition to trauma, fasting and reduced activity have been shown to cause muscle protein loss through changes in synthesis and breakdown. Many of the effects of these states are mediated by alterations in the concentrations of insulin, glucagon, steroids and catecholamines. Branched-chain amino acids also appear to have specific effects in improving protein synthesis. Recently, prostaglandins have been identified as having a central role as mediators in the control of protein metabolism by many hormones and pathological states.

Identification of factors which control muscle protein synthesis leads to the possibility that the metabolic response to illness and injury and its attendant muscle protein loss could be open to pharmacological manipulation. Inhibition of prostaglandin synthesis by non-steroidal anti-inflammatory drugs can improve muscle protein turnover, but their clinical usefulness may be limited by side-effects. Hormonal manipulation may offer the possibility of abolishing the metabolic response. For example, inhibition of adrenal secretion in surgical patients by spinal anaesthesia appears to modify many of the metabolic effects of injury.

A variety of other treatments have been used to minimize the metabolic derangements of injury. Some of these have considerable potential, but as yet clinical benefits from their use have not been positively identified. It is likely that a pharmacological approach to the nutritional disorders of stress and injury will prove to be of major interest in the future.

REFERENCES

Adibi SA (1980) Roles of branched-chain amino acids in metabolic regulation. *Journal of Laboratory and Clinical Medicine* **95:** 475–484.

Allison SP, Tomlin PJ & Chamberlain MJ (1969) Some effects of anaesthesia and surgery on carbohydrate and fat metabolism. *British Journal of Anaesthesia* **41:** 588–593.

Askanazi J, Nordenshom J & Rosenbaum SH (1981) Nutrition of the patient with respiratory failure. *Anaesthesiology* **54:** 373–377.

Asoh T, Shirasaka C, Uchida I & Tsuji H (1987) Effects of indomethacin on endocrine responses and nitrogen loss after surgery. *Annals of Surgery* **106:** 770–776.

Baillie AGS, Maltin CA & Garlick PJ (1988) The effect of fasting and insulin infusion on muscle protein synthesis in immature and adult rats. *Proceedings of the Nutrition Society* **47:** 114A.

Baracos V, Rodemann HP, Dinarello CA & Goldberg AL (1983) Stimulation of muscle protein degradation and prostaglandin E2 release by leukocytic pyrogen (interleukin 1). A mechanism for the increased degradation of muscle proteins during fever. *New England Journal of Medicine* **308:** 553–558.

Bates PC, Chew LF & Millward DJ (1987) Effects of the anabolic steroid stanozolol on growth and protein metabolism in the rat. *Journal of Endocrinology* **114:** 373–381.

Beatty CH, Peterson RD, Bocek RM, Craig NC & Weleber R (1963) Effect of glucagon on incorporation of glycine-C14 into protein of voluntary skeletal muscle. *Endocrinology* **73:** 721–726.

Bessey PQ, Watters JM, Aoki TT & Wilmore DW (1984) Combined hormone infusion simulates the metabolic response to injury. *Annals of Surgery* **200:** 264–281.

Blamey SL, Garden OJ, Shenkin A & Carter DC (1984) Modification of nitrogen balance following surgery with a pre-operative anabolic steroid. *Clinical Nutrition* **2:** 187–192.

Booth FW & Watson PA (1985) Control of adaptations in protein levels in response to exercise. *Federation Proceedings* **44:** 2293–2300.

Brackett DJ, Schaefer CF & Wilson MF (1985) The effects of H1 and H2 histamine receptor antagonists on the development of endotoxaemia in the conscious, unrestrained rat. *Circulatory Shock* **16:** 141–153.

Brandt MR, Kehlet H, Binder C, Hagen C & McNeilly AS (1976) Effect of epidural analgesia on the glycoregulatory endocrine response to surgery. *Clinical Endocrinology* **5:** 107–114.

Brandt MR, Kehlet H, Faber O & Binder C (1977) C-peptide and insulin during blockade of the hypoglycaemic response to surgery by epidural analgesia. *Clinical Endocrinology* **6:** 167–170.

Brandt MR, Fernandes A, Mordhorst R & Kehlet H (1978) Epidural analgesia improves postoperative nitrogen balance. *British Medical Journal* **1:** 1106–1108.

Brennan MF, Cerra F, Daly JM et al (1986) Branched chain amino acids in stress and injury. *Journal of Parenteral and Enteral Nutrition* **10:** 446–452.

Brevet A, Pinto E, Peacock J & Stockdale FF (1976) Myosin synthesis increased by electrical stimulation of skeletal muscle cell cultures. *Science* **193:** 1152–1154.

Brown JG & Millward DJ (1983) Dose response of protein turnover in rat skeletal muscle to tri-iodothyronine administration. *Biochimica et Biophysica Acta* **757:** 182–190.

Brown JG, Bates PC, Holliday MA & Millward DJ (1981) Thyroid hormones and muscle protein turnover. *Biochemical Journal* **194:** 771–782.

Burns HJG, Galloway DJ & Ledingham IMcA (1981) The effect of naftidrofuryl on the metabolic response to surgery. *British Medical Journal* **283:** 7–8.

Buse MG & Reid SS (1975) Leucine: a possible regulator of protein turnover in muscle. *Journal of Clinical Investigation* **56:** 1250–1261.

Buse MJ, McMaster J & Buse J (1965) The effect of denervation and insulin on protein synthesis in the isolated rat diaphragm. *Metabolism* **14:** 1220–1232.

Cameron CM, Kostyo JL, Adamafio NA et al (1988) The acute effects of growth hormone on amino acid transport and protein synthesis are due to its insulin-like action. *Endocrinology* **122:** 471–474.

Cheng KN, Pacy PJ, Dworzak F, Ford GC & Halliday D (1987) Influence of fasting on leucine and muscle protein metabolism across the human forearm determined using L-[$^{1-13}$C,^{15}N] leucine as the tracer. *Clinical Science* **73:** 241–246.

Clowes GHA Jr, George BC, Villee CA & Saravis CA (1983) Muscle proteolysis induced by a circulating peptide in patients with sepsis or trauma. *New England Journal of Medicine* **308:** 545–552.

Cooper GM, Holdcroft A, Hall GM & Alaghband-Zadeh J (1979) Epidural analgesia and the metabolic response to surgery. *Canadian Anaesthetic Society Journal* **26:** 381–385.

Cosgrove DO & Jenkins JS (1974) The effect of epidural anaesthesia on the pituitary–adrenal response to surgery. *Clinical Science and Molecular Medicine* **46:** 403–407.

Crile GW (1910) Phylogenetic association in relation to certain medical problems. *Boston Medical and Surgical Journal* **703:** 893–904.

Cuthbertson DP (1930) The disturbance of metabolism produced by bony or non-bony injury, with notes on certain abnormal conditions of bone. *Biochemical Journal* **24:** 1244–1263.

Dinarello CA & Wolff SM (1982) Molecular basis of fever in humans. *American Journal of Medicine* **72:** 799–819.

Dohm GL, Tapscott EB & Louis TM (1979) Skeletal muscle protein turnover after testosterone administration in the castrated rat. *IRCS Medical Science* **7:** 40.

Duke JH, Jorgensen SB, Broell JR, Long CL & Kinney JM (1970) Contribution of protein to caloric expenditure following injury. *Surgery* **68:** 168–174.

Eagle H, Oyama VI, Levy M, Horton CL & Fleischman R (1956) The growth response of mammalian cells in tissue culture to L-glutamine and L-glutamic acid. *Journal of Biological Chemistry* **218:** 607–616.

Engquist A, Fog-Moller F, Christiansen C, Thode J, Vester Andersen T & Nistrup Hodsen S (1980) Influence of epidural analgesia on the catecholamine and cyclic AMP responses to surgery. *Acta Anaesthesiologica Scandinavica* **24:** 17–21.

Emery PW, Rothwell NJ, Stock MJ & Winter PD (1984) Chronic effects of β-adrenergic agonists on body composition and protein synthesis in the rat. *Bioscience Reports* **4:** 83–89.

Fagan JM & Goldberg AL (1985) Muscle protein breakdown, prostaglandin E2 production, and fever following bacterial infection. In Kluger M, Openheim J & Powanda W (eds) *The Physiologic, Metabolic and Immunologic Actions of Interleukin-1*, pp 201–210. New York: Alan R. Liss.

Fahmy NR & Battit GE (1975) Effects of pentolinium on blood sugar and serum potassium concentrations during anaesthesia and surgery. *British Journal of Anaesthesia* **47:** 1309–1313.

Fern EB, McNurlan MM & Garlick PJ (1985) Effect of malaria on the rate of protein synthesis in individual tissues of rats. *American Journal of Physiology* **249:** E485–E493.

Flaim KE, Li JB & Jefferson LS (1978) Protein turnover in rat skeletal muscle: effects of hypophysectomy and growth hormone. *American Journal of Physiology* **234:** E3843.

Fournell A, Wilhelmy B, Falke K, Sandmann W & Bohmer G (1980) Kontineurlische Messing der Sauerstofaufnalime bei postoperativer Periduralanalgesie. In West HJ & Zindler M (eds) *Nene Asperkte in der Regionalanaesthesie 1*, p 54. Berlin: Springer Verlag.

Frayn KN & Maycock PF (1979) Regulation of protein metabolism by a physiological concentration of insulin in mouse soleus and extensor digitorum longus muscles. *Biochemical Journal* **184:** 323–330.

Fulks RM, Li JB & Goldberg AL (1975) Effects of insulin, glucose and amino acids on protein turnover in rat diaphragm. *Journal of Biological Chemistry* **250:** 290–298.

Gann ME, McNurlan MA, McHardy KC, Milne E & Garlick PJ (1988) Non-steroidal anti-inflammatory agents and protein turnover in the elderly. *Proceedings of the Nutrition Society* **47:** 133A.

Garber AJ, Karl IE & Kipnis DM (1976) Alanine and glutamine synthesis and release from skeletal muscle; β-adrenergic inhibition of amino acid release. *Journal of Biological Chemistry* **251:** 851–857.

Garlick PJ & Grant I (1988) Amino acid infusion increases the sensitivity of muscle protein synthesis in vivo to insulin: effect of branched chain amino acids. *Biochemical Journal* **254:** 579–584.

Garlick PJ, Fern M & Preedy VR (1983) The effect of insulin infusion and food intake on muscle protein synthesis in postabsorptive rats. *Biochemical Journal* **210:** 669–676.

Garlick PJ, Grant I & Glennie RT (1987) Short-term effects of corticosterone treatment on muscle protein synthesis in relation to feeding. *Biochemical Journal* **248:** 439–442.

Gelfand RA & Barrett EJ (1987) Effect of physiologic hyperinsulinemia on skeletal muscle protein synthesis and breakdown in man. *Journal of Clinical Investigation* **80:** 1–6.

Gibson JNA, Halliday D, Morrison WL et al (1987) Decrease in human quadriceps muscle protein turnover consequent upon leg immobilization. *Clinical Science* **72:** 503–509.

Goldberg AL (1967) Work induced growth of skeletal muscle in normal and hypophysectomized rats. *American Journal of Physiology* **213:** 1193–1198.

Goldberg AL, Jablecki C & Li JB (1974) Effects of use and disuse on amino acid transport and protein turnover in muscle. *Annals of the New York Academy of Sciences* **228:** 190–201.

Goldspink DF (1976) The effects of denervation on protein turnover of rat skeletal muscle. *Biochemical Journal* **156:** 71–80.

Goldspink DF (1977) The influence of activity on muscle size and protein turnover. *Journal of Physiology* **264:** 283–296.

Goldspink DF (1978a) The influence of passive stretch on the growth and protein turnover of the denervated extensor digitorum longus muscle. *Biochemical Journal* **174:** 595–602.

Goldspink DF (1978b) The effects of food deprivation on protein turnover and nucleic acid concentrations of active and immobilised extensor digitorum longus muscles of the rat. *Biochemical Journal* **176:** 603–606.

Goldspink DF, Garlick PJ & McNurlan MA (1983) Protein turnover measured in vivo and in vitro in muscles undergoing compensatory growth and subsequent atrophy. *Biochemical Journal* **210:** 89–98.

Goodman MN, Larsen PR, Kaplan MM, Aoki TT, Young VR & Ruderman NB (1980) Starvation in the rat II. Effect of age and obesity on protein sparing and fuel metabolism. *American Journal of Physiology* **239:** E277–E286.

Gordon NH, Scott DB & Percy Robb IW (1973) Modification of plasma corticosteroid concentrations during and after surgery by epidural blockade. *British Medical Journal* **1:** 581–583.

Grigsby JS, Bergen WG & Merkel RA (1976) The effect of testosterone on skeletal muscle development and protein synthesis in rabbits. *Growth* **40:** 303–316.

Hakansson E, Rutberg H, Jorfeldt L & Martenson J (1985) Effects of extradural administration of morphine or bupmucaine on the metabolic response to upper abdominal surgery. *British Journal of Anaesthesia* **57:** 394–399.

Hallberg D & Oro L (1965) Free fatty acids of plasma during spinal anaesthesia in man. *Acta Medica Scandinavica* **178:** 281–290.

Halliday D, Pacy PJ, Cheng KN, Divorzak F, Gibson JNA & Rennie MJ (1988) Rate of protein synthesis in skeletal muscle of normal man and patients with muscular dystrophy. *Clinical Science* **74**: 237–240.

Hansell DT, Davies JWL, Shenkin A, Garden OJ, Burns HJG & Carter DC (1987) The effects of an anabolic steroid and naftidrofuryl on the metabolic response to surgery. *Nutrition* **3**: 249–255.

Hirata F (1983) Lipomodulin: a possible mediator of the action of glucocorticoids. *Advances in Prostaglandin, Thromboxane and Leukotriene Research* 73–78.

Holly RG, Barnett JG, Ashmore CR, Taylor RG & Mole PA (1980) Stretch-induced growth in chicken wing muscles: a new model of stretch hypertrophy. *American Journal of Physiology* **238**: C62–C71.

Jansson JO, Eden S & Isaksson O (1983) Sites of action of testosterone and oestradiol on longitudinal growth. *American Journal of Physiology* **244**: E135–E140.

Jaspers SR & Tischler ME (1984) Atrophy and growth failure of rat hind limb muscles in tail cast suspension. *Journal of Applied Physiology* **57**: 743–759.

Jaweed MM, Alam I, Herbison GJ & Ditunno JF Jr (1981) Prostaglandins in denervated skeletal muscle of the rat; effect of direct electrical stimulation. *Neuroscience* **6**: 2787–2792.

Jeejeebhoy KN, Anderson GH, Nakhooda AF, Greenberg GR, Sanderson I & Marliss EB (1976) Metabolic studies in total parenteral nutrition with lipid in man. Comparison with glucose. *Journal of Clinical Investigation* **57**: 125–136.

Jefferson LS, Li JB & Rannels SR (1977) Regulation by insulin of amino acid release and protein turnover in the perfused rat hemicorpus. *Journal of Biological Chemistry* **252**: 1476–1483.

Jepson MM, Pell JM, Bates PC & Millward DJ (1986) The effects of endotoxemia on protein metabolism in skeletal muscle and liver of fed and fasted rats. *Biochemical Journal* **235**: 329–336.

Johnston DJ, Brooks DC, Pressler VM et al (1986) Hypothermic anaesthesia attenuates postoperative proteolysis. *Annals of Surgery* **204**: 419–429.

Johnston IDA & Chenneour R (1963) The effect of methandienone on the metabolic response to surgical operation. *British Journal of Surgery* **50**: 924–928.

Kehlet H (1984) Epidural analgesia and the encodrine–metabolic response to surgery. Update and perspectives. *Acta Anaesthesiologica Scandinavica* **28**: 125–127.

Kehlet H & Schulze S (1986) Modification of injury response. In Little RA & Frayn KN (eds) *The Scientific Basis of the Care of the Critically Ill*, pp 153–168. Manchester: Manchester University Press.

Kostyo JL & Nutting DF (1974) Growth hormone and protein metabolism. In Sawyer WH & Knobil E (eds) *Handbook of Physiology*, sect. 7, vol. 4, Washington DC: American Physiological Society.

Laurent GJ, Sparrow MP, Bates PC & Millward DJ (1978a) Muscle protein turnover in the adult fowl. I. Rates of protein synthesis in fast and slow skeletal cardiac and smooth muscle of the adult fowl (Gallus domesticus). *Biochemical Journal* **176**: 393–405.

Laurent GJ, Sparrow MP & Millward DJ (1978b) Muscle protein turnover in the adult fowl II. Changes in rates of protein synthesis and breakdown during hypertrophy of the anterior and posterior latissimus dorsi muscles. *Biochemical Journal* **176**: 407–417.

Lautt WW (1983) Afferent and efferent neural roles in liver function. *Progress in Neurobiology* **21**: 323–487.

Ledingham IMcA & Watt I (1983) Influence of sedation on mortality in critically ill multiple trauma patients. *Lancet* **i**: 1270.

Lewis L, Dalm M & Kirkpatrick JR (1981) Anabolic steroid administration during nutritional support: a therapeutic controversy. *Journal of Parenteral and Enteral Nutrition* **5**: 64–66.

Li JB & Jefferson LS (1977) Effect of isoproterenol on amino acid levels and protein turnover in skeletal muscle. *American Journal of Physiology* **232**: E243–E249.

Li JB & Jefferson LS (1978) Influence of amino acid availability on protein turnover in perfused skeletal muscle. *Biochimica et Biophysica Acta* **544**: 351–359.

Li JB, Higgins JE & Jefferson LS (1979) Changes in protein turnover in skeletal muscle in response to fasting. *American Journal of Physiology* **236**: E222–E228.

McGrath JA & Goldspink DF (1982) Glucocorticoid action on protein synthesis and protein breakdown in isolated skeletal muscles. *Biochemical Journal* **206**: 641–645.

Mackova E & Hnik P (1973) Compensatory muscle hypertrophy induced by tenotomy of synergists is not true working hypertrophy. *Physiologia Bohemoslovaca* **22:** 43–49.

McMillan DN, Reeds PJ, Lobley GE & Palmer RM (1987) Changes in protein turnover in hypertrophying plantaris muscle of rats: effect of fenbufen, an inhibitor of prostaglandin synthesis. *Prostaglandins* **34:** 841–852.

McNurlan MA, McHardy KC, Broom J et al (1987) The effect of indomethacin on the response of protein synthesis to feeding in rats and man. *Clinical Science* **73:** 69–75.

Maltin CA, Reeds PJ, Delday MI, Hay SM, Smith FG & Lobley GE (1986) Inhibition and reversal of denervation-induced atrophy by the β-agonist growth promoter, clenbuterol. *Bioscience Reports* **6:** 811–818.

Martinez JA, Buttery PJ & Pearson JT (1984) The mode of action of anabolic agents: the effect of testosterone on muscle protein metabolism in the female rat. *British Journal of Nutrition* **52:** 515–521.

Mayer M & Rosen F (1977) Interactions of glucocorticoids and androgens with skeletal muscle. *Metabolism* **26:** 937–962.

Michelsen CB, Askanazi J, Kinney JM, Gump FE & Elwyn DH (1982) Effect of an anabolic steroid on nitrogen balance and amino acid patterns after total hip replacement. *Journal of Trauma* **22:** 410–413.

Millward DJ, Garlick PJ, Nnanyelogo DO & Waterlow JC (1976) The relative importance of muscle protein synthesis and breakdown in the regulation of muscle mass. *Biochemical Journal* **156:** 185–188.

Millward DJ, Odedra B & Bates PC (1983) The role of insulin, corticosterone and other factors in the acute recovery of muscle protein synthesis on refeeding food-deprived rats. *Biochemical Journal* **216:** 583–587.

Moldawer LL, O'Keefe SJD & Bothe A Jr (1980) In vivo demonstration of nitrogen sparing mechanism of glucose and amino acids in injured rats. *Metabolism* **29:** 173–180.

Moller IW, Hjortoo E, Krantz T, Wandall E & Kehlet H (1984) The modifying effect of spinal anaesthesia on intra- and postoperative adrenocortical and hyperglycaemic response to surgery. *Acta Anaesthesiologica Scandinavica* **28:** 266–269.

Moncada S & Vane JR (1980) Inter-relationships between prostacyclin and thromboxane A2. *CIBA Foundation Symposium* **78:** 165–177.

Nakao K & Miyata M (1977) The influence of phentolamine, an adrenergic blocking agent, on insulin secretion during surgery. *European Journal of Clinical Investigation* **7:** 41–45.

Odedra BR & Millward DJ (1982) Effect of corticosterone treatment on muscle protein turnover in adrenalectomised rats maintained on insulin. *Biochemical Journal* **204:** 663–672.

Odedra BR, Bates PC & Millward DJ (1983) Time course of the effect of catabolic doses of corticosterone on protein turnover in rat skeletal muscle and liver. *Biochemical Journal* **214:** 617–627.

O'Shaughnessy L & Slome D (1934) Aetiology of traumatic shock. *British Journal of Surgery* **22:** 589.

Pain VM & Garlick PJ (1974) Effect of streptozotocin diabetes and insulin treatment on the rate of protein synthesis in tissues of the rat in vivo. *Journal of Biological Chemistry* **249:** 4510–4514.

Pain VM, Albertse EC & Garlick PJ (1983) Protein metabolism in skeletal muscle, diaphragm and heart of diabetic rats. *American Journal of Physiology* **245:** E604–E610.

Palmer RM & Wahle KWJ (1986) Protein synthesis and degradation in isolated muscle. Effect of w3 and w6 fatty acids. *Biochemical Journal* **242:** 615–618.

Palmer RM, Reeds PJ, Atkinson T & Smith RH (1983) The influence of changes in tension on protein synthesis and prostaglandin release in isolated rabbit muscles. *Biochemical Journal* **214:** 1011–1014.

Palmer RM, Bain PA & Reeds PJ (1985) The effect of insulin and intermittent mechanical stretching on rates of protein synthesis and degradation in isolated rabbit muscle. *Biochemical Journal* **230:** 117–123.

Palmer RM, Bain PA & Reeds PJ (1986) Time dependent effect of indomethacin on the stimulation of protein synthesis in isolated rabbit muscle by insulin. *Bioscience Reports* **6:** 485–491.

Pell JM & Bates PC (1987) Collagen and non-collagen protein turnover in skeletal muscle of growth hormone-treated lambs. *Journal of Endocrinology* **115:** R1–R4.

Pflug AE & Halter JB (1981) Effect of spinal anaesthesia on adrenergic tone and the neuro-endocrine response to surgical stress in humans. *Anaesthesiology* **55:** 120–126.

Pomposselli JJ, Palombo JD, Hamaury KJ, Bistrian BR, Blackburn GL & Moldawer LL (1985) Comparison of different techniques for estimating rates of protein synthesis in vivo in healthy and bacteraemic rats. *Biochemical Journal* **226:** 37–42.

Powell-Tuck J, Fern EB, Garlick PJ & Waterlow JC (1984) The effect of surgical trauma and insulin on whole-body protein turnover in parenterally fed patients. *Human Nutrition. Clinical Nutrition* **38C:** 11–22.

Preedy VR & Garlick PJ (1983) Protein synthesis in skeletal muscle of the perfused rat hemicorpus compared with rates in the intact animal. *Biochemical Journal* **214:** 433–442.

Preedy VR & Garlick PJ (1985) The effect of glucagon administration on protein synthesis in skeletal muscles, heart and liver in vivo. *Biochemical Journal* **228:** 575–581.

Preedy VR & Garlick PJ (1986) The response of muscle protein synthesis to nutrient intake in postabsorptive rats: the role of insulin and amino acids. *Bioscience Reports* **6:** 177–183.

Preedy VR & Garlick PJ (1988a) Inhibition of protein synthesis by glucagon in different rat muscles and protein fractions in vivo and in the perfused rat hemicorpus. *Biochemical Journal* **251:** 727–732.

Preedy VR & Garlick PJ (1988b) The biochemical actions of phentolamine and papaverine on rat perfused skeletal muscle. *Journal of Pharmacy and Pharmacology* **40:** 267–271.

Reeds PJ & Palmer RM (1983) The possible involvement of prostaglandin F2a in the stimulation of muscle protein synthesis by insulin. *Biochemical and Biophysical Research Communications* **116:** 1084–1090.

Reeds PJ & Palmer RM (1984) Changes in prostaglandin release associated with inhibition of muscle protein synthesis by dexamethasone. *Biochemical Journal* **219:** 953–957.

Reeds PJ & Palmer RM (1986) The role of prostaglandins in the control of muscle protein turnover. In Butter PJ, Haynes NB & Lindsay DB (eds) *Control and Manipulation of Animal Growth*, pp 161–185. London: Butterworths.

Reeds PJ, Hay SM, Glennie RT, Mackie WS & Garlick PJ (1985) The effect of indomethacin on the stimulation of protein synthesis by insulin in young postabsorptive rats. *Biochemical Journal* **227:** 255–261.

Reeds PJ, Hay SM, Dorward PM & Palmer RM (1986) Stimulation of muscle growth by clenbuterol: lack of effect on muscle biosynthesis. *British Journal of Nutrition* **56:** 249–256.

Reeds PJ, Hay SM, Dorward PM & Palmer RM (1988) The effect of β-agonists and antagonists on muscle growth and body composition of young rats. *Comparative Biochemistry and Physiology* **89C:** 337–341.

Renck H (1969) The elderly patient after anaesthesia and surgery. *Acta Anaesthesiologica Scandinavica* **34:** 44.

Rennie MJ, Hundal HS, Babij P et al (1986) Characteristics of a glutamine carrier in skeletal muscle have important consequences for nitrogen loss in injury, infection and chronic disease. *Lancet* **ii:** 1008–1012.

Rodemann HP & Goldberg AL (1982) Arachidonic acid, prostaglandin E2 and F2a influence rates on protein turnover in skeletal and cardiac muscle. *Journal of Biological Chemistry* **257:** 1632–1638.

Rodemann HP, Waxman L & Goldberg AL (1982) The stimulation of protein degradation in muscle by Ca^{2+} is mediated by prostaglandin E2 and does not require the calcium-activated protease. *Journal of Biological Chemistry* **257:** 8716–8723.

Rodemann HP, Baracos VE & Goldberg AL (1983) The regulation of protein breakdown by prostaglandins. In *New Aspects of Clinical Nutrition*, pp 310–318. Basel: Karger.

Ruff RL & Secrist D (1984) Inhibitors of prostaglandin synthesis or cathepsin B prevent muscle wasting due to sepsis in the rat. *Journal of Clinical Investigation* **73:** 1483–1486.

Shangraw RE & Turinsky J (1984) Altered protein kinetics in vivo after single limb burn injury. *Biochemical Journal* **223:** 747–753.

Shaw JHF & Wolfe RR (1988) Metabolic intervention in surgical patients. An assessment of the effect of somatostatin, ranitidine, naloxone, diclophenac, dipyrimadole or salbutamol on energy and protein kinetics in surgical patients using stable and radio-isotopes. *Annals of Surgery* **207:** 274–282.

Shaw JHF, Galler L, Holdaway IM & Holdaway CM (1987) The effect of extradural blockade upon glucose and urea kinetics in surgical patients. *Surgery, Gynecology and Obstetrics* **165:** 260–266.

Smith R & Elia M (1983) Branched chain amino acids in stress and injury. *Journal of Parenteral and Enteral Nutrition* 10: 446–452.

Smith RH, Palmer RM & Reeds PJ (1983) Protein synthesis in isolated rabbit forelimb muscles. The possible role of metabolites in arachidonic acid in the response to intermittent stretching. *Biochemical Journal* 214: 153–161.

Stanley RH, Berman L, Green O & Robertson D (1980) Plasma catecholamine and cortisol responses to fentanyl-oxygen anaesthesia for coronary artery operations. *Anaesthesia* 53: 250–253.

Taggart DP, Preston T, McMillan D, Wheatley DJ, Shenkin A & Burns HJG (1988) Profound intra-operative hypothermia modifies protein metabolism after cardiac surgery. *Clinical Nutrition* 7 (supplement 36).

Templeton GH, Padalino M & Moss R (1986) Influences of inactivity and indomethacin on soleus phosphatidylethanolamine and size. *Prostaglandins* 31: 545–559.

Tischler ME, Desautels M & Goldberg AL (1982) Does leucine leucyl-tRNA or some metabolite of leucine regulate protein synthesis and degradation in skeletal and cardiac muscle? *Journal of Biological Chemistry* 257: 1613–1621.

Tomas FM, Murray AJ & Jones LM (1984) Interactive effects of insulin and corticosterone on myofibrillar protein turnover in rats determined by N-methylhistidine excretion. *Biochemical Journal* 220: 469–479.

Tsuji H, Asoh T, Shirasaka C & Takenchi Y (1980) Inhibition of metabolic responses to surgery with beta-adrenergic blockade. *British Journal of Surgery* 67: 503–505.

Turner LV & Garlick PJ (1974) The effect of unilateral phrenicectomy on the rate of protein synthesis in rat diaphragm in vivo. *Biochimica et Biophysica Acta* 349: 191–246.

Tweedle D, Walton C & Johnston IDA (1973) The effect of an anabolic steroid on post-operative nitrogen balance. *British Journal of Clinical Practice* 27: 130–132.

Vernon BG & Buttery PJ (1978) Protein turnover in rats treated with trenbolone acetate. *British Journal of Nutrition* 36: 575–579.

Walser M (1984) Therapeutic aspects of branched-chain amino and keto acids. *Clinical Science* 66: 1–15.

Ward HC, Halliday D & Sim AJW (1987) Protein and energy metabolism with biosynthetic human growth hormone after gastrointestinal surgery. *Annals of Surgery* 206: 56–61.

Ward MWN, Halliday D, Matthews SM et al (1983) The effect of enteral nutritional support on skeletal muscle protein synthesis and whole body protein turnover in fasted surgical patients. *Human Nutrition. Clinical Nutrition* 37C: 453–458.

Waterlow JC, Garlick PJ & Millward DJ (1978) *Protein Turnover in Mammalian Tissues and in the Whole Body*. Amsterdam: North Holland.

Williams PEV (1987) The use of β-agonists as a means of altering body composition in livestock species. *Nutrition Abstracts and Reviews*.

Williams PEV, Pagliani L, Innes GM, Pennie K, Harris CI & Garthwaite P (1987) The effects of the β-agonist (clenbuterol) on growth, carcass composition, protein and energy metabolism of veal calves. *British Journal of Nutrition* 57: 417–528.

Wilmore DW (1976) Hormonal responses and their effect on metabolism. *Surgical Clinics of North America* 56: 999–1018.

Wilmore DW, Long JM, Mason AD, Skreen RW & Pruit BW (1974a) Catecholamines: mediation of the hypermetabolic response to thermal injury. *Annals of Surgery* 180: 653–669.

Wilmore DW, Moglan JA, Bristow BR, Mason AD & Pruitt BA (1974b) Anabolic effects of human growth hormone and high caloric feedings following thermal injury. *Surgery, Gynecology and Obstetrics* 138: 875–884.

Woolfson AMJ, Heatley RV & Allison SP (1979) Insulin to inhibit protein catabolism after injury. *New England Journal of Medicine* 300: 14–17.

Young GA, Yule AG & Hill GL (1983) Effects of an anabolic steroid on plasma amino acids, proteins and body composition in patients receiving intravenous hyperalimentation. *Journal of Parenteral and Enteral Nutrition* 7: 221–225.

Yule AG, Macfie J & Hill GL (1981) The effect of an anabolic steroid on body composition in patients receiving intravenous nutrition. *Australian and New Zealand Journal of Surgery* 51: 280–284.

12

Nutritional pharmacology in the treatment of neoplastic disease

K. C. H. FEARON

Current cancer chemotherapy commonly involves the use of cytotoxic agents to inhibit cell division within the tumour. These agents are non-selective since they also inhibit cell division within the tissues of the host. Their use is based upon the assumption that the rate of cell division within the tumour is greater than that of the majority of host tissues. Clearly this is not always a valid assumption (Calman et al, 1980) and such treatment is limited by host toxicity, some of which is manifested by deterioration in the nutritional status of the patient (Kokal, 1985). In the cancer patient, anti-neoplastic therapy should be effective yet non-toxic. A more selective and thus less toxic approach to the treatment of cancer might be based on differences between tumour and host cells. One such difference is the altered energy metabolism and substrate requirements of many tumour cells. The aim of this chapter is to review selected aspects of tumour energy metabolism and show how such knowledge has led to various nutritional and pharmacological approaches to the management of cancer.

MITOCHONDRIA OF NORMAL CELLS

Every eukaryotic cell contains mitochondria. The Greek words from which mitochondria get their name (mitos—thread; chondros—granule) character-ize the appearance of these organelles under the light microscope. However, under the electron microscope, mitochondria have a highly organized structure. Two membranes surround the inner matrix. The smooth outer membrane is porous to molecules up to a molecular weight of 8000 (Zalman et al, 1980). The inner membrane is plicated to form cristae and acts as a semipermeable membrane. The primary function of mitochondria is to couple the degradation of various organic compounds to the formation of ATP. Hence, they have been regarded as the 'power houses' of the cell. Mitochondria are also remarkable because they are in possession of their own genetic system (Kroon and Saccone, 1980) and replicate in a manner similar to that of the binary fission of bacteria. However, although mitochondria are able to synthesize some of their own constituent proteins (mainly those bound to the inner membrane), the nuclear genetic system is responsible for the majority of the proteins within these organelles.

Mitochondria contain numerous enzymes which provide the cell with reducing equivalents and metabolic intermediates. They contain a system for the oxidative degradation of fatty acids, the β-oxidation pathway (Greville and Tubbs, 1968), and also possess enzymes for the oxidative decarboxylation of some amino acids. In addition, mitochondria contain the Krebs cycle enzymes (Lowenstein, 1969) which degrade acetyl CoA. Acetyl CoA is formed as a result of the oxidative degradation of lipids, some amino acids and carbohydrates. The processing of these substrates along such catabolic pathways leads to the production of reducing equivalents in the form of NADH and reduced flavins. The availability of reducing equivalents is required for the formation of ATP during oxidative phosphorylation.

The respiratory chain is a multienzyme system which is firmly embedded in the inner mitochondrial membrane. The chain is composed of flavoproteins, iron–sulphur proteins, ubiquinone and several cytochromes. Reducing equivalents, formed during various oxidation reactions occurring inside as well as outside the mitochondria, are transferred along this chain to molecular oxygen. The hydrogen atoms, or the electrons, are thus passed from the negative redox potential of their initial acceptors to the positive potential of oxygen. This fall of free energy of electrons is the primary force for ATP synthesis (oxidative phosphorylation).

MITOCHONDRIA OF TUMOUR CELLS

Almost 60 years ago Warburg hypothesized that damage to respiration, i.e. a deficiency in the respiratory chain, causes the transformation of normal cells into tumour cells (Warburg, 1930). However, tumour mitochondria generally contain normal, functional respiratory chains. It is possible to quantify the efficiency of ATP synthesis by mitochondria. If a known amount of ADP is added to isolated mitochondria, the amount of oxygen consumed in order to convert the ADP to ATP can be determined and is known as the P/O ratio. Carefully isolated tumour mitochondria show normal P/O ratios and normal respiratory control indices (Pederson, 1978). A general disorder of tumour mitochondria is therefore unlikely to be the major underlying factor in the neoplastic transformation process (Weinhouse, 1982). Nonetheless, an extensive literature has accumulated to show that tumour cell mitochondria have aberrations of one kind or another. These include deficiencies of enzymes involved in the metabolism of ketone bodies (Tisdale and Brennan, 1983), alterations in inner membrane components, particularly phospholipids (Reitz et al, 1977), abnormal adenine nucleotide translocation (Lau and Chan, 1984), and alteration of respiratory chain components (Nelson et al, 1984).

Whatever the significance of these mitochondrial alterations in terms of carcinogenesis, it is clear that in a great many cancers the organelle is defective. From the viewpoint of cancer chemotherapy, this would seem to be a weak spot in cancer cells and could be the focal point of therapy using antimitochondrial agents. Indeed, various anticancer drugs have been shown to inhibit mitochondrial function (Gosalvez et al, 1976; Bernal et al, 1982) and several inhibitors of mitochondrial function have been demonstrated to have selective antineoplastic effects (Wilkie, 1979). However, as yet the use of such agents to selectively inhibit mitochondrial function and thereby reduce tumour growth rate has received little or no attention in clinical cancer chemotherapy.

HIGH GLYCOLYTIC CAPACITY OF TUMOUR CELLS

An increased rate of anaerobic and aerobic glycolysis has been demonstrated repeatedly in rapidly growing tumours (Warburg, 1930; Weber et al, 1961). Moreover, many tumours have been shown to have a high rate of glucose consumption and to be susceptible to carbohydrate deprivation (Demetrakopoulos et al, 1978). The increased glycolysis of some tumours has been linked to enhanced levels of glycolytic enzymes (Weber and Morris, 1963). These appear largely as fetal-like isoenzymes (Ibsen, 1977; Weber, 1977) which are less prone to produce inhibition (Bustamante and Pederson, 1977). Alternatively tumour architecture may play a role in the choice of metabolic substrates. Large solid tumours tend to have a poor blood supply and a large fraction of tumour cells is consequently hypoxic. Under such conditions glucose may be the only substrate which can be utilized, since the Embden–Meyerhoff pathway is the only means of ATP production which does not require oxygen.

INHIBITION OF TUMOUR ENERGY METABOLISM BY PHARMACOLOGICAL METHODS

The increased glycolysis of tumour cells has prompted several attempts to reduce carbohydrate availability or utilization in the hope that such intervention might preferentially impair malignant cells. The glucose antimetabolite 2-deoxyglucose competes with glucose for transport and phosphorylation by hexokinase. The 2-deoxyglucose 6-phosphate is subsequently dephosphorylated by a phosphatase, creating a cycle of ATP utilization and depletion. Incubation of tumour cells with 2-deoxyglucose results in rapid depletion of ATP, although normal cells also suffer a similar or less rapid loss in ATP, thus limiting its usefulness (Demetrakopoulos and Brennan, 1982). Nevertheless, 2-deoxyglucose has been shown to reduce the growth rate of various rodent tumours in vivo (Sokoloff et al, 1955; Ball et al, 1957).

An alternative method of reducing glycolysis could be to induce a state of hypoglycaemia. This can be achieved by inhibiting gluconeogenesis in the fasting state. In tumour-bearing rats, inhibition of gluconeogenesis with hydrazine sulphate has been shown to have antineoplastic activity (Gold, 1971). Furthermore, hydrazine sulphate can enhance the efficacy of conventional cytotoxic therapy (Gold, 1975). However, although both 2-deoxyglucose (Landau et al, 1958) and hydrazine sulphate (Lerner and

Regelson, 1976) have been administered to cancer patients, clinical efficacy has not been demonstrated conclusively.

A series of experiments involving the mitochondrial dye Rhodamine 1,2,3 has recently given new impetus to the use of tumour energy metabolism as a target for systemic therapy in cancer. Rhodamine 1,2,3 and Rhodamine 6G (R6G) are two related compounds which have been shown to be cytotoxic in vitro (Zigman and Gilman, 1980; Johnson et al, 1982; Wilkie and Fearon, 1985). They belong to a series of permeant cationic fluorochome dyes with a high negative reduction potential which inhibit both protein and DNA synthesis in intact cells and also delay mitosis (Zigman and Gilman, 1980). Both agents are potent inhibitors of mitochondrial oxidative phosphoryla- tion (Higuti et al, 1980; Lampidis et al, 1983) and it has been suggested that their cytotoxic activity is related to an inhibition of ATP production (Darzynkiewicz et al, 1982).

Rhodamine 1,2,3 is taken up into the mitochondria of both normal and tumour cells but is retained for much longer in those of the tumour cells. This retention is associated with the cytotoxic action of the dye. In addition, Rhodamine 1,2,3 has been shown to be selectively cytotoxic against numerous malignant cell lines (Lampidis et al, 1983). This selectivity is thought to be related to a transformation-dependent abnormality of mitochondrial membrane potential (Nadakavukaren et al, 1985). If the glucose antimetabolite 2-deoxyglucose is administered simultaneously, the two agents have been shown to have synergistic antitumour activities both in vitro (Lampidis et al, 1983) and in vivo (Bernal et al, 1983). Thus it would appear that much greater efficacy can be achieved if both glycolysis and oxidative phosphorylation, the two main intracellular sources of ATP, are inhibited simultaneously.

The Walker 256 tumour is a rodent tumour which has been frequently used in studies of tumour energy metabolism. It has been shown that the growth rate of the Walker 256 tumour in rats can be reduced by administra- tion of the glucose antimetabolite 2-deoxyglucose (Ball et al, 1957) or by administration of hydrazine sulphate (Gold, 1971), which inhibits gluconeo- genesis. This suggests that the Walker 256 tumour is largely dependent on glucose as an energy substrate. Walker 256 cells have been shown to possess few mitochondria, and those that are present have abnormal morphology and a reduced complement of enzymes (Pederson, 1978).

A recent study from our own laboratory (Fearon et al, 1987) has shown synergistic inhibition of the Walker 256 in rats when the mitochondrial inhibitor R6G was administered during a period of hypoglycaemia induced by the gluconeogenic inhibitor 6-mercaptopicolinic acid (6MPA). In this study it is possible that the synergy between R6G and hypoglycaemia was the result of R6G inhibiting an already restricted capacity for ATP pro- duction via oxidative phosphorylation. Thus, the tumour would be even more dependent on glycolysis for energy production. In this situation even a small decrease in the substrate available for glycolysis might lead to sub- stantial reduction in intracellular ATP concentration, thereby reducing cell viability.

Under normal circumstances, when 1 mole of glucose is fully oxidized to carbon dioxide and water, 2 moles of ATP are produced via glycolysis, and 36 moles are produced from oxidative phosphorylation. Therefore, in terms of ATP production it is much more efficient if glucose is fully oxidized via oxidative phosphorylation rather than partially oxidized to lactate via glycolysis. The AS-30D hepatoma is similar to the Walker 256 tumour in that it is a rapidly growing rodent tumour which is known to exhibit high rates of aerobic glycolysis and lactate production in vitro (Pederson, 1978). It has been demonstrated that when glucose is supplied to AS-30D cells as the exogenous energy source, 60% of total ATP production is derived from glycolysis and only 40% from oxidative phosphorylation (Nakashima et al, 1984). However, in the absence of added glucose, glutamine alone can maintain the same ATP production rates. Thus, although these hepatoma cells rely predominantly on the inefficient glycolytic mode for energy production in vitro, in the absence of glucose other substrates which enter the Krebs cycle directly are able to maintain ATP production.

In our study a selective antineoplastic effect was demonstrated by administration of an inhibitor of oxidative phosphorylation (R6G) during a period of hypoglycaemia. Neither treatment was effective on its own. This suggests that, for the Walker 256 tumour in vivo, both glycolysis and oxidative phosphorylation are important in the maintenance of cellular ATP levels. Furthermore, cancer cell lines exhibit a broad spectrum of aerobic glycolytic activity. Slow-growing, well differentiated tumours resemble normal cells in that they exhibit low rates of glycolysis and high rates of oxidative metabolism for energy production (Pederson, 1978; Weinhouse, 1982). Previous attempts to use tumour energy metabolism as a target for antineoplastic therapy have used single agents aimed at inhibiting either glycolysis or oxidative phosphorylation (Ball et al, 1957; Wilkie, 1979). Since most tumour cells use both pathways for energy production, this approach is unlikely to succeed. The results of current studies (Bernal et al, 1983; Lampidis et al, 1983; Fearon et al, 1987) indicate that simultaneous manipulation of both sources of intracellular ATP may be used to achieve a more selective control of tumour growth. The results of further studies are awaited.

INHIBITION OF TUMOUR ENERGY METABOLISM BY DIETARY MANIPULATION

As mentioned previously, several studies have suggested that certain tumours are dependent on glucose as their principal substrate for energy metabolism. In order to maintain a glucose supply to the tumour, it has been suggested that host muscle protein is broken down to supply amino acids for an increased de novo synthesis of glucose in the liver (Gold, 1968). This hypothesis is supported by several studies that have demonstrated increased rates of gluconeogenesis in humans and animals with cancer (Waterhouse, 1974; Waterhouse et al, 1979; Lundholm et al, 1982). Thus the tumour grows at the expense of the host and this process is thought to contribute to the syndrome of cancer cachexia.

Ketone bodies are fat-derived energy substrates which may act to reduce gluconeogenesis by inhibiting muscle protein degradation. Several tumour cell lines have been shown to be deficient in the mitochondrial enzymes which allow the cell to use ketone bodies for energy production (Tisdale and Brennan, 1983; Fearon et al, 1985). Moreover, it has been suggested that the in vitro growth rate of certain tumour cell lines may be reduced by the presence of 3-hydroxybutyrate at a concentration which is observed in simple starvation (Magee et al, 1979). Thus, the induction of systemic ketosis in the cancer-bearing host has been suggested as a method of selectively feeding the host while restricting the supply of glucose to the tumour and reducing tumour growth rate (Conyers et al, 1979; Williams and Matthaei, 1981; Tisdale, 1982).

The evidence which supports the hypothesis that ketone bodies reduce protein breakdown in skeletal muscle is controversial. The initial studies by Sherwin et al (1975) suggested that the release of alanine from skeletal muscle may be reduced by ketone bodies, thereby accounting for nitrogen conservation in starvation. Subsequently, Pawan and Semple (1983) demonstrated that administration of DL-3-hydroxybutyrate to obese subjects on very low energy diets significantly reduced net protein loss and increased the fat/lean ratio of tissue loss. However, the latter study was criticized because the administration of salts of organic acids has a protein-sparing effect by reducing the need for ammonium ion excretion by the kidneys, and the same result can be achieved with an equal amount of sodium bicarbonate (Miles and Hammond, 1983). Thus, the current literature does not support a direct effect of ketone bodies on proteolysis (Miles et al, 1983). This has been confirmed in a recent study of cachectic cancer patients (Fearon et al, 1988), where a 70% medium-chain triglyceride diet supplemented with $4\,\mathrm{mmol\,kg^{-1}\,day^{-1}}$ D-3-hydroxybutyrate did not significantly influence nitrogen balance or turnover when compared with an isocaloric, isonitrogenous non-ketogenic diet.

The effect of systemic ketosis on tumour growth rate is similarly controversial. The growth rate of the Walker 256 tumour in rats was uninfluenced by the presence of systemic ketosis induced by a 70% medium-chain triglyceride diet (Fearon et al, 1985). In contrast, Tisdale et al (1987) have shown that both weight loss and tumour weight are reduced in animals bearing the MAC-16 tumour when they are fed a ketogenic diet. These contrasting results may simply reflect the different substrate requirements of different tumours. Alternatively, the response of host metabolism to the induction of ketosis may be different, depending on the tumour type involved.

SUMMARY

The altered energy metabolism and substrate requirements of tumour cells can provide a target for selective antineoplastic therapy. The supply of substrates for tumour energy metabolism can be reduced by dietary manipulation (e.g. ketogenic diet) or by pharmacological means at the cellular level (e.g. inhibitors of glycolysis or oxidative phosphorylation). Both these approaches are examined with a view to the development of selective and therefore non-toxic methods of controlling tumour growth in vivo.

REFERENCES

Ball HA, Wick AN & Sanders C (1957) Influence of glucose antimetabolites on the Walker tumour. *Cancer Research* **17**: 235–239.

Bernal SD, Shapiro HM & Chen LB (1982) Monitoring the effect of anticancer drugs on L1210 cells by a mitochondrial probe, Rhodamine-123. *International Journal of Cancer* **30**: 219–224.

Bernal SD, Lampidis TJ, McIsaac RM & Chen LB (1983) Anticarcinoma activity in vivo of Rhodamine 1,2,3, a mitochondrial specific dye. *Science* **222**: 169–172.

Bustamante E & Pederson PL (1977) High aerobic glycolysis of rat hepatoma cells in culture: role of mitochondrial hexokinase. *Proceedings of the National Academy of Sciences of the USA* **74**: 3735–3739.

Calman, Smyth & Tattersall (1980) *Basic Principles of Cancer Chemotherapy.* London and Basingstoke: Macmillan Press.

Conyers RAJ, Need AG, Durbridge T, Harvey NDM, Potenzy N & Roffe AM (1979) Cancer, ketosis and parenteral nutrition. *Medical Journal of Australia* **1**: 398–399.

Darzynkiewicz K, Traganos F, Coico-Staiano L, Kapuscinski J & Melamed MR (1982) Interactions of Rhodamine 1,2,3 with living cells studied by flow cytometry. *Cancer Research* **42**: 799–806.

Demetrakopoulos GE & Brennan MF (1982) Tumoricidal potential of nutritional manipulations. *Cancer Research* **42**(supplement): 7565–7695.

Demetrakopoulos G Ev, Linn B & Amos H (1978) Rapid loss of ATP in malignant cells deprived from glucose in contrast to normal cells. *Biochemical and Biophysical Research Communications* **82**: 787–794.

Fearon KCH, Tisdale MJ, Preston T, Plumb JA & Calman KC (1985) Failure of systemic ketosis to control cachexia and the growth rate of the Walker 256 carcinosarcoma in rats. *British Journal of Cancer* **52**: 87–92.

Fearon KCH, Plumb JA, Burns HJG & Calman KC (1987) Reduction of the growth rate of the Walker 256 tumour in rats by Rhodamine 6G together with hypoglycaemia. *Cancer Research* **47**: 3684–3687.

Fearon KCH, Borland W, Preston T, Tisdale MJ, Shenkin A & Calman KC (1988) Cancer cachexia: influence of systemic ketosis on substrate levels and nitrogen metabolism. *American Journal of Clinical Nutrition* **47**: 42–48.

Gold J (1968) Proposed treatment of cancer by inhibition of gluconeogenesis. *Oncology* **22**: 185–207.

Gold J (1971) Inhibition of Walker 256 intramuscular carcinoma in rats by administration of hydrazine sulphate. *Oncology* **25**: 66–71.

Gold J (1975) Enhancement by hydrazine sulphate of antitumour effectiveness of cytoxan, mitomycin C, methotrexate and bleomycin in Walker 256 carcinoma in rats. *Oncology* **31**: 44–53.

Gosalvez M, Garcia-Canero R, Blanco M & Gurucharri-Lloyd C (1976) Effects and specificity of anticancer agents on the respiration and energy metabolism of tumour cells. *Cancer Treatment Reports* **60**: 1–8.

Greville GD & Tubbs PK (1968) The catabolism of long chain fatty acids in mammalian tissues. *Essays in Biochemistry* **4**: 155–212.

Higuti T, Niimi S, Saito R et al (1980) Rhodamine 6G, inhibitor of both H^+-ejections from mitochondria energised with ATP and with respiratory substrates. *Biochimica et Biophysica Acta* **539**: 463–467.

Ibsen KH (1977) Interrelationships and functions of the pyruvate kinase isoenzymes and their variant forms: a review. *Cancer Research* **37**: 341–353.

Johnson LV, Summerhayes IC & Chen LB (1982) Decreased uptake and retention of

Rhodamine 1,2,3 by mitochondria in feline sarcoma virus transformed mink cells. *Cell* **28:** 7–14.

Kokal WA (1985) The impact of antitumour therapy on nutrition. *Cancer* **55:** 273–278.

Kroon AM & Saccone C (eds) (1980) *The Organisation and Expression of the Mitochondrial Genome*. Amsterdam: Elsevier/North Holland.

Lampidis TJ, Bernal SD, Summerhayes IC & Chen LB (1983) Selective toxicity of Rhodamine 1,2,3 in carcinoma cells in vitro. *Cancer Research* **43:** 716–720.

Landau BR, Laszlo J, Stengle J & Burk D (1958) Certain metabolic and pharmacologic effects in cancer patients given infusions of 2-deoxy-D-glucose. *Journal of the National Cancer Institute* **21:** 485–494.

Lau BWC & Chan SH (1984) Efflux of adenine nucleotides in mitochondria from rat tumour cells of varying growth rates. *Cancer Research* **44:** 4458–4464.

Lerner HJ & Regelson W (1976) Clinical trial of hydrazine sulfate in solid tumours. *Cancer Treatment Reports* **60:** 959–960.

Lowenstein JM (ed.) (1969) *Citric Acid Cycle. Control and Compartmentation*. New York and London: Marcel Dekker.

Lundholm K, Edstrom S, Karlberg I, Ekman L & Schersten T (1982) Glucose turnover, gluconeogenesis from glycerol and estimation of net glucose cycling in cancer patients. *Cancer* **50:** 1142–1150.

Magee BA, Potenzy N, Rafe AM & Conyers RAJ (1979) The inhibition of malignant cell growth by ketone bodies. *Australian Journal of Experimental Biology and Medical Science* **57:** 529–539.

Miles JM & Hammond MW (1983) 3-Hydroxybutyrate to conserve protein during therapeutic starvation. *Lancet* **1:** 409.

Miles JM, Nissen SL, Rizza RA, Gerich JE & Haymond MW (1983) Failure of infused β-hydroxybutyrate to decrease proteolysis in man. *Diabetes* **32:** 197–205.

Nadakavukaren KK, Nadakavukaren JJ & Chen LB (1985) Increased Rhodamine 1,2,3 uptake by carcinoma cells. *Cancer Research* **45:** 6093–6099.

Nakashima RA, Paggi MG & Pedersen PL (1984) Contributions of glycolysis and oxidative phosphorylation to adenosine S^1-triphosphate production in AS-30D hepatoma cells. *Cancer Research* **44:** 5702–5706.

Nelson BD, Kabir F, Kalarov J et al (1984) Immunochemical analysis of the membrane proteins of rat liver and Zajdela hepatoma mitochondria. *Archives of Biochemistry and Biophysics* **234:** 24–30.

Pawan S & Semple SJG (1983) Effect of 3-hydroxybutyrate in obese subjects on very low energy diets and during therapeutic starvation. *Lancet* **1:** 15–17.

Pederson PL (1978) Tumour mitochondria and the bioenergetics of cancer cells. *Progress in Experimental Tumour Research* **22:** 190–273.

Reitz RC, Thomson JA & Morris HP (1977) Mitochondrial and microsomal phospholipids of Morris Hepatoma 7777. *Cancer Research* **37:** 561–567.

Sherwin RS, Hendler RG & Felig P (1975) Effect of ketone infusion on amino acid and nitrogen metabolism in man. *Journal of Clinical Investigation* **55:** 1382–1390.

Sokoloff B, Eddy WH, Saelhof CC & Beach J (1955) Glucose antagonists in experimental cancer. *Archives of Pathology* **59:** 729–732.

Tisdale MJ (1982) Tumour and host nutrition. *Cancer Topics* **3:** 113.

Tisdale MJ & Brennan RA (1983) Loss of acetoacetate coenzyme A transferase activity in tumours of peripheral tissues. *British Journal of Cancer* **47:** 293–297.

Tisdale MJ, Brennan RA & Fearon KC (1987) Reduction of weight loss and tumour size in a cachexia model by a high fat diet. *British Journal of Cancer* **56:** 39–43.

Warburg O (1930) *Metabolism of Tumours*. London: Arnold Constable.

Waterhouse C (1974) Lactate metabolism in patients with cancer. *Cancer* **33:** 66–71.

Waterhouse C, Jeanpretre N & Keilson J (1979) Gluconeogenesis from alanine in patients with progressive malignant disease. *Cancer Research* **39:** 1968–1972.

Weber G (1977) Enzymology of cancer cells. *New England Journal of Medicine* **296:** 486–493, 541–551.

Weber G & Morris HP (1963) Comparative biochemistry of hepatomas. 111. Carbohydrate enzymes in liver tumours of different growth rates. *Cancer Research* **23:** 987–994.

Weber G, Banerjee G & Morris HP (1961) Comparative biochemistry of hepatomas. 1. Carbohydrate enzymes in Morris hepatoma 5123. *Cancer Research* **21:** 933–937.

Weinhouse S (1982) Changing perceptions of carbohydrate metabolism in tumours. In Arnott MS, Van Eys J & Wang YM (eds) *Molecular Interrelations of Nutrition and Cancer*, pp 167–181. New York: Raven Press.

Wilkie D (1979) Antimitochondrial drugs in cancer chemotherapy: preliminary communication. *Journal of the Royal Society of Medicine* **72:** 599–601.

Wilkie D & Fearon K (1985) Mitochondria and cancer. In Quagliariello E (ed.) *Achievements and Perspectives of Mitochondrial Research*, vol. II, pp 437–444. Amsterdam: Elsevier Science Publishers.

Williams JF & Matthaei KI (1981) Cancer induced body wasting. A review of cancer cachexia and a hypothesis concerning the molecular basis of the condition. *Asean Journal of Clinical Science* **2:** 158–166.

Zalman LS, Nikaido H & Kagawa Y (1980) Mitochondrial outer membrane contains a protein producing nonspecific diffusion channels. *Journal of Biological Chemistry* **255:** 1771–1774.

Zigman S & Gilman P (1980) Inhibition of cell division and growth by a redox series of cyanine dyes. *Science* **208:** 188–191.

Index

Note: Page numbers of article titles are in **bold** type.